"Dr. McKnight's efforts and her own harrowing account have helped to bring important attention to the root causes of these avoidable tragedies. I commend her advocacy and efforts to raise awareness about the impacts of healthcare-related infections involving hepatitis C and other potentially life-threatening illnesses."

—Shelley Berkley, congresswoman, Nevada

"This will be the wake-up call to doctors, nurses and to patients. Everyone's concerns for patient safety should be resolved, reporting systems should be immediately linked and swift action should be encouraged to protect all patients. This book will be the text for all ethical healthcare providers."

—Joe Hardy, MD, Nevada State Assembly

"Evelyn McKnight has taken a courageous step in telling her personal experience of being infected with hepatitis C. Her story has provided encouragement and hope to people across the nation and to the patients in Nevada who are coping with an all too similar outbreak."

—Lawrence Sands, DO, MPH

"This is a 'must-read' for hospital and clinic administrators, providers, and especially patients. It is up to each of us in our respective roles to proactively assure that what happened to Evelyn McKnight and is happening in alarming numbers to other patients across the country, doesn't happen under our watch or in our personal care situation."

—Charles Stokes, president and CEO, CDC Foundation

A Never Event

Exposing the Largest Outbreak
of Hepatitis C
in American Healthcare History

A Never Event

Exposing the Largest Outbreak
of Hepatitis C
in American Healthcare History

Evelyn V. McKnight
and
Travis T. Bennington

Arbor Books, Inc.

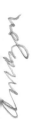

A Never Event:
Exposing the Largest Outbreak of Hepatitis C in American Healthcare History
Copyright © 2008 Evelyn V. McKnight and Travis T. Bennington
Published by Arbor Books, Inc.

For more information, please contact:
www.HONOReform.org

Book design by:
Arbor Books, Inc.
www.arborbooks.com
19 Spear Rd., Suite 301
Ramsey, NJ 07446

Printed in the United States of America

A Never Event:
Exposing the Largest Outbreak of Hepatitis C in American Healthcare History
Evelyn V. McKnight and Travis T. Bennington

1. Title 2. Author 3. Healthcare transmission of Hepatitis C

Library of Congress Control Number: 2008929036

ISBN 10: 0-9800582-8-7
ISBN 13: 978-0-9800582-8-4

AUTHOR BIOGRAPHIES

■

EVELYN VINDUSKA MCKNIGHT

Evelyn is a wife, mother and audiologist who lives in Fremont, Nebraska. She is one of a hundred cancer survivors who contracted hepatitis C through health-care transmission at the Fremont Cancer Center in 2000–2001. Using the money from her settlement against the oncology clinic, she co-founded the patient advocacy foundation HONOReform, which has been recognized by CBS, CNN's *American Morning, USA Today,* The Associated Press and *Newsday.* She is married to Dr. Thomas McKnight, a family physician who helped uncover the Nebraska outbreak.

TRAVIS THORNE BENNINGTON

A practicing civil trial attorney, Travis was one of the attorneys who represented victims of the Nebraska outbreak in their civil actions against Dr. Tahir Ali Javed, the nurses who worked for him, the Fremont Cancer Center and the Fremont Area Medical Center. Nineteen of the Nebraska Outbreak victims were his clients, neighbors and friends. Mr. Bennington is also a co-founder of HONOReform.

TABLE OF CONTENTS

■

The Lawsuit to Stop You From Reading This Book

As authors of this manuscript, we took great pains to make sure that we told the truth. Along the way, we were very careful to keep the contents of our manuscript confidential.

In the first week of June 2007, Travis threw away a nearly complete copy of our manuscript. We were shocked to learn that several days later, on June 21, 2007, the Fremont Area Medical Center (our local hospital) filed a lawsuit to prevent us from publishing this book. The hospital's attorneys allegedly "received a copy of [the] book in a brown paper envelope" on June 12, 2007. The hospital's lawsuit essentially claimed that the book contained some statements that were "inaccurate, false, malicious, negligent, salacious, scandalous, untrue and defamatory," although none of these "false" statements were satisfactorily specified in the legal complaint.

We wrote the book to honor the victims of the outbreak, and to make sure that the wrongs that led to the outbreak would be fixed and that no one else would suffer the same fate. Hiding the events that led to this tragedy would only ensure future healthcare transmissions of diseases.

Within a couple of days, we hired a First Amendment specialist to defend the lawsuit against us. After two and a half months, and $37,000 in legal fees, the court dismissed the lawsuit, and we were finally able to tell this story.

PREFACE

■

In the fall of 2002, the largest hepatitis C outbreak in American history was uncovered in the small, Midwestern town of Fremont, Nebraska. One hundred people were infected with the potentially life-threatening virus, which is carried through the blood and affects the liver.

The Nebraska outbreak was a shock to the farming community of Fremont and to the state of Nebraska. One of the most devastating things was the way in which these people were infected. All 100 were patients of Tahir Ali Javed, MD, and were infected in his clinic during their chemotherapy treatments. Just before the outbreak became public, Dr. Javed fled to his native Pakistan, where he serves as the minister of health for Punjab province. The legal and moral quagmire that he left behind resulted in one of the largest series of lawsuits in Nebraska history.

A Never Event: Exposing the Largest Outbreak of Hepatitis C in American Healthcare History is the story of how the Nebraska outbreak occurred and how it changed the lives of its victims. As we wrote this book, we told this story as honestly and objectively as possible. We hope *A Never Event* exposes the lessons of the Nebraska outbreak, promotes long-overdue healing, and advances positive change. Our intention in writing this book was not to damage the reputation of the participants but to learn from the outbreak so that no one will ever repeat its mistakes. We hope that it can be a starting point for positive change in the medical and legal systems in the United States.

We have changed the names of some participants for various reasons. The first time these changed names are used, they are italicized.

In some instances, we have made deductions from the evidence that we realize are subject to debate. We were not present for some of the conversations reconstructed in this book. We have stated them as we believe they must have taken place, based upon evidence. Our sources of information were court documents, witness depositions and interviews, newspaper articles, and interviews with other participants. We recognize that some of the people identified in this book will not agree with our retelling of the story and our opinions. When possible, we have tried to include the relevant documents upon which we relied. We implore the readers of this book to look at the evidence and make up their own minds.

We dedicate this book to the victims of the Nebraska hepatitis C outbreak. Their story needed to be told. We sincerely hope that this book will bring to light their physical and emotional suffering. In doing so, we hope that the systemic short-comings that led to and resulted from the outbreak will be corrected so that no one else will ever suffer these same injustices.

ACKNOWLEDGMENTS

■

We would like to thank all the people who have contributed to our understanding of the Nebraska outbreak and its aftermath. Specifically, we acknowledge Bob Ridder, Glenn Doescher, Jill Watson, Byron Schafersman, *Monica Weber, Valerie Wheaton* and the dozens of other outbreak survivors who granted us interviews. We sincerely hope that this book does justice to their plight. We also thank the legal and medical professionals who provided us insight and information. We thank Dr. Tom McKnight for use of his photographs to illustrate the improper procedures.

Fremont, Nebraska (the site of the Nebraska outbreak) was named after General John C. Fremont. He was commissioned to explore and survey the Great American West in the 1830s and '40s. For his contribution to the nation's knowledge of the West, he was given the nickname "The Pathfinder." We want to specifically acknowledge Dan McGill and Cheryl Gentry, who were the Nebraska outbreak's "Pathfinders." Through treating Dan and Cheryl, the first victims to die because of the outbreak, doctors expanded their understanding of the hepatitis C virus. The victims of the Nebraska outbreak, as well as hepatitis C patients everywhere, owe them a debt of gratitude.

We would also like to thank our families and friends who steadfastly supported our intentions and our efforts throughout the writing of this book. Without your unwavering encouragement, this book wouldn't have been written.

"All sorrows can be borne if you put them into a story or tell a story about them."

—*Isak Dinesen*

BOOK I

■

The Nebraska
Hepatitis C Outbreak

CHAPTER 1

Evelyn Describes the New Doctor in Town

September 1997

"Hello?" I answered the telephone.

"Mornin', Evelyn," Tom said. "Did you get the boys off to school?"

"Yeah," I answered. "But with difficulty. Curt couldn't find his shoes. Alex needed to bring a sack lunch for his class field trip, but we didn't have anything in the fridge, so we had to stop at the grocery store before school. Luke called and wanted a new tennis racquet. The usual chaos, and 'Mom, we're going to be late and it's *his* fault.' What about you?"

"Pretty good. I had to see an earache in the ER at six o'clock this morning, so I just stayed at the hospital and did my rounds. I have a really nice elderly patient on the fourth floor. She has heart failure and bad pneumonia, so we had to put her on the ventilator. I don't know if she is going to make it, but her family won't let her go. They want every possible test and treatment to keep her alive. It's a sad situation for everyone." Tom took a deep breath and mentally shifted gears. "Then, when I got to the office, I found that Medicare is cutting reimbursement. On top of all that, the front receptionist and the bookkeeper are having a catfight and both are threatening to quit."

It was a pretty typical morning conversation between my husband and me. He was a family practice physician and I was an audiologist in Fremont, Nebraska. We had three sons—one in elementary school, one in junior high and one in high school. Our lives were busy and very blessed.

"Anyway," Tom continued, "there is a group of doctors and hospital people going out to eat tonight. The hospital is recruiting an oncologist and it is an opportunity to convince the doc that he should move to Fremont. As president of the medical staff, I should probably join them. What do you think?"

"Uh, let's see." I pondered his question. "Luke has a tennis match tonight. You don't want to miss that, do you?"

"No, I forgot about that. Well, I'll meet the new doc some other time. Sounds like the hospital really wants him. He's pretty high-powered. He has a lot of impressive credentials and trained at Albert Einstein. It's surprising he would want to come to Fremont after a prestigious appointment like that. I guess he has a great bedside manner and an infectious grin. He has an unusual name—Jamed or Javed or something like that."

"Why is the hospital recruiting an oncologist?" I asked. "We already have one."

"They want one here full-time," he answered. "The oncology coverage we have now is part-time. The hospital thinks they are losing too much business to Omaha hospitals. They can admit more cancer patients here if we have a full-time oncologist on staff."

Tom took a deep breath and let it out slowly.

"Times are changing, Ev," he continued. "The hospital is expanding services and adding on at every turn. It's not the small-town hospital that it was when we first came here. I miss the small-town feel," he lamented.

"Yeah, nothing stays the same. Life is full of change," I remarked, not realizing how prophetic my words were. I didn't know it at the time but in the years to come, this new doctor would change my life—and the lives of many others—forever.

"Well, I'll see you at the tennis match," I said as I hung up.

"See you then," I heard him answer.

Tom and I had come to Fremont sixteen years earlier with high hopes and big dreams. We had been twenty-eight and twenty-six years old respectively, had a nine-month-old baby and more student loan debt than I care to remember. Tom had started a solo family medical practice located in the hospital. Now it is called Fremont Area Medical Center but then, it was known as the Memorial Hospital of Dodge County. I had stayed home with the new baby, had two more, and begun an audiology practice.

In Fremont, our dreams were realized. We found that it was a good place to raise our children and to earn a fair living. We knew our neighbors, had true and lasting friends and made a comfortable home for our family.

Fremont, Nebraska, is located almost directly in the center of the United

States. In 1997, it had approximately 23,000 residents, many with families who had lived there for generations. Everyone knew each other and liked it that way. The people were hard-working, trusting, salt-of-the-earth souls. Farmland surrounded the community and gave it a wide buffer from big-city Omaha. The chamber of commerce worked hard to attract new industries into the community but growth was slow. For rural Nebraska, Fremont was a big small town.

For years, the hospital had been the second-largest employer in Dodge County. The Hormel packing plant was the only other big industry in town, making Fremont the canned SPAM capital of the world. Officially, the hospital was a county hospital but it was administered by its own board of trustees and did not take from, nor contribute to, the county treasury. In recent years, the hospital had been doing very well, expanding services, building large additions and winning awards for patient care.

Expanding cancer services in Dodge County made healthcare more convenient for patients. Given the choice, most patients, especially those with very taxing diseases, opted to stay close to home. It was much easier than driving the forty miles to Omaha and fighting city traffic. The Fremont Area Medical Center wanted to be the first choice for hospital care in Dodge County and the surrounding areas. By recruiting Dr. Javed, it could reach that goal.

Dr. Tahir Ali Javed

Tahir Ali Javed was born on April 26, 1965 in the Punjab province of Pakistan. He attended school in Pakistan, receiving a medical degree from King Edward Medical College in Lahore, Pakistan in 1988. After a one-year residency at Mayo Hospital in Lahore, he completed a three-year residency in Internal Medicine at Flushing Hospital Medical Center and the Albert Einstein College of Medicine in New York. From 1993 to 1996, he pursued further training in hematology and oncology at the Medical University of South Carolina in Charleston. At the time that he was recruited to Fremont, he was section chief of hematology and oncology in the Department of Medicine in the Guthrie Clinic in Sayre, Pennsylvania. He was board-certified in internal medicine and hematology and was working toward board certification in medical oncology. He was licensed to practice medicine in Pennsylvania, New York, South Carolina and Arizona. Tahir was married to the gorgeous Fouzia, who was also a Pakistani physician. They had three small children. The Javeds had dual US/Pakistan citizenship.

At first glance, it seemed a bit surprising that the highly educated and well-trained Dr. Javed would be interested in a position in Fremont, Nebraska. He had always been in large, challenging practices in prestigious settings. The family had always lived in large cities with many cultural advantages that were not available in Fremont. Likely, they would be the only Pakistani Muslims in Fremont. They would have to travel to Omaha to find any ethnic or religious affiliation.

However, the recruitment package offered to Dr. Javed was very attractive. Dr. Javed would not be employed by the hospital but would start a new practice and run it as he wanted. The practice would be conveniently located on the main floor of the hospital. If things went well, the practice could even support a partner. In the meantime, several oncologists from Omaha were willing to cover Dr. Javed's occasional call. In addition to all of this, there was one enticement larger than all the rest: money.

The Fremont Area Medical Center offered Dr. Javed a lot of money to lure him to Fremont and to keep him there. He received a $50,000 signing bonus to initiate an oncology practice, and another $14,000 in relocation expenses. There was an additional $50,000 business start-up loan, which would be forgiven if he practiced in Fremont for four years. The hospital purchased his office furnishings and equipment. In addition, the hospital gave him an income guarantee of $600,000 per year for at least two years. The income guarantee terms outlined that if Dr. Javed's gross income was less than $50,000 *per month*, the hospital would pay him the difference. The only way he was required to pay any of the money back was if he left before four years. In short, with the assurances of the hospital administration that an oncology practice would quickly build, the practice opportunity in Fremont would likely be very lucrative.

Although he did not negotiate the contract, president of Fremont Area Medical Center Mike Leibert denied that the recruitment package offered to Dr. Javed was extraordinary. In sworn testimony given in conjunction with the hepatitis C lawsuits in 2004, Mr. Leibert called the agreement "…A fairly standard recruiting package and recruiting agreement." Given Dr. Javed's credentials, specialty and marketplace factors, the hospital felt that the recruitment package was not excessive.

However, at the time, other new physicians in Fremont did not receive even a portion of the benefits offered to Dr. Javed by the hospital. When a new obstetrician/gynecologist was recruited by the hospital in 2001, the recruitment package was a $5,000 signing bonus, a $5,000 moving allowance and a payoff of the physician's student loans of about $35,000. Altogether, the recruitment package totaled $45,000. Dr. Javed, on the other hand, was offered over $1.3 million in potential incentives, with the possibility of earning even more if his practice was successful.

CHAPTER 2

The Foundation
for an Outbreak

*"...This doctor [Javed] has been brought on board, brought within the four walls
of [the] hospital to be a director of oncology service, and oversee and assume responsibilities as a director. He is not renting a room to sell shoes. He is representing the
hospital as the Director of Oncology."*

—Dr. Michael A. McIlroy, MD
(Expert witness testimony, February 21, 2006)

January 9, 1998

Dr. Javed walked through the main doors of Fremont Area Medical Center with
a hop in his step. It was the first week of his new practice in Fremont. He smiled
broadly and nodded at the volunteer at the information desk. Curiously, she
watched this well-dressed, dark-featured stranger turn at the elevator and
proceed down the hall toward the cafeteria. "Who was that?" she asked the other
grey-haired volunteer. "I've never seen him before."

"That's the new cancer doctor, Dr. Javed. He's opening a new oncology
practice. I met him at his welcome reception," the woman in the pink volunteer's
jacket answered. "He was so nice. He's foreign, but that doesn't matter these
days. I told him my husband is being treated for prostate cancer now and he
asked all about him and offered to help in any way he could. If I ever need a
cancer doctor, I'm going to go to him," she gushed. "And besides," she added
with a wink, "he's so handsome."

By now, Javed had reached the door off the hospital corridor marked
"Cancer Center." He cut though the large waiting room and passed the chairs
that lined the far wall. On the other side of the waiting room was the check-in
for the radiation oncology clinic, and again he smiled warmly at the receptionist. He opened the door to his new office, the Fremont Cancer Center.

"Good morning, Doctor," a middle-aged, blond nurse said as he entered
the receptionist area.

"Morning, Linda," he answered as he passed her. "Are you ready to start work after all the holiday festivities? I'll show you a few nursing procedures. I'm going to step into my office for a minute, and then I'll meet you in the infusion room," he directed politely as he turned down the main hallway of the cancer center and headed past the doors leading into the exam rooms.

"Yes, Doctor," she answered.

It was Nurse Linda Prochaska's first day as a chemotherapy nurse. Javed had called her in the fall of 1997 at the recommendation of another Fremont physician. A native Nebraskan, Linda had worked at the hospital as a registered nurse from 1982 to 1986. Since that time, she had worked in several Omaha hospitals. She had wanted the nursing position at the Fremont Cancer Center because it was full-time and the regular daytime work schedule would allow her to have more time with her young son. Even though Linda had no experience in oncology nursing, or any kind of private office nursing, Dr. Javed had called her at home after he'd heard of her interest. He described the job to her, and within a few weeks, offered her the position. Although she was inexperienced in oncology nursing, she seemed eager to learn and was willing to work for modest wages. As a result, Javed thought she was perfect for the job.

Even with an empty patient schedule, starting the new medical practice was surprisingly busy. The first days were filled with ordering supplies, furnishing the office and setting up an accounting system. Today was no less hectic. Today, he would begin the task of training Nurse Prochaska in the nursing duties of an oncology practice.

Following her orders, Nurse Prochaska headed down the hallway to the chemotherapy infusion room to await Javed. She turned as she entered and passed the eight chemotherapy recliner chairs, which had been provided by the hospital. She stopped and leaned against the countertop in the nurse's work area, beneath the cupboards.

"Okay, Linda," he broke the silence when he entered. "I know you are a skilled nurse, but as we talked about in your interview, we need to catch you up on some oncology procedures. You'll see that they are really very simple. Today, I want to go over accessing and flushing ports, obtaining blood draws, admixing chemotherapy infusions and infusing chemotherapy. Basically, everything you will need to know as an oncology nurse."

Over the course of the next hour, Javed worked with Linda, training her for her new job.

"Okay, Doctor," Linda said. "What do I do if a patient requires, say, twenty-six milligrams of Taxotere? Each vial only holds twenty milligrams. Do I open another vial to get the last six milligrams? How do we store that opened vial?"

"Oh, don't open another vial," he answered without even hesitating. "Just use the twenty milligrams. When the chemo is all mixed up, it turns out to be a little more than what the package says, so you can go ahead and note in the chart that you gave the full amount. That way, the patient's medical records are complete and we don't have to open and store another vial."

He was outlining a procedure that would compromise patient treatment. He was also instructing her to falsify patients' medical records to cover it up.

"Oh," Linda answered slowly. "Is that how it's done with chemotherapy drugs?"

"Oh, yes," he answered confidently as he continued his instruction. "Alright," he went on. "Most of the patients we will be seeing will already have venous access devices or ports surgically implanted just below their collarbones. These ports make it easier to administer chemotherapy, but we need to flush them out with saline from time to time or else the patients' blood will coagulate in them and clog them up."

She had never worked with chemotherapy ports before, but nodded her head in understanding.

"Now, we use disposable syringes when we administer chemotherapy and flush patient ports. And, you know that they are supposed to be used only once and disposed of. But from time to time, in certain situations, it's okay for us to reuse them."

Linda looked quizzically at Javed. He was giving her so much new information that it was hard to take it all in.

"For now, we are going to flush ports with single-use saline vials, but we will use larger, multi-dose saline bags as we see more patients. They are cheaper," Javed instructed.

The conversation had just taken a deadly turn. The saline was to be injected directly into patients' ports at nearly every office visit. Reusing blood-contaminated syringes to access a community saline bag meant that patients would be exposed to each other's blood. It was not a question of *whether* a patient would be getting injected with other patients' unscreened blood; it was just a question of *how many* patients' blood they would get. It was a concept that should have been repugnant to a doctor who had as much training and experience as Dr. Javed. The acts they were now discussing had escalated from unethical to deadly.

"Once you have given treatment to a patient, you should note it in the patient's medical records and identify it on the patient's superbill. The superbill will go to our billing service, where it will be filed with the patient's insurance, Medicaid, or Medicare for payment. And," he added in passing, "you're not going to have to give all the injections to patients. I will give some of them myself, and in those instances, I will document the injections in the patient's medical record, and I'll mark the superbill." In reality, he likely had something else in mind altogether. By setting up the office system in this way, it would be possible for him to make notations of treatments into patient's medical records even though the patient had never received the treatment—as he would later be accused of doing by dozens of his patients. This could create a paper trail to justify fraudulent billing to the patient's insurance, Medicare and/or Medicaid. Allegations of such criminal fraud were raised by his patients after the Nebraska outbreak became known. It was investigated by federal authorities, but apparently, no charges were ever filed.

CHAPTER 3

Blood on Her Hands

"As a hospital staff [they] have knowledge that…a nurse…is sticking pointsettia plants in a [chemotherapy mixing] hood, and who is drawing blood without gloves and has blood on her hands… This is not 1940. It's absolutely astounding that they would say, 'Well, we can't do anything about it.' I mean, it just—it makes me weep."

—Stephen Anderson
(Expert witness on healthcare quality assurance testimony, October 8, 2004)

August 5, 1999

"Tahir," Dr. Rodney Koerber said as he waived Javed into his private office.

It had been eighteen months since Javed's cancer center had opened. The clinic had grown from having only a few patients to hundreds. However, there had been frequent signs of danger.

"Listen, there's *another* problem with the blood draws coming from your office," Rod began. "One of my people just told me that your Nurse Prochaska came to the lab with a handful of lab sample vials and then took a marker and labeled them with patient's names before she handed them to the technician. Apparently, she just labeled them with the names as she remembered them. I guess ultimately, it doesn't matter if she labeled them correctly or not, because all the samples were compromised and we can't accept them anyway. Just call your last five patients and have them go directly to the lab for another draw, will you?"

"Sure, Rod. Be glad to," Javed responded in his usual congenial manner.

Dr. Koerber had been the supervising pathologist of the hospital's laboratory for years, and Javed wasn't about to contest him.

"Everything else going okay?" Javed asked as he sat down.

"No," Koerber answered flatly. "Prochaska just refuses to take constructive criticism. As gently as possible, the lab technicians try to instruct her on the proper collection and labeling of specimens. But she flies off the handle and says 'That's not the way Javed taught me.' Now I know you wouldn't have taught her improper methods, but she sure isn't following proper procedures."

"I'll talk to her, Rod. We'll get this straightened out," Javed answered with as much surprise as he could muster. "I'll make sure she understands proper procedure."

Dr. Koerber took a deep breath.

"You know, Tahir." Rod paused as he sighed. "I understand there is a learning curve for everyone when a new clinic opens. I've called you three or four times a week for more than a year to talk about these issues. I've even offered in-service training to your staff. But these same problems keep happening over and over. I don't know what else I can do to help you."

"Yeah, I appreciate all you've done, Rod." Javed smiled convincingly. "You've been such a help to us. I know Linda's a little stubborn but she's making progress, really." He leaned forward to emphasize his confidence. "I really believe she's becoming a good nurse."

"Well, I hope you're right, Tahir," Koerber replied hopefully. "Oh, and one other thing. I've noticed recently you're not sending nearly as many specimens to the lab. Is your business down?"

"Oh, no, I'm just sending more lab work to the med center. They're cheaper, you know." He winked.

The "med center" to which he referred was the University of Nebraska Medical Center in Omaha.

"Well, I can work with you on the cost, if that's what it is. I just don't want you to switch labs because of a few personality issues between my people and yours."

"Oh, no," Javed insisted. "It's not a personality issue. We can talk about cost some other time. The important thing is good communication between you and me. And we've always had that, haven't we, Rod? That's not going to change." Javed smiled with conviction. "Well." He stood and walked to the door. "I'd better get back to work."

Dr. Koerber nodded silently and gave a halfhearted wave as Dr. Javed disappeared around the corner. He turned his attention to a stack of papers on his desk, confident that Javed would solve all the lab collection problems in his clinic.

It did seem that way because as time went on, there were fewer lab collection errors coming from the Fremont Cancer Center that demanded Dr. Koerber's attention. However, the explanation for fewer collection errors may have been that Dr. Javed sent a major portion of his lab work to Omaha.

August 6, 1999

Gerri Means, RN, sat in Dr. Koerber's private office, waiting for him to return from lunch. Gerri was the hospital's infection control practitioner. She had worked at the hospital for many years. At first, she'd worked on the in-patient floors, but for the last ten years she'd worked as the infectious disease practitioner. Her job was to investigate in-hospital patient infections and give infection control continuing education to the hospital staff. She reported to Dr. Koerber, and consulted with him frequently. She had a number of things to discuss with him that day, and several of the discussion points centered on the Fremont Cancer Center.

"Hi, Gerri. Sticky out, isn't it? Typical August day in Nebraska," Dr. Koerber greeted her as he entered his office and tossed his keys on the desk. "What's on your mind today?"

"Two things." She cut to the chase. "I got an email from Deb Wohlenhaus' secretary last week."

Deb Wohlenhaus was the clinical operations manager at the hospital. She oversaw the risk management, quality assurance and infection control and safety programs.

"The email said that there is a pointsettia plant in the chemo hood in Dr. Javed's office," Gerri continued. "Why would they have a poinsettia in the chemo hood? How can they mix their infusions?"

"I have no idea, Gerri. I don't know. But I'll call Javed and talk to him. I'm sure he'll deal with it," Koerber replied. "Anything else, Gerri?"

"One of your lab technicians, Kay, came over to talk to me," Gerri continued to report. "Yesterday, she had to go over to Dr. Javed's office to transport a specimen to the lab because the cancer clinic was short-staffed. Well, when she got there, she asked the nurse, Linda, for some gloves and Linda said, 'We don't use them.' And then Linda drew the lab through the port bare-handed and with visible blood on her hands. She had *blood on her hands!*"

Koerber just shook his head in disbelief. "*Blood on her hands?* I'll talk to Javed, Gerri. I'll see him at the next vascular access device committee meeting on August twentieth. I'm sure he will take care of everything. You know, what makes this whole Fremont Cancer Center thing so tricky is that it is rented space. It is Javed's own private practice, and the hospital bylaws do not give the hospital any jurisdiction over private-practice employees, unfortunately. The only thing I can do is talk to him about the problems. If he doesn't ask for our help in correcting the problems, there is nothing more we can do. I can't even take the issue up with the hospital infection control committee."

All the physicians on the medical staff at the hospital were appointed to a committee. The medical staff committee system was a self-policing mechanism. The duty of the various committees was to give input on policies and procedures within the hospital. They were also empowered to police patient safety concerns at the hospital, investigate problems regarding physicians' behavior within their hospital practice, and potentially impose sanctions on physicians if warranted. Sanctions could range from a discussion of the problem to removing the physician's hospital admitting privileges. There was a hierarchy of the committee structure so that a question or complaint was initially brought to an entry-level committee (for example, the infection control committee). It would be discussed and possibly referred to a higher-level committee (for example, the executive committee).

Dr. Koerber believed that he could not take the "blood on her hands" and the "poinsettia in the chemo hood" report to the infection control committee for discussion because the medical staff committees had jurisdiction only within the hospital setting and not over a physician's private practice.

Dr. Koerber and Gerri did not report the Fremont Cancer Center to the Occupational Safety and Health Administration (OSHA). OSHA's purpose was to protect workers' safety and health in the workplace. When Linda Prochaska had patients' blood on her skin, the Fremont Cancer Center was in violation of OSHA regulations. Linda's health and safety was at risk because if she had a scratch on her hand when she was exposed to patients' blood, she could have contracted a blood-borne disease through exposure to the patients' blood.

The vascular access device committee meeting that Dr. Koerber referred to was part of an investigation that had been initiated in the hospital. There had been an uncommonly high number of patients having difficulty with clogged chemotherapy ports during 1999 and the purpose of this newly formed committee was to examine the problem.

A "port" was a type of rubber stopper implanted just below the skin, below the patient's collarbone. It had a small tube that led to the patient's subclavian vein. The port would allow the patient to have chemotherapy and blood draws without having to be stuck over and over again with a needle. Infusions and blood draws through a port were easier on the veins than if done directly through veins in the arms or hands. However, when something went wrong with a port, such as blood clotting, it was a very serious, potentially life-threatening problem.

The vascular access device committee (VADC) was made up of doctors and nurses from many departments throughout the hospital. Dr. Javed and

Linda Prochaska were also members of the committee. The VADC studied surgical implantation techniques, the various vascular access devices and the different techniques for accessing and flushing ports. They found that the nurses who administered chemotherapy used several different techniques for flushing ports. Although one goal of the VADC was to standardize the port-flushing procedure between the hospital and the cancer center, Nurse Prochaska refused to adopt the recommended procedure. The VADC did not take action to determine if Javed's clinic adopted the new standardized procedure.

The number of clotted ports did decrease after the vascular access device committee released its recommendations. One recommendation was that all patients implanted with a port at the hospital be put on a blood-thinning drug. The decreased number of clotted ports was likely the result of the blood thinning drug, since the standardized port flush was not adopted by Javed's cancer center. Their goal having been reached, the vascular access device committee disbanded.

November 8, 1999

Trouble continued to brew in the Fremont Cancer Center. In early November 1999, Peg Kennedy, the vice president and chief nursing officer at the hospital, sent Dr. Javed a letter. She told Javed that Nurse Prochaska had been drawing blood from patients in the outpatient department of the hospital. Hospital staff had told Linda three times that she was not allowed to draw blood outside of the Fremont Cancer Center, since she was not a hospital employee. Peg asked Javed to intervene and admonish Linda not to draw blood outside the walls of the Fremont Cancer Center.

Later in November, Javed received a resignation letter from his receptionist, Karla.

"There are many things that are not done to OSHA codes and I know you are aware of them but don't seem to make her [Linda] accountable," Karla wrote. "I also know many people and administration from the hospital have questioned her ways."

CHAPTER 4

The Fremont Cancer Center— A Growing Cancer

A String of Improper Waste Management Reports

The Fremont Cancer Center contracted with the hospital housekeeping services for cleaning under terms of its lease with the hospital. Housekeeping services staff was untrained in medical procedures and biohazard disposal. They were, however, required to report all questionable incidences of waste management to hospital supervisor Diane Sukstorf. Between April 19, 2000 and March 5, 2002, Diane received ten reports from housekeeping staff warning that the cancer center was disposing of hazardous waste improperly. The reports contained evidence that the cancer center was throwing away patients' blood into community garbage cans and other unsafe practices. The reports were faithfully documented and passed along the hospital chain of command. Altogether, twelve hospital employees received the reports. In addition, a number of other hospital employees had witnessed the apparent dangers in Javed's clinic. Employees at all levels of the hospital hierarchy, from entry level janitors to high-level administrators, were aware of the growing *cancer* at Javed's clinic. However, because of the clinic's status as a private practice and not a hospital practice, hospital employees felt the hospital had no authority to compel altered procedures in the clinic.

Improper Waste Management Report—April 20, 2000

At the close of 1999, Gerri Means, RN, was confident that the hazardous conditions in Javed's clinic would be remedied. She believed that Dr. Koerber could persuade Dr. Javed to improve his patient care. Shortly into 2000, she received more reports that improvements in Javed's patient care in his clinic had not taken place.

"Diane Sukstorf called me this afternoon," Gerri typed in an email to Deb Wohlenhaus, the safety officer at the hospital. "…In Dr. Javed's office there was a small tube with a plastic apparatus laying on…the chemo chair."

Diane had received a report regarding suspicious tubing lying on a chemo chair in Dr. Javed's clinic, and forwarded it to Gerri, who passed the report further up the administrative chain. It was a potentially dangerous situation. Chemotherapy tubing was kept in plastic, sealed containers prior to use. Once opened, the tubing was to be utilized by one patient immediately. Once used, the tubing was contaminated with dangerous medication and patient blood. Anyone exposed to it was at risk. If the tubing had not yet been used there was a risk that it had been contaminated by the cleaning crew, or simply by the chair itself.

Gerri sent her email off to Deb, but did not hear from her until the next day.

"Not much else Diane can do but report through that manner, and note for her own records," the hospital's safety officer responded. "We have no jurisdiction in that office, but I can pass info on to John Hughes [the vice president of the hospital]…"

Improper Waste Management Report—November 30, 2000
A syringe filled with liquid was left on the floor of Javed's clinic.

Improper Waste Management Report—December 27, 2000
Glass vials of blood were found in trash cans located within the hospital. The vials were broken and blood had leaked onto the hospital floor. Diane Sukstorf investigated and found that the trash bag came from the cancer center.

Improper Waste Management Report—December 28, 2000
Vials of blood were found sitting out on the cancer center counter overnight.

Improper Waste Management Report—January 2, 2001
A vial of blood was, once again, left on the counter overnight.

Improper Waste Management Report—October 31, 2001
Used needles and syringes were found in a coffee can rather than a biohazard container.

New Nursing Staff Added

As the Fremont Cancer Center practice grew, Linda Prochaska was not able to keep up with patient-care demands. She asked Dr. Javed to hire a second nurse to assist her, but he refused.

"At this point, I simply cannot afford to hire another RN," he explained.

In December of 1998, Javed hired *Raegene Lawson*, a certified nursing assistant (CNA) whom he met working on the general medicine floor of the hospital. Raegene's training consisted of a seventy-two hour course on bathing, walking, transferring and feeding patients, and taking patients' vital signs. Her training did not include drawing blood, giving injections, vascular access skills or giving oral medications. When Raegene first started at the Fremont Cancer Center, her duties were limited to escorting patients to the exam rooms, taking their vital signs, getting them ready for examination by Dr. Javed and then escorting them to the chemotherapy room. Despite her limited formal training, Raegene's duties expanded within a few months. Linda taught her how to run lab tests, give growth factor shots and flush the patients' ports.

The Fremont Cancer Center practice continued to grow and needed more staff. In December of 2000, Javed hired Heather Schumacher, RN, on a part-time basis. Like Linda, Heather did not have any training in oncology nursing before her employment with the Fremont Cancer Center. As with Raegene, Linda Prochaska was responsible for training Heather.

"Okay," Linda said as Heather followed her through the clinic, to the reception desk, on Heather's first day on the job. "The patient checks in with the receptionist and then is escorted to an exam room by the nursing assistant."

Heather nodded as she scratched down a few notes in her note pad. They had a busy day ahead of them, so Linda decided to go over office protocol early that morning, before many patients arrived.

"Once the patient is in the exam room," Linda went on as she quickly led Heather down the hall to an empty exam room, "the nursing assistant will take the patient's vital signs."

"Okay." Heather nodded again in understanding as she continued to take notes.

"At this point, Dr. Javed will come in to examine the patient," Linda said, pointing through the open exam room doorway to the exam table. "It's a pretty standard exam, like in any general medical practice. He will review the patient's recent test results, answer questions the patient may have, and then ask how they are handling the side effects of chemotherapy."

Linda quickly turned and led Heather back down the hallway, to the chemotherapy room.

"Then the patient will be escorted to the chemotherapy treatment room and be seated in a recliner, where we will administer the patient's chemo," Nurse Prochaska explained as the two women entered the chemo room. "Okay," she continued as she picked up the small tote basket of medical supplies behind her on the counter. "You will have a tote like this one. As you can see, it has all the tubing, needles and other supplies you need to give chemotherapy to a patient."

Heather scribbled in her notes as they quickly inventoried the basket.

"Okay," Linda said once they were done. "Let's step over here so you can see how infusions are done."

Linda led the way as they approached the first patient of the day.

"Good morning, *Mrs. Jones*," Linda began and then continued instructing Heather. "Mrs. Jones is not here today for chemotherapy. Today, she is just here to have some blood work done, to make sure she is handling chemo okay. So we will just flush her port and collect some blood."

"Hello, Mrs. Jones," Heather said, since Linda hadn't taken the time to introduce them.

"So, you start your procedure by setting the basket down where you can reach it," Linda said. "I like to set it right in the patient's lap. Each patient has a port. If you're not familiar with ports, when a patient is diagnosed with cancer, they are taken into surgery at the hospital, and the port is implanted under their skin. It is surgically attached to the patient's clavicle," she added, reaching down to touch her own collarbone as a demonstration. "The port has a rubber face on it, so that when the needle pierces the patient's skin just under their clavicle, the needle slides into the port."

"So the other end of the port is surgically inserted into the patient's subclavian artery?" Heather asked.

"Right. This way we have an easy access point to give the patients chemotherapy, without having to constantly stick them with needles in their arms or hands," Linda explained. "Alright, so once the patient is seated in the chemo recliner we begin by wiping the patient's skin over their port with alcohol and Betadine. That will sterilize the skin."

As she spoke, Linda pulled an alcohol swab and a Betadine swab from her tote and cleaned the area above Mrs. Jones' port.

"Once the Betadine and alcohol dry on the patient's skin you will go back to the tote and pull out a sterile Huber needle. Now," Nurse Prochaska said as she pulled the seal open and removed the needle, "you take the Huber needle and introduce it into the patient's port."

Linda pierced it the elderly woman's skin with the needle to access the port.

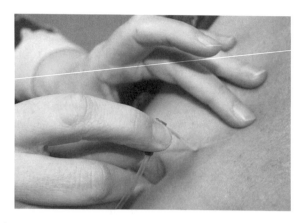

"What about latex gloves?" Heather whispered quietly. "Or hospital gowns, or masks?"

Linda stopped for a moment and gave Heather a sharp glance.

"We don't use them here," she retorted.

There was an awkward moment of silence.

"I'm sorry for interrupting," Heather finally apologized, nodding to the elderly woman. "Please go on."

"Next," Linda continued as she left the Huber needle hanging from the woman's chest, "we get a syringe. They are disposable and individually wrapped in their own sterile packages as well. We will call this 'syringe A.'"

She quickly retrieved the syringe package from her tote and opened it as she continued.

"Now, we take a 500cc bag of saline and couple the syringe to the bag. Once it is attached, you open the stopcock on the bag and draw back 10cc of saline into syringe A. Then you close the stopcock and disconnect the syringe from the bag."

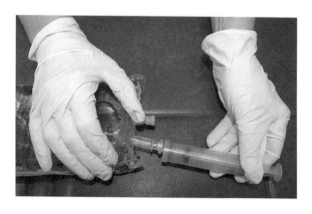

Heather watched intently.

"Next," Linda said as she connected the syringe to the Huber needle, which still hung from the patient, "you simply inject the 10cc of saline in syringe A into the patient to flush the port.

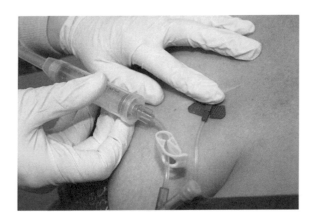

"While syringe A is still attached to the Huber needle, we draw back 10cc of the patient's blood. This blood is 'discard blood,'" she explained. "In between treatments, a patient's blood will pool in the port and begin to coagulate. It will clog up the port if we are not careful."

Linda disconnected the syringe from the Huber needle and set it on the patient's chart.

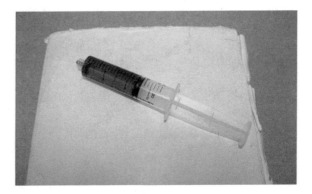

"Now." She turned back to face Heather and the patient as she withdrew a second syringe from her tote. "We take a new sterile syringe. We'll call this one 'syringe B.'"

Heather nodded in understanding as she jotted it down in her notebook.

"We couple syringe B to the Huber needle, which is still attached to the patient. Again, we draw back 10cc of blood. Syringe B," she said as she unhooked it and held it up to show Heather, "is now full of 10cc of the patient's blood. That is enough for us to run two tests."

Linda reached into her tote, which still sat in the patient's lap, and retrieved two small, sterile vials.

"The first 5cc will be run through our own CBC machine here in the clinic," she added as she attached a needle to syringe B and then injected 5cc of Mrs. Jones' blood into one of the vials. "The CBC machine will tell us the patient's complete blood count. We have to make sure the patient's blood count is high enough to withstand chemotherapy. The in-house CBC machine lets us test the patient's blood right here, before we administer the chemo."

"That's very handy." Heather nodded again as she smiled down at Mrs. Jones.

Mrs. Jones just smiled back. She didn't want to interrupt the training session.

"The second 5cc of blood will be put into this second vial," Linda said as she emptied syringe B into the second vial.

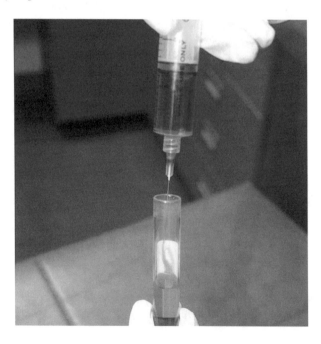

"This vial will be sent to the hospital lab for more detailed testing. That testing will tell us the patient's complete metabolic profile. We won't get that test result back until tomorrow."

Nurse Prochaska sealed the rubber stoppers onto the vials and dropped them, unlabeled, into the pocket on the front of her nursing scrubs.

"Okay," she continued as she laid syringe B down on the counter and picked up syringe A. It was still filled with Mrs. Jones' partially coagulated discard blood. "We simply reconnect syringe A to the Huber needle and re-infuse the discard blood into the patient."

Heather's eyes opened wide with surprise as she watched Nurse Prochaska re-inject the discard blood into Mrs. Jones. Heather had not anticipated that. It seemed odd to inject something called "discard blood" back into the patient. Heather was right. It was extremely dangerous. The discard blood was partially coagulated. It could have instantly stopped Mrs. Jones' heart. Thankfully, it did not.

"Now," Linda said as she unhooked syringe A from the patient, "syringe A is thrown away."

She reached to the countertop beside them and dropped it into a biohazard container.

"Lastly, we wipe the saline bag down with alcohol," she said as she picked up syringe B off the countertop, where it had been laying. She unhooked the needle from syringe B, dropped it, too, into the biohazard container and then attached a new sterile needle. "We use syringe B to withdraw 10cc more saline from the saline bag so we can flush the patient's port once more."

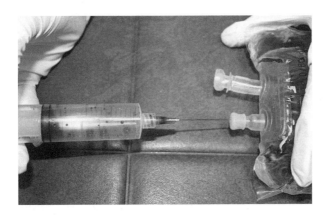

Heather watched the needle on syringe B pierce the rubber stopper on the saline bag. Something didn't feel right. Syringe B had just been filled with Mr.

Jones' blood. She could still see the droplets of the patient's blood in the syringe. Now, the very same syringe was attached to the 500cc *community* saline bag—the same *community* saline bag that would be used for all the cancer center patients. Heather was certain that she must have missed something. Certainly, she couldn't be seeing what she saw. She watched as the blood-laden syringe filled with saline. The saline in the syringe had a pink hue as the saline mixed with the blood droplets that still remained inside. Time slowed down, and she thought she could see traces of blood floating into the community saline bag. If small droplets of Mrs. Jones' blood were now floating around in the community saline bag, that meant that the next patient to come along would be injected with Mrs. Jones' blood. Consequently, the third patient of the day would be injected with both Mrs. Jones' blood and that of the patient after her. It was suddenly apparent that if this was right, the last patient of the day would be injected with the blood of *every* prior patient.

"Umm," Heather interjected softly, but then stopped herself. She was already beginning to learn Linda's impatience with questions. Clearly, there must have been something she didn't understand. There was no need to make a fool of herself by asking a stupid question on her first real day on the job.

Linda disconnected syringe B from the saline bag and reattached it to the Huber needle in Mrs. Jones' port. Heather stood quietly as Linda squeezed the syringe. The saline rushed through the Huber needle and into Mrs. Jones. Heather watched as Linda finished the procedure by injecting the Mrs. Jones with an anti-clotting drug, again using syringe B.

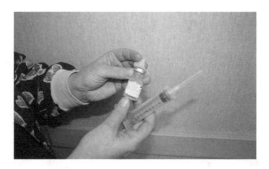

"If Mrs. Jones were here today for chemo," Linda added, "we would also give her some anti-nausea drug."

Linda finally pulled the Huber needle from Mrs. Jones' port and taped a cotton ball over the port to stop the bleeding.

"Thank you, Mrs. Jones," Heather said as Linda picked up her tote and the two nurses turned and walked away.

"I'm sorry to ask," Heather apologized to Linda. "But should we be reusing syringes to access the saline bag?"

Linda stopped and glanced down at the community saline bag, which still lay in her nursing tote, and then looked back to Heather. "Sure, it's okay. It's not like we are using them on different patients. We use a syringe on the same patient."

"But wouldn't reusing the syringe introduce blood into the saline bag?" Heather protested.

Linda's eyes narrowed as she glanced quickly at the saline bag. A long moment went by as she considered the question. She returned her gaze to Heather and said sharply, "That is the way we do it in this office." She gathered up her tote and walked away briskly.

Heather watched her retreat. She was puzzled by the exchange but decided to let it go for now. She didn't want to cause a rift between her and Linda on her first day.

Heather Seeks Information

Heather was not satisfied with the explanation Linda had given her. Over the next few weeks, she studied oncology nursing manuals. Her intuition was right. The contaminated community saline bag was endangering the life of each and every cancer center patient.

She approached Linda again.

"I looked it up," she began. "Using the blood-tainted syringe to access the community saline bag is improper procedure. It contaminates the saline bag."

Once again, Linda did not like having her authority challenged.

"That is the way Dr. Javed wants it done," she declared.

Heather looked at her doubtfully.

"Look." Linda took a deep breath. "When the needle pierces the rubber stopper on the saline bag, the rubber stopper acts like a filter, to filter out the blood from the syringe. And like I said before, our procedure is how Dr. Javed taught me, and *that is how he wants it done!*"

Linda was the head nurse, and Heather didn't feel comfortable challenging her further, so she dropped the issue. In her research, she had also found that the cancer center regularly violated several other standard nursing practices, such as not using gloves and gowns for administration and mixing of chemotherapy. She decided to ask Dr. Javed about it.

"If you would like to wear the space suit," he replied sarcastically, "we'll get it for you."

However, the gowns and gloves were not brought into the cancer center for another six months.

"Doctor," Heather continued, "my uncle—who is a patient with us—asked if it was safe for us to use a common flush bag for all the patients. In the hospital, each patient has their own separate saline bag for flushes. And, one other thing… I don't think it is safe for us to—"

"You are not working in the hospital," he finally cut her off. He was annoyed with her questions. He wished Heather were more like Linda, who did what she was told without question. "We don't follow the same rules as the hospital," he explained as patiently as he could. "The way that we do it here is acceptable. In the future, if anyone ever has a question about what you're doing, then I would like you to direct them to me. *I* am the doctor. *I* am the expert in oncology."

Heather was silent. There was nothing else to be said. Dr. Javed had an outstanding reputation in the medical community as a well-educated oncologist, and Heather was only in her second month of oncology nursing. He should know what he was talking about. Still, the port flush procedure just didn't look safe. However, Javed was her boss and she didn't want to jeopardize her employment by irritating him with her questions. She decided the best course of action was not to challenge Javed or Linda any further, but to quietly adopt the proper nursing techniques she learned from her independent reading.

■

CHAPTER 5

A Possible Suicide Attempt

Over the next two years, Javed's clinic continued to grow at an astonishing rate. Javed's nursing staff quickly had its hands full handling the patient demand, even when the *entire* staff was present. When one of them was absent because of illness or vacation, it was impossible to attend to all the new cancer center patients. From time to time, some of the hospital's nurses helped out at the cancer center on their own time, when it was short-staffed. As they returned to their nursing duties in the hospital, rumors of Javed's personal life began to spread. He had been increasingly absent from his office during work hours, taking long lunch breaks, coming in late and leaving early. His staff began complaining that sometimes, they could not even reach him by telephone to ask questions about patient treatment. When he was in the office, he had begun spending more and more time locked in his private office on long, drawn-out phone calls with an unidentified woman. It was becoming well-understood around gossip circles that Javed was having an affair and that he refused to fire Nurse Prochaska, despite her ill demeanor and repeated protocol violations, because she allowed him to conduct his affair at her cabin on Lake Okoboji. More importantly, however, he was obviously letting it get in the way of treating patients.

August 9, 2000—12:32 P.M.

"Why? Why? You can't do this!" Javed screamed as he slammed the phone on the kitchen countertop in his house in Fremont. "Don't say those things! I need you! You can't leave me!" he shouted as he held the phone out at arm's length.

His face was dark red as tears poured down his cheeks.

"I don't care," he cried aloud, putting the phone back to his ear. "No! No! You cannot say that!"

He cradled the phone to his ear with his shoulder as he fumbled with a pill bottle.

"Alright, fine! I can't live without you!" He slammed the telephone receiver down and wrestled with the pill bottle.

August 9, 2000—1:05 P.M.

"*Dr. Aronson,*" a voice over the intercom interrupted the silence. "There is a call from the ER on line two."

Dr. Marvin Aronson had been an internal medicine physician in Fremont and the chairman of the medicine committee at the hospital for years. He picked up the phone in his private practice office, hoping he wouldn't have to make a trip over to the hospital emergency room. He had a lot of patients to see that afternoon and didn't want to get behind schedule.

"Aronson," he said.

"Marvin, we have an odd situation in the ER," the voice began.

In previous years, the hospital had not had regular ER physicians on staff. Instead, Dr. Aronson and the other primary care physicians were regularly called to see the emergency room patients. Dr. Aronson had seen all the horrors that an ER had to offer, so whatever it was, he could handle it.

"What have you got?" He sighed.

"The squad just brought in a possible suicide attempt in handcuffs."

Aronson calmly nodded his head as he looked back down to the paper-work on his desk.

"Yes?" he asked as he went back to signing the documents before him.

"It's one of the medical staff."

"What?" Marvin asked, puzzled.

"It's Dr. Javed."

"It's a suicide attempt? Are you sure?" he quizzed.

"The EMT is calling it is a possible suicide attempt. Would you come over and see him? He asked for you."

"Sure, I'll be right there."

Puzzled by the news, Aronson made his way across the street, from his office to the ER. He had never known Javed to have emotional problems in all his many encounters with him over the past two years.

"How is he?" he asked the attending nurse as she met him just outside the patient room door.

"He's stable," she answered, handing him updated medical records.

"Hello, Tahir," Aronson said, almost as a question, as he entered and began to look him up and down.

Javed sat on the exam table before him. His hair was in disarray, and he tried to comb through it with his fingers.

"Marvin, sorry to bother you," he apologized. "I'm fine. My friend just got a little excited and called 911."

"How are you feeling?" Dr. Aronson said, leaning in closer as he shined a small light into Javed's eyes. Javed looked okay. His eyes were bloodshot, although Aronson did not note it in his report. Javed had already confessed to the paramedic that they were red because he had been having personal problems.

"Have you been drinking or taking drugs?"

"No." Javed blinked reflexively at the light. "I've just, umm… I had a heated and emotional discussion with a friend earlier. That's all. It was all just a mistake, you know?"

Dr. Aronson was silent.

"You know, it was all just a misunderstanding. I have been crying because I was upset over some personal issues. I don't know if you know this, but Fouzia left me. I miss her and the kids so much I can't stand it. I'm just crazy with loneliness for them. I decided to take my mind off of them by transferring some meds from sample packets to a pill bottle. I was so upset that I spilled the pills all over the floor. My friend came by to check on me because she knows I am so miserable. When she walked in she saw me crying and sitting on the floor with all these pills around me and she assumed that I was trying to overdose. But I wasn't. I was just transferring pills from sample packets to a pill bottle. So, it was really just a big misunderstanding, you know? I should be going now, I have patients to see."

"Look, Tahir," Aronson cut him off, putting his hand on Javed's shoulder to stop him from climbing down off the exam table. "I know you've had some increased stress of late, but you have to take care of yourself. Your patients need you. We all need you here in Fremont."

"Don't worry, I'm fine," Javed declared. "Look, I'll show you. I'll take a drug test. I'll take a urine screen. I'll prove I didn't take anything."

Javed brushed his hand over his eyes and took a deep breath as he waited for Dr. Aronson to respond. Dr. Aronson could report the possible suicide attempt to the hospital physician health committee for review. The physician health committee was a division of the hospital medical staff committees. Its purpose was to review reported concerns about physicians' health, and how their health issues affected their ability to safely practice medicine. If Dr.

Aronson reported the possible suicide attempt to the physician health committee, there was the chance that the committee would find Javed too emotionally distraught to safely practice medicine. In that case, Javed would lose his admitting privileges to the hospital. If he lost his admitting privileges, his office practice would be greatly hampered. He simply could not care for oncology patients effectively if he could not admit patients to the hospital. Javed had to convince Dr. Aronson that he had not attempted suicide if he was to continue to practice medicine in Fremont.

Tahir sat up straight.

"Marvin, I'm fine," Javed repeated as he took a deep breath and spoke earnestly. "Things have turned around for me. I spoke to Fouzia last night and she is considering coming home," he lied. "You know, I love her. When she and the kids come back, then everything will be back to normal. But whether she is here or not, I will continue to be devoted to my patients here in Fremont."

There was silence as Dr. Aronson carefully examined Javed. He found no physical abnormalities. He took his stethoscope out of his ears and looked Javed over one last time as he pondered the situation. He had never had a reason to doubt Javed's truthfulness in the past. Javed's offer to take a urine screen was persuasive. Once it came back negative, all the physical evidence showed that Javed was not an immediate danger to himself or others. Dr. Aronson flipped open the patient chart and started making a few notes.

"All right, Tahir, I can see this was a misunderstanding," he said as he wrote. "I won't do an alcohol assessment, and I'm not going to interview the young lady who called the rescue squad. I suggest you go home and get some rest. Alright?"

Dr. Aronson did not report Javed's possible suicide attempt to the hospital's physicians health committee. Javed weathered the situation unscathed.

April 1, 2001

Dr. Javed was having an affair. It is unknown if this woman was the one who called in the possible suicide attempt a year earlier. Years later, in the state's investigation, she would be identified as "Individual #7." Her real name was withheld from the public for her own protection. She didn't know it then, but she was going to become a victim of Dr. Javed.

"Hey, babe," Javed spoke softly into the telephone.

"Oh," she paused. "Tahir. Hi," she answered unenthusiastically. She had become tired of their relationship, but didn't have the will to tell him it was over. In the past couple of months she had repeatedly given him signals that she wanted to break it off altogether, but the hints fell on deaf ears.

"Hey, listen," he began after an awkward pause in the conversation. "Let's get together tonight—"

"You know, Tahir, I've been meaning to talk to you—"

"—at my office," he cut her off, sensing her reluctance.

He caught her off-guard and it broke her train of thought.

"Your office?" she was puzzled.

"Well, I've noticed something that worries me, and I'd like to run a couple of tests. But I'm sure it's nothing."

She was confused by his request.

"What are you talking about, Tahir?"

"Just relax, honey," he tried to calm her.

"What are you talking about?"

"I don't want to worry you, like I said, I'm sure it's nothing. I just want to make sure."

"Make sure of what? What is it? Do you think I have cancer? Is this a sick April Fool's joke?"

"No, no. I wouldn't joke about something as serious as this. Just meet me at my office around seven tonight. No one will be around and I'll check you over. Just remember that I love you, and I'll take care of you. Okay, babe?"

She had begun the phone call determined to end the relationship but the suggestion that she might be ill drove the thought out of her mind.

"Alright." She paused. "I'll be there at seven."

The hours of the day passed with endless worry. When the time finally arrived to meet him at his office, she was riddled with anxiety. Her inclination to break off their relationship seemed trivial compared to the idea of dying a long and horrible death from cancer. When they finally met at his office door that night he greeted her with a quick peck on the cheek, and then led her back to a patient room. With the skillful hands of a trained oncologist, he carefully carried out the charade of examining her, making notes along the way. He even drew a vial of blood to send to the pathology lab. She was naïve to the process. She had no idea it was all a deception.

"Well?" she asked as she was getting dressed after the exam. "Tell me what is going on, Tahir. Level with me."

"I won't know anything for sure until I get the lab results back. I'll put a rush order on it and we should know soon," he said as he finished his note in her medical record. "But for now, the best thing to do is take your mind off our worries. Let's go out and have some fun. We can eat at the restaurant that you like, and you can stay at my house tonight. Tomorrow, I'll get the results back from the lab and then likely, we can celebrate your good health." He smiled as he looked into her eyes and then kissed her passionately. She didn't resist him.

In the morning, he woke up just after seven o'clock and left her sleeping in his bed to go into the office. Casually, he had his cup of coffee and went over some office charts.

"Dr. Javed," his receptionist finally interrupted his morning routine. "There is a call for you on line one."

He knew who it was without asking.

"Hey, babe," he answered the phone after closing the door for privacy.

She could tell something was wrong by the sad tone in his voice.

"What did you find out?" she whimpered.

"I'm sorry to have to tell you this," he said somberly. "You have a very rare type of cancer. It's fast-moving, but thankfully, we caught it early on."

There was silence on the other end of the phone.

"Honey?" he continued. "This is a terrible thing, but it is treatable. We can get through this together."

The news hurt so deeply that she struggled to breathe as tears began to roll down her face.

"Is…is it terminal?"

He paused again for effect.

"Well, I'm not going to sugarcoat it for you. It is a very aggressive type of cancer. But there have been a few recorded cases where people have overcome it. And there are some new, easier techniques and treatments. You won't have to even go though traditional chemo. If you do have any side effects I can prescribe medications that will make them go away. You won't even know you have cancer."

There was no answer, only a faint sobbing.

"The only downside to the treatment is that it is extremely expensive. If you even turn a request for this drug over to your insurance they will likely cancel you altogether, and no other health insurance provider will be willing to pick you up. But you don't have to worry about that as long as I am around. I'll pay for every dime of this myself, babe. We will get you through this together. I love you," he said as he took the notes from the night before and tossed them into the trashcan by his desk.

She swallowed hard and found herself saying, "I love you, too."

June 2001

Two months had come and gone since Individual #7 had begun her "treatment regimen," which was billed to her insurance company. As time went on, she began to question the entire situation. She was suspicious that an aggressive type of cancer could be treated so easily. Javed was evasive when she asked him questions about the cancer and her prognosis. She decided to seek a second opinion.

Javed felt threatened when he found out that she was going to see another oncologist. He acted hurt by her lack of confidence and argued that she was gambling with her life by seeking care from anyone else. But she didn't care. She wasn't going to live with the uncertainties anymore. She needed to know the truth. After many sleepless nights of debating, she finally told him that their doctor/patient relationship was over. Shortly thereafter, their romantic relationship ended as well.

Eighteen days passed before she finally got in to see her new physician. The story she told him of Javed's treatment regimen didn't sound right, but it was hard to believe that Javed would concoct such a story to take advantage of the young woman. After all, this was immoral and unethical behavior. If he was found out, it would certainly be the end of his medical career, and no one would be foolish enough to take such a risk. Nevertheless, with an abundance of caution, her new physician ordered tests and sent them to a laboratory in Omaha.

July 19, 2001

Javed was nervous as he paced the floor of his office. With the door closed, he was able to think over the situation. Once those results came back, he could be in serious trouble. His options were limited but he thought about them over and over again. Finally, he sat behind his desk and reached for the phone.

He held his breath as he heard the phone ringing on the other end of the line.

"Hello," he began once a voice answered. "I'm calling about some tests I ordered yesterday for a young lady," he lied. "I'd like to cancel those labs tests."

"Let me check that for you, Doctor," the voice replied.

When the voice came back on, it brought bad news for Javed. The laboratory would not cancel the tests.

July 23, 2001

Desperate to stop the lab tests, Javed called the Omaha laboratory again four days later. This time, he impersonated another local physician. Again, he had the same result. The lab tests could not be cancelled. This time, it was because he was too late—the lab tests had already been run. However, the lab did agree to send him a copy of the results.

Impersonating another physician, sexual misconduct with a patient, falsifying medical records and insurance claims were all grounds to lose a medical license. Tahir Javed was on a downward spiral. It was only a matter of time.

CHAPTER 6

∎

Evelyn Recalls
Her First Cancer Diagnosis

October 16, 2000

"Good morning, Evelyn!" one of the other parents called to me as I pulled my car up to the curb.

"Good morning," I answered as Alex leaned over and kissed me on the cheek.

"Bye, Mom."

"Bye, Sparky. Good luck with your presentation." I smiled to myself. Alex was fourteen years old and still kissing his mother goodbye. I was blessed beyond measure.

I turned the car west on Military Avenue. The street had recently been lined with flags to mark Columbus Day. Every year on Memorial Day, Flag Day, July Fourth and Columbus Day, the local veterans put up hundreds of American flags, which lined Military Avenue from one end of town to the other.

I drove into the Fremont State Lakes and parked the car near Victory Lake. The lakes were always brimming with people in the summer but that day, it was deserted except for an occasional walker. I strapped on my Rollerblades and took a quick spin around the park. The October sun made the falling cottonwood leaves look like drops of gold falling into the blue water.

Ah, it's going to be a special day, I thought to myself. I could feel it. I was forty-five years old, in excellent health, had three fine sons and a wonderful husband. Life was good.

The five-minute drive to my office was not long enough for me to catch my breath. Gathering up my business suit and duffle bag, I walked across the McDonald's parking lot to my husband's office. His building had an on-call room with an adjoining bathroom. It was empty at that time of day, so I could use the shower to get ready for the day.

"Morning, Evie. The doctor's looking for you," Jean, the office manager, said as I entered the back door.

"Hi, Jean. Is he in his office?"

"I don't know. But I know he wants to talk to you."

I walked down the back hall, looking for Tom. Although it was only a little after eight o'clock in the morning, there were already patients waiting in the hall for lab work and X-rays.

"Evie, Doctor wants to see you," a staff member informed me.

"Doctor's in an exam room right now but he wants to talk to you," another said.

Every few yards, a different staff member delivered the same message. I was beginning to feel embarrassed because all the patients were looking at me, wondering what Tom wanted to say to me. I was beginning to wonder myself.

"Would you tell him I am downstairs taking a shower and then after that, I'll be at my office?" I told Robin when she, too, passed on the message. It was hard to know how long he would be in the exam room with a patient and I had my own patients to see in half an hour.

As I soaped up in the shower, I ran through the possibilities of what was on Tom's mind. I had just dropped off Alex. Maybe he had forgotten the poster presentation he was to give today and had called Tom to relay the message to me.

Perhaps there was a different family issue. We had talked to our two older sons, Luke and Curtis, at the university the night before and they'd seemed fine. Our parents were fine when we last talked to them—although with all of them in advanced age, anything could happen.

Probably just an employee problem, I thought as I rinsed off in the shower, being careful to avoid the bandage on my right breast.

Tom's family practice employed more than twenty employees. Quite a few of them had been with him more than ten years and were more like family members than employees.

When I opened the door of the shower room, my dear husband of twenty-one years appeared. His face was serious, with a hint of fear around his eyes.

"What's the matter?" I demanded. The concern on his face made me anxious.

"Let's go to your office. I'll tell you there," he said as he turned and led the way up the stairs.

He couldn't wait any longer to give me the news, however, and he stopped as we stepped outside.

"Ev, I have something to tell you. Your biopsy was positive." His face crumpled into tears. "Dr. Koerber called me this morning and told me."

"What? What are you saying?" I demanded, perplexed and fearful.

"Your breast biopsy. It was positive. You have breast cancer. I'm so sorry." Tears were streaming down his face.

"Oh, my God. I'd forgotten about the biopsy. Are you sure? Could there be a mistake? The other biopsies were negative," I said anxiously. "Maybe we should do another biopsy to make sure," I suggested.

"No, they're sure. But we can ask Dr. Javed when we see him. I already talked to him and he said we could come over any time."

"Wait a minute—you're going too fast. See Javed? Don't you think I should see Dr. Soori? He's rented office space from us for years."

"No, Soori is a fine oncologist but he is only in Fremont two days a week. It will be easier for you to have chemotherapy at Javed's Fremont office than to travel to Soori's office in Omaha. And, if you have a problem, it will be more convenient to see Javed right here in town."

"WAIT! Chemotherapy! I'm *not* having chemotherapy. I'll just have surgery and maybe radiation—but *no* chemotherapy."

Tom closed his eyes and slowly shrugged his shoulders.

"That's why we need to talk to the oncologist. We need to get all the information and options. We can go over and see Javed now if you want," he said in almost a whisper.

"Are you sure I should see Javed? What will I say to Dr. Soori when I see him in the hall?"

"Don't worry about that. I'll talk to Soori. He will want us to do what is best for us. When can you see Javed?"

Tom was being strong and helpful even though he was truly miserable inside.

"I don't know," I finally answered after a moment's pause. "I'll call you after I check my schedule."

I folded into his arms.

"Everything will be okay, honey," Tom whispered through my hair. "I love you."

"I love you too," I whispered back.

36

We lingered a bit before parting, bravely smiling at each other before turning away. In a daze, I slowly walked across the McDonald's parking lot to my office building.

I couldn't believe breast cancer had happened to *me*. I had always taken good care of myself. I exercised regularly, I never smoked or drank. I had breastfed each of our three sons for well over a year. I never dreamed that I would end up with cancer.

Inside my private office, I tried to collect my thoughts.

Okay, what do I have to do? Check my schedule... What am I looking for? An opening so we can see Dr. Javed... Dr. Javed? Oh my God, I've got breast cancer... I can't believe it... What am I going to do? Oh, check my schedule... What am I looking for?

The cycle of thoughts went round and round in my head until I finally forced my hand to pick up the phone and buzz my receptionist.

"Are there any openings in my schedule today? Would you bring me the appointment book?" I asked her.

My receptionist immediately knew there was a problem. She had been my right-hand woman for the past ten years. She could read my body language easily. She knew that I'd had a breast biopsy the previous week and at this point, there was no need to tell her the results. She could tell by the sound of my voice.

"You've got a couple of rechecks this morning. Mrs. Arnold is already here. But I'll call the others and see if I can catch them. I can have you done this morning by ten o'clock at the latest," she replied.

"Thanks, but Tom's not taking off the afternoon. I'm sure I won't have any doctor's visits this afternoon, and I don't want to sit at home by myself. I'll see patients after lunch. Just schedule me out from ten to one."

I wanted to be at work. I was too shocked and frightened to be alone with my thoughts. I desperately wanted the comfort that I've found working with patients. As we sat together in the hearing aid fitting room, patients generously shared their life stories with me. They talked about their marriages, families and occupations. They gave their first-person accounts of the Depression, World War II and the Cold War. They told me about their health problems. In the recounting of their stories, I witnessed their gracious acceptance of life's assaults as well as their dogged bravery to carry on as best they could. Today, more than ever, I needed to be with my patients, who were my mentors in courage.

At ten o'clock, Tom and I dodged cars as we walked across busy 23rd Street to Fremont Area Medical Center. Once we checked in with the receptionist at Fremont Cancer Center, we were immediately ushered into Dr. Javed's private office. Tom knew Dr. Javed well through mutual patients and respected his medical expertise. Today was my first introduction to him and he immediately put me at ease with his warmth and compassion.

"Well, you have been given a bit of bad news. But your tumor is very small and you have an excellent prognosis. With a tumor that small, you have a ninety-six percent chance of a five-year survival. If we can get you to that five-year point without a reoccurrence, you will have a normal life expectancy. You have several options for treatment and there are lots of good medicines now to keep you comfortable and keep your blood counts up so that you can complete therapy. Let's go over your options."

He smiled sincerely and picked up a pad and pen. He outlined all the surgical and radiation options. His presentation was thorough, clear and empathetic. When he finished his discussion and had answered all our questions, he walked us to the door.

"Cancer is challenging physically, emotionally and spiritually. But we are going to help you as much as we can. And I believe that you will come through it all very well."

He smiled again as he shook our hands. For the first time in several hours, I felt a bit of confidence.

For the next ten days, Tom and I searched for information on the Internet and spoke to breast cancer survivors. We consulted with the radiation oncologist, general surgeon, plastic surgeon, physical therapist, mental health counselor, spiritual advisor and a hairdresser/wigmaker. After carefully weighing all the considerations, we decided on a modified mastectomy with auxiliary node dissection and eight rounds of chemotherapy.

"Well, it's a good thing I gave up my aspirations of becoming a movie star a long time ago," I commented to Tom after we made our decision.

"Why? I think you can still be a movie star if you want to," he replied.

"No, after all of this, I don't think anyone would buy a movie ticket to see me nude."

"Not all movie stars are nude."

"Name one female movie star who hasn't been in a nude scene."

"Well, I can't name one right off hand but I'll do a Google search for 'fully clothed female movie stars' and see what I find. Or better yet, I'll Google 'nude movie stars' and then apply the process of elimination. There will be better illustrations that way," he teased. "And sweetheart," he gently continued, "I hate to be the one to break the news to you, but really, I'm not sure many people would have paid money to see you nude *before* all of this."

We both laughed. It felt good to laugh after so many intense conversations about cancer.

The mastectomy was done on November 1, 2000. The resulting lab report showed a disappointing finding. I had one positive lymph node out of the sixteen that were removed. Once again, Dr. Javed was positive and encouraging.

"Since the tumor was so small and because it is an estrogen-positive tumor, you still have an excellent prognosis. You'll do fine," he reiterated.

I believed him with all my heart. He was compassionate but upbeat. Moreover, he was able to quote pertinent research and statistics off the top of his head. I thought he was an intelligent man and an excellent physician. I was certain that I was receiving the very best medical care.

Chemotherapy

My first chemotherapy infusion was on November 16, 2000. Through the next six months, I lost my hair, had nausea, vomiting, fatigue, "swimmy" eyesight, low blood counts and joint aches from the growth factor shots—all par for the course.

Tom and I developed a friendly relationship with Tahir through the course of the chemotherapy. We asked him about his children and he asked us about ours. He never mentioned that he was separated from his wife and children and we had not heard about the split through the hospital grapevine. Dr. Javed was very attentive to me and even called me on the weekend immediately after each chemotherapy infusion to inquire about nausea and the other side effects.

I had a chemotherapy infusion every three weeks. Tom would meet me at Dr. Javed's office on the appointed Thursday morning. After we checked in with his receptionist, *June*, the medical assistant, Raegene, would escort me to an exam room and take my vitals. My routine lab work was drawn the day before and processed through my primary care physician, *Dr. Vincent Osborn*. When Dr. Javed entered the room, he would review the lab results and briefly examine me. He would ask me about the nausea, bone pain and fatigue, and offer treatment options if I needed more help with side effects.

When the clinic visit was over, Tom would either go back to work or he would follow me to the infusion room. On the days he went with me to the infusion room, he would sit with me until chemotherapy was underway, then return to work. I always had my blood drawn at my primary care physician's office. As a result, the cancer center nurses never drew my blood, and therefore, Tom did not witness their reuse of blood-tainted syringes.

Chemotherapy was administered in a large room with eight recliners. A TV was bracketed to the wall on one end of the room. On the other end there was a counter where the nurses kept their supplies. The lab tests were run in a smaller, glass room off to the side.

The recliners were usually full of cancer patients in various stages of sickness and treatment. Often, patients developed camaraderie and talked among themselves. At that point, I was too tired and depressed to visit with the other patients. I didn't want to compare notes with the other cancer patients about side effects, lab reports, or whether the tumor was growing or shrinking. I just wanted to close my eyes and sleep during chemo and dream about better times.

Chemotherapy was difficult but not defeating. Throughout, there was a wonderful outpouring of love, concern, prayers, gifts, meals and favors from family, friends and the community in general. I received over 200 get-well cards—many from people I didn't know.

My last chemotherapy treatment finally took place on April 10, 2001. Tom came as I was finishing and then we were called into Dr. Javed's private office. We chatted a minute about the plan for follow-up and how often I needed to have my port flushed. Dr. Javed smiled charmingly and congratulated us on the completion of chemotherapy.

"Now we just have to sit back and wait for the good results," he predicted.

It was nearly noon and the cancer center was all but deserted. As we walked past the front desk to exit, Linda, Raegene and June jumped up from where they had crouched down below the counter and threw handfuls of confetti at us.

"CONGRATULATIONS, EVELYN!" they yelled.

Tom and I were bursting with optimism as we brushed off the confetti. Our hope was so warm it felt like the spring sun was shining on us inside the Fremont Area Medical Center.

I had a conversation that night with our son, Alex.

"Glad to be done with chemo, Mom?" he asked as he set the table.

"Oh, yeah. Very glad. Very, very glad," I answered while stirring soup at the stove. "Only thing, though, I like the word 'swimmy,' as in 'my eyes are swimmy.' I won't have the opportunity to say that any more."

"Hmm," Alex considered this thoughtfully. "Well, you could say, 'Tadpoles are swimmy.'"

"Well, true, but it's a little difficult to work into a conversation."

He thought as he put a spoon at each place setting.

"Well, my friend Jeff likes to fish. You could call him and tell him."

I watched him as I considered that option.

"So, how would this conversation go?" I formed my fingers into an imaginary telephone receiver and put it to my ear. "Hello, Jeff? This is Alex's mom. Did you know that tadpoles are swimmy?"

We both laughed. A little silliness was good for our souls. Even though everyone was optimistic, I still had five years of waiting to see if the cancer stayed in remission. At that moment, I knew that no matter what happened to me, though, my boys would be okay. Whether the chemo worked or not, the boys had grown in maturity and independence as they'd supported me through my cancer journey. In addition, Tom was an excellent father. Whatever further parenting was needed, Tom could handle it if I was not around to help him. The realization gave me great comfort.

Several weeks later, I had a checkup with Dr. Javed. He briefly examined me and reviewed my lab results.

"I see your liver enzymes are elevated," he noted. "I'm going to order a hepatitis C screen."

"That will come back negative," Tom insisted, rather surprised at the suggestion. "She has never had any exposure to hepatitis C. She has never had a blood transfusion. She has never abused drugs."

"Let's just go ahead and make sure," Javed said, looking unconcerned.

Tom called me several days later. "Your hepatitis C screen came back negative. I knew it would," he rejoiced.

"Oh, good" I said. "What is hepatitis C, anyway?"

I didn't listen to his answer, though. I was thinking about our future. I was confident that our future included a return to excellent health.

■

CHAPTER 7

The Dan McGill Story

March 25, 2001

Kay McGill had just arrived at her office at the Arbor Manor Nursing Home when a voice interrupted her.

"Are you Kay? I have flowers for you," said the elderly flower deliveryman with a carnation pinned on his lapel. "I hope you enjoy them."

Kay turned from hanging her coat in the closet to see the man put a large bouquet of red roses on her desk. She carefully took the card from its holder so as not to disturb the roses' fragile beauty.

"Thank you for forty wonderful years—Love, Dan," the card read.

Kay breathed in the flowers' fragrance while tears filled her eyes. It was their wedding anniversary. She and Dan had stuck together for better or worse, in sickness and in health, for forty years. Lately, sickness had been more predominant in their lives than health. Dan had been diagnosed with colon cancer in the fall of 1999. He'd had several difficult surgeries, months of taxing chemotherapy and a cycle of radiation that caused excruciating burns. Just recently, Dr. Javed had called them to say that the latest round of tests showed no evidence of cancer. To celebrate their anniversary and his apparent return to good health, Kay and Dan were going to spend the weekend at a casino resort in Council Bluffs, Iowa.

Even though it was their anniversary, Kay was surprised to receive flowers from Dan. He had never sent flowers to her in all their years together. Dan was loving and considerate, but he usually kept his feelings to himself. As a truck salesman, he had been a good provider for her and their two daughters. His happy-go-lucky attitude and his fun-loving nature were what first attracted Kay to him. Even during the worst of the cancer treatment, Dan would steer conversations away from his illness and on to some funny joke or story.

Yes, it has been forty wonderful years, Kay thought as she wiped the tears from her eyes. *I hope the cancer is really gone and we will have many more wonderful years together.*

They did have a wonderful weekend at the casino. It was delightful to have a happy, carefree time together without worrying about sickness or the possibility of cancer shortening their lives together.

The day after their casino weekend, Dan woke up feeling ill. His stomach was distended and he felt nauseous. He went to see his family physician, who immediately admitted him to the hospital. His blood pressure dropped dangerously low. His stomach became hugely distended and very hard. It all happened within just a few hours.

"What's going on?" Kay questioned the doctor. "He felt so well over the weekend. How could he get so sick so quickly?"

"I don't know, Kay," the doctor replied. "I'm worried about him. I suggest we transfer him to the med center in Omaha and let the gastroenterologists take over his care."

At the University of Nebraska Medical Center (UNMC), Dan was assigned to the care of Dr. Hemant Roy. Dr. Roy ordered blood tests and scans and determined that Dan was infected with hepatitis C. Dr. Roy carefully questioned Dan and Kay about Dan's risk factors. Dan had had a blood transfusion at age seventeen because of a ruptured appendix. However, he had passed Red Cross screening tests to be a regular blood donor for most of his adult years. He had never used recreational drugs.

"I'm sorry, Dan," Dr. Roy admitted. "We just can't give you the cause of your hepatitis C. And at this point, I can't even give you a prognosis. Right now, we are working very hard to get your blood pressure stable, reduce the fluid in your abdomen and stop the diarrhea. Generally, hepatitis C progresses very slowly, over decades. Usually, people don't even know they have it until the disease is very advanced. You are having so many symptoms now that it leads me to believe that there is something additional going on here. One explanation could be alcohol abuse. How much alcohol are you drinking these days?"

Dan's voice was too weak to be heard, so Kay answered for him.

"He is only a social drinker, and has drunk even less since the cancer diagnosis.

He did have a glass of wine with dinner during our weekend at the casino, but that has been nearly two weeks ago now," Kay answered. "Dr. Roy, why hasn't the hepatitis C shown up before now? He has had blood tests over the past year as part of his cancer treatments. They never showed anything. How is it that he sailed through cancer treatment and now this 'insignificant' disease is making him so sick?"

"Well, hepatitis C is only diagnosed if a specific test is ordered," Dr. Roy answered. "If Dan's doctors did not see anything in his history or lab results to suggest hepatitis C, they would not have ordered a test to see if he had it. And I didn't mean to suggest that hepatitis C is always a benign disease. It can be fatal in very advanced cases. But again, it usually does not progress rapidly unless there are other factors, such as alcoholism. Now, how many drinks per week would you say Dan has?" Dr. Roy reiterated.

Kay gave the same answer. He was not, nor had he ever been, an alcoholic. Nevertheless, it was a question she would have to answer repeatedly over the course of the next year. Although many questions about Dan's health did not have answers, that one question had a very clear and consistent answer. Dan was only a social drinker. For the past eighteen months, he'd rarely drank. He was not drinking any alcohol at all since the latest health crisis.

Several days were devoted to evaluating Dan for a liver transplant in June 2001. Again, many questions were asked regarding his medical history, including the question that had now becoming quite annoying: "How much alcohol does Dan drink?"

In early July 2001, Dr. Roy called Kay at work.

"Kay," he began, "we are going over all of the information about Dan to determine if and when he should be placed on the liver transplant list. There is a report here from your family doctor that says, 'Dan is drinking alcohol heavily and excessively.' I don't understand that. When I've asked you, you've told me he does not drink alcohol at all. Can you explain this to me?"

"Dr. Roy, as I have said many times before, Dan is not now, nor has he ever drank heavily and excessively. He has not had any alcohol to drink since our anniversary in March. And he drank very little before then. We saw the physician's assistant in our primary care doctor's office recently. He asked me if Dan was drinking. I thought he meant was he drinking his nutritional supplement. I said 'No, I'm having a terrible time trying to get him to drink any.' He didn't ask me about alcohol at all that I remember. And if he had, the answer is, as before, 'Dan is not drinking alcohol.'"

"Well, Kay, I suggest you call your family doctor and ask him to change the report," Dr. Roy responded flatly.

Dr. Roy had no way of knowing how Dan had contracted hepatitis C. He didn't know of the dangerous nursing practices at the Fremont Cancer Center. He did know, however, that hepatitis C could advance very rapidly in alcoholics, and Dan's disease was advancing rapidly. That fact shaped the way he and other healthcare providers questioned Dan.

"If Dan is drinking at all," Dr. Roy added, "there is very little likelihood that he will be placed on the transplant list. For the time being, the transplant team is going to recommend that Dan be cancer-free for five years before we transplant him. Now, how long has he been cancer-free?"

Kay counted backwards in her head.

"He has been cancer-free for about eighteen months now. So, he can't get a new liver for three and a half years?"

"Yes, we'll revisit the idea then. The simple fact is that there are not enough livers to go around. The transplant team wants to make sure a patient will have a long-term chance of survival before the patient will be put on the list. We don't want someone to get one of the precious few available livers if their life will be shortened through cancer or alcoholism. We'll continue to work real hard to get his diarrhea, internal fluid buildup and blood pressure under control. Once we do, I'm sure the three and a half years will go by quickly and uneventfully."

The Course of Dan's Hepatitis C: March 2001–April 2002

Dan's doctors were not able to get his symptoms under control. Dan's liver began to fail and he developed cirrhosis. As the hepatitis C virus destroyed his liver, previously healthy liver tissue was replaced by scar tissue. His liver could no longer function properly. The scar tissue blocked the normal flow of blood through the liver. Fluid seeped from his liver into his abdominal cavity. The accumulated fluid (known as "ascites") distended his abdomen. To relieve his discomfort, doctors drained the fluid through a needle inserted into his abdomen. Often, as much as two liters of fluid would be removed from Dan's abdomen. Frequently, he developed low blood pressure in response to the removal of such a large quantity of fluid. Intravenous fluids and medications were then given to Dan to combat his low blood pressure.

Dan's life became a cycle of tapping his abdomen to drain off the fluid, then giving him IV fluids and albumin (a type of protein) to counteract his resulting low blood pressure. He became weaker and weaker. Fluid began to accumulate not only in his abdomen, but also in his legs and organs. Within a year, Dan went from a big, strapping, six-foot tall, 230-pound man to an emaciated skeleton weighing less than ninety pounds. His suffering was relentless.

Watching Dan deteriorate was heartbreaking for Kay and their family. She called her family physician's office in January of 2002, seeking help. She told the clinic nurse that Dan's diarrhea had become uncontrollable.

"Is he back on the booze again?" the nurse asked.

Kay was so outraged that she hung up without dignifying the question with an answer.

Dan entered the hospital for the last time in mid-April 2002. He knew he wasn't going to live much longer. His wife and daughters lovingly sat by his bedside and tended to his needs. He lost his stoic demeanor and readily offered weak hugs and kisses to his family.

On April 15, 2002, their family physician visited his room. He asked Kay to step into a consultation room so he could speak to her privately. He gently told her that Dan's organs were shutting down and that there was no hope for survival. All they could do was to make him as comfortable as possible.

While Kay was out of the room, a dark-complexioned man in a business suit entered. He greeted Dan's daughters and looked Dan over briefly before he asked to speak to Kay. He made small talk with Dan's two daughters while he waited for Kay but he had to leave before she returned to the room.

"Who was that?" daughter Susanne asked the staff nurse after the man left the room.

"That was Dr. Javed," the nurse answered.

"Well, that was nice of him to stop by. Mom will be disappointed she didn't get to speak to him. She and Dad think so highly of him," Susanne told her sister.

Dan died shortly thereafter, in the company of his loving family. His year-long battle with hepatitis C was over. It was unknown at the time, but the first victim of the Nebraska outbreak had been claimed.

■

CHAPTER 8

Some Alarming Patient Reports

"I'm dumbfounded that when something like this is occurring that people in these roles didn't seek advice from knowledgeable people in the field to handle the situation properly."

—Dr. Michael A. McIlroy, MD
(Expert witness testimony, February 21, 2006)

February 5, 2001

"Hello, Dr. Javed? This is *Ralph Dinsdale*. One of my breast cancer patients that you have been treating has elevated liver enzymes. I did some tests and it turns out she has hepatitis C. She's a real nice older lady and has no risk factors. She has never had a blood transfusion—nothing. What do you make of it?"

Dr. Ralph Dinsdale had been practicing internal medicine in Fremont since 1973. As a seasoned primary-care physician, he had seen some unusual things. However, a new diagnosis of hepatitis C in a white-haired pillar of the Baptist Church was more than unusual—it was unheard of.

"Really?" Javed questioned with a surprised tone. "Who is it?"

"*Priscilla Green*," Dinsdale answered.

"Oh, really? I don't know, Ralph," Javed answered. "I suppose she has probably had it for a long time and this is just the first time she was tested for it. She probably got it years ago during a surgery or an IV. Women of her generation often contracted it through blood transfusions after childbirth, you know."

"But she has never had any blood transfusions," Dr. Dinsdale insisted. "Actually, she has never even had an IV other than when she was receiving chemo at your clinic."

"Well, drug abuse has existed for years," Javed smoothly replied. "Who knows what's in her past? I have several cases of hepatitis C in my clinic. We think the good folks of Nebraska are angels in overalls, but temptation has always existed, no matter where people live."

"I assure you, this lady was no drug abuser," Dinsdale replied firmly. "I've been taking care of her for thirty years and she never had elevated liver enzymes until this December."

"Hmm. Well, chemo does some strange things to the immune system. Maybe her chemo is the reason for the elevated liver enzymes," Javed explained. "Other than that, I just don't know. I'm sorry, Ralph. I have no idea where she may have gotten it. I'm sure it won't be much of a problem for her, though. I would tell her not to worry about it, if I were you."

Dinsdale was not satisfied, but the conversation with Javed was fruitless.

"Alright," he finally replied. "Well, thanks for your time."

"Anytime," Javed said as they hung up.

Javed stood up from behind his desk and walked down the hall to the chemo room.

"Hello, Doctor." One of his patients waved to him from where she sat in a chemo chair across the room.

"Hi, *Mrs. Hawver.*" He waved back politely, with a smile, as he opened one of the cupboard doors.

A sticky note was stuck to the inside of the cabinet door. Without hesitation, he withdrew his ballpoint pen from his white coat pocket and scribbled down a name.

"Priscilla Green," he wrote below the other names.

Dr. Dinsdale was puzzled when he hung up the phone. He had seen one, maybe two cases of hepatitis C in over thirty years of medical practice. Now, he had just diagnosed a new case and Javed had told him of "several" other cases in his practice. His conversation with Javed had raised more questions than answers.

What is the world coming to if hepatitis C was showing up in innocent, elderly people in Middle America? he thought to himself.

Unsatisfied, he dialed Gerri Means, the infection control nurse at Fremont Area Medical Center.

"Hello, Gerri? Ralph Dinsdale," he began once she answered. "I just diagnosed a nice, older lady with hepatitis C, but there is something not right about it. She has no risk factors. She has no history of drug use or promiscuous sex. She had never had an IV until she started seeing Dr. Javed for chemotherapy. I'm just perplexed how she may have gotten it. Do you have any ideas?"

"No risk factors?" Gerri repeated.

"No."

"So she doesn't have tattoos, either? Hepatitis C can be passed through unclean tattoo needles."

"No," Dinsdale interjected. "She doesn't have any tattoos."

"No transfusions, IV drugs or promiscuity?"

"No," he repeated.

"Has she ever lived with someone with hepatitis C?" Gerri continued to question him.

"No, nothing. She has *no* risk factors, except that she is currently on chemo. But I can't imagine that she could have gotten it there."

Even though Javed's clinic was the obvious answer, it was inconceivable to Dr. Dinsdale that the clinic would have infected one of its own patients.

"Did you talk to Dr. Javed?" Gerri asked.

"Yes, he can't figure it out either," Dinsdale continued. "He said he had several other cases of hepatitis C. Have you come across other cases? Are you seeing a general increase in the numbers?"

"I'll look at my line log," Gerri answered. "Right off hand, I don't remember that there is an increase."

"Are you going to look into these cases, Javed's and mine and any others? Are you going to run an investigation?"

"When I look at my line log, I'll see if there are any patterns or any red flags," Gerri promised. "I'll keep my eyes open, but you know I don't have access to Dr. Javed's records since his clinic is not part of the hospital. Thanks for letting me know, Dr. Dinsdale. I'll keep a lookout."

One of Gerri's responsibilities was to keep a record of the communicable diseases that were diagnosed in the hospital. When a communicable disease was reported to her, she would enter it into her "line log." By law, Gerri was required to report some of the diseases—like AIDS, hepatitis C and polio—to the Nebraska Department of Health and Human Services. She was also required to report "...clusters, outbreaks or unusual events or epidemics of any health problem." If several cases of an unusual disease, like hepatitis C, were diagnosed within a short time period, Gerri would consult with Dr. Koerber (chairman of the infection control committee) to determine if the diseases were connected. She would examine the infected patients' medical records to determine if the infections were linked.

At this time, Gerri's line log only reflected a few hepatitis C diagnoses. In fact, there were more. For some time, Dr. Javed had been sending some of his clinic's blood collections to the University of Nebraska Medical Center (UNMC) laboratory for testing. Gerri didn't have access to the lab results from UNMC. As a result, Gerri's line log showed only a portion of the hepatitis C diagnoses from Javed's clinic. The other outbreak victims were listed in UNMC's line log.

February 14, 2001

When Gerri went to lunch on Valentine's Day, 2001, she ran into Monica Weber. Monica was a long-term, unlicensed employee of the hospital.

"Gerri, could I talk to you a few minutes?" Monica asked as she stopped Gerri in the hallway. "Did you know I recently finished chemotherapy for breast cancer at Dr. Javed's office?"

Gerri didn't have time to answer before Monica continued.

"I want to talk to you about their procedures."

"Oh," Gerri finally answered. "What about them?"

"Well, I've also had chemotherapy as an inpatient at the hospital, and the hospital does it a lot differently than Javed's office. I don't think they are doing it right at Javed's clinic."

"Let's step over here," Gerri said as she pulled Monica out of the cafeteria traffic. "What's going on?"

"Well," Monica continued once she glanced around to make sure no one was listening. "When I was taking chemo at Javed's clinic, I wasn't like the other patients. Most of them slept through their chemo treatments. But for some reason, the chemo had the opposite effect on me. I was restless, and I just couldn't sleep. So I sat there and watched everything that was going on. There are some big differences between the way the hospital gives chemo and the way the cancer center does."

Gerri leaned in curiously. "What differences?" she asked.

"Well, you know Nurse Prochaska, right?" Monica continued. "First off, Linda seldom wears gloves when working on patients. Sometimes, she will go from patient to patient without even washing her hands. I know that can't be right," she insisted. "The nurses in the hospital *always* wear gloves."

It was a story that was all sickeningly familiar.

"After she accessed my port, she injected the discard blood back into me," Monica said as she mimicked the syringe next to her port. "Then, she used the very same needle and syringe to draw off saline from a large saline bag that was also used for other patients. How can that be safe? A bloody needle being inserted into our group saline bag! She doesn't even wipe the rubber dam on the saline bag with alcohol before she inserts the needle into it."

Gerri drew in a deep breath. "Did you ever talk to Dr. Javed about these issues?" she asked.

"As a matter of fact, I did," Monica replied indignantly. "I complained to Dr. Javed at every clinic visit about Linda's unfriendly demeanor and poor technique, but Dr. Javed would always just dismiss whatever I said, like he didn't believe me. One time, I got a burn on my back from a heating pad and had to be hospitalized. When I was in the hospital, the hospital nurses had to give me one of my chemo treatments. Right then, I knew something was wrong. They do the procedure a whole lot differently than they do at Javed's clinic. I even brought that up to Dr. Javed. But he said the way Linda does it is fine and he wasn't the least bit concerned." Monica paused for a moment. "Anyway, I thought I'd let you know."

"Thanks for letting me know," Gerri said as they parted. "You should try to talk to Dr. Javed again, and perhaps even report this to the hospital vice presidents, Peg Kennedy and John Hughes. I'll see you later."

"Okay," Monica agreed as she turned to leave. "I will."

As Monica walked away, she wondered if it had been wise to tell her fears to Gerri. Monica was not simply a patient; she was also a hospital employee. She worried that reporting Dr. Javed would endanger her job. Despite her fears, she had felt compelled to report what she'd seen to Gerri. She was certain that Javed's clinic was endangering its patients. It would take almost another two years before Monica would learn just how dangerous Javed's clinic was. As she made her report to Gerri Means, Monica had no way of knowing that she was already an outbreak victim herself.

Gerri immediately walked down the hall to tell Dr. Koerber. Dr. Koerber listened and then asked Gerri to make a memo about the report. Gerri was not satisfied to simply make a memo. After meeting with Koerber, she went to meet with Peg Kennedy, vice president of clinical operations. As she entered Peg's office, she was glad to see that Deb Wohlenhaus, the safety officer, was already sitting across the desk from Peg. Gerri told them both what Monica had reported.

"Well, Gerri," Peg replied. "I appreciate the report, but as you know, there is nothing we can do about this. It's outside our jurisdiction. It's not our place to tell Dr. Javed how to run his office."

"But Peg, to me, this is a *red alert*! It's a major deviation from infection control practice!" Gerri protested.

"Look, Gerri," Peg explained. "First of all, we don't know that any of this is true. All this is second-hand knowledge. You haven't witnessed anything yourself. We don't know if this is just a biased report by a disgruntled patient who doesn't like a particular nurse," Peg insisted. "I don't think we have grounds to do anything."

"Well, how about if I go in and observe personally? I'm sure Dr. Javed won't mind. I'll call him first," Gerri offered.

"Gerri," Peg cut her off. "Listen. We can't go in unless Dr. Javed invites us. Let me put it this way. Say we're in Fremont Shopping Mall, okay? The hospital is Penney's and Fremont Cancer Center is Sears. Penney's can't go into Sears and inspect them and ask to see their fire drill plan or their daily receipts or their inventory or anything else. The hospital simply cannot go into the cancer center and nose around and tell them what they are doing wrong. If you feel it's necessary, go talk to Dr. Javed about the complaint. Go talk to Dr. Koerber and he will speak to Dr. Javed, too. Explain everything and then I'm sure Javed will fix the problem. Just make sure you have everything in writing so Dr. Koerber has a clear understanding of what is being alleged."

"Okay, Peg," Gerri agreed. "I understand. I will put everything in writing. I'll have Monica review it to make sure that I have her explanation of the procedure correct. Then I'll give it to Dr. Koerber. I know he is going on vacation soon, so I will have the report ready for him as soon as he gets back."

Gerri stood and left the room, leaving Deb and Peg alone once again.

"I know we can't investigate Javed's clinic," Deb finally spoke. "But shouldn't we report him to the state? *They* can do an investigation."

"I don't think so, Deb," Peg replied. "We don't have first-hand knowledge. We are not mandated to report anything to the state unless we have first-hand knowledge."

"But Monica Weber is a hospital employee," Deb replied. "Other employees have noticed things too. Isn't *that* first-hand knowledge?"

"I don't think so. Tell you what. I'll call the state and ask them what is required to make a report, and I'll let you know. Alright?" Peg concluded the conversation.

"Okay," Deb said as she stood and left Peg's office.

Peg picked up the phone and called Nebraska Health and Human Services' Division of Investigations. When a woman's voice answered, Peg got right to the point.

"I'm calling about the mandatory reporting law concerning medical malpractice," she said. "Is it true that a licensed professional needs to have first-hand knowledge of an incident when making a report?"

"Well, umm, yes." the woman replied, slightly caught off-guard.

"Okay, thank you." She concluded the short conversation. "Goodbye."

Peg hung up the phone and quickly jotted off a memo to Deb, stating that they would not report the Fremont Cancer Clinic to the Nebraska Health and Human Services' Division of Investigations because they did not have "first-hand knowledge." She did not ask the hospital's legal counsel or medical staff ethics committee for advice on the situation. For Peg, the question was settled—there was nothing further that could be done.

Monica Weber followed Gerri's suggestion and scheduled a visit with John Hughes, the hospital vice president for professional services. She knew him personally and felt sure that John would take action to correct the dangers.

For an hour, John listened carefully. He made notes and asked questions. He seemed genuinely surprised and concerned. He encouraged Monica to bring her concerns directly to Dr. Javed. He thanked Monica for the report and then made the short trip down the hall to Dr. Javed's office to relay his concerns.

February 21, 2001

Gerri carefully put together her written report for Dr. Koerber. She noted her findings of two recent diagnoses of hepatitis C from her line log. As could be guessed, both hepatitis C cases were patients of Dr. Javed. She outlined the Dinsdale report and "a person's" (Monica Weber's) description of nursing practices in the Fremont Cancer Center.

"Hearing about this office practice," she wrote in the memo, "I am concerned there *might* be contamination of saline and/or heparin if these multidose products have had a needle/syringe with blood introduced into them."

She even went so far as to enclose a medical article (Widell A, Christensson B, Wiebe T, Schalen C, Hansson HB, Allander T, Persson MA. Epidemiologic and molecular investigation of outbreaks of hepatitis C virus infection on a pediatric oncology service. Ann Intern Med. 1999 Jan 19;130(2):130-4) about how hepatitis C was spread through a hospital ward in exactly the same way as described by Monica Weber.

April 24, 2001

Two months had passed since John Hughes had spoken to Dr. Javed about the dangers in his clinic. When the phone rang in Gerri's office that day, Gerri knew that the unsafe practices continued.

"This is Gerri," she said as she answered the phone.

"Hi, Gerri. This is *Gina Cline*."

Gina was a nurse at the hospital.

"I want to make a report about Dr. Javed's clinic," she continued. "One of his patients came to me and explained the port-flushing procedures they are using over there. There are some real dangers going on."

Gerri took a deep breath as she picked up a note pad from her desktop.

"Go on," she sighed.

April 27, 2001

Three days later, Gerri received yet another report.

"Gerri?" a voice questioned as Gerri answered her office phone.

"Yes," she answered as she sat down behind her desk.

"This is *Nurse Tilson*. I'm a nurse in the outpatient department."

"Yes," What can I do for you?"

"One of Dr. Javed's patients came to me with a complaint that I thought I should pass on to you. It sounds pretty serious."

"Go on," Gerri sighed.

"The patient reported the use of a blood-tainted syringe to draw off saline from a common saline bag."

Gerri listened to yet another retelling of the story.

"I'll pass it on," she said. "Would you tell the patient to talk to Dr. Javed?"

Once again, Gerri made another memo describing the new report, and forwarded it Dr. Koerber. She then went to speak with Dr. Koerber and Deb Wohlenhaus directly.

Several Days Later

"Tahir? This is Rod Koerber," Dr. Koerber said once Javed answered his phone. "Listen, there have been some complaints by patients about improper port flushing in your clinic. Ralph Dinsdale reported to Gerri Means that he shares a patient with you who has no risk factors, but who now has hepatitis C. Gerri's concerned that hepatitis C could spread through your clinic through improper port flushes."

"Yeah, I've talked to Ralph," Javed answered. "He said the patient remembers going to a movie in Omaha. She threw away some trash and in the process was pricked with something sharp. It could have been a hypodermic needle. So I think *that* must be our explanation of how she got hepatitis C."

"Well, I know about needle sticks," Rod admitted. "I stuck myself this morning during an autopsy. I ordered a stat hepatitis C test on the decedent and I'm very worried about the result."

"Be careful, Rod. I think hepatitis C is on the increase," Javed warned. "I've got several cases coming through my clinic."

"Really? Gosh, that makes me even more worried," Rod lamented. "But anyway, what about the port-flushing procedure? The patient alleges that Linda reuses a blood-tainted syringe to draw saline out of a common bag."

"Oh, don't believe everything you hear, Rod," Javed said with disgust. "I know who the patient is and she has had a personality conflict with Linda since the first day she came into the clinic. She's wrong about Linda reusing tainted syringes. The patient just doesn't like Linda."

"You know, you've had a lot of problems with Linda over the years. She's slow to change. Are you sure she is doing the port flushes properly?" Rod questioned.

"Rod, the patient has a misperception of the port flush procedure. It simply isn't happening the way she describes it. But *if* there had been any problems with port flushing in the past, we've corrected them long ago, I assure you," Javed stated adamantly. "Linda may have rinsed the needle in the saline bag, but that couldn't possibly have been a cause of any case of hepatitis."

"Well, okay, that's good to hear," Rod responded. "I'll talk to you later."

Dr. Koerber hung up the phone believing that nursing practices were safe at the Fremont Cancer Center. It was inconceivable to him that a registered nurse was flushing ports in the way described by several patients. In addition, Javed was a highly trained and respected physician. As a highly trained and respected physician himself, Rod Koerber trusted that Javed supervised the Fremont Cancer Center's practices closely, as Koerber carefully supervised his own pathology lab. Unfortunately, this was not the case. The unsafe nursing practices continued unchecked at Fremont Cancer Center.

CHAPTER 9

∎

The Missouri Valley Cancer Consortium

"We're talking about life and death, all right… Sometimes you go outside a bylaw if you're talking about life or death… Sometimes you have to go outside the bylaws for what's in the best interests of the patients and community at large."
—Stephen Anderson
(Expert witness testimony, October 8, 2004)

"Alright, last item for our agenda…" Javed paused as he glanced down at his meeting notes. It was early 2001, and the hospital cancer committee was meeting. Since Dr. Javed was the only full-time oncologist, the hospital had appointed him as the committee chairman. The meeting was being held in the Fireside Room at the Fremont Area Medical Center. In addition to Javed, many other departments of the hospital were represented, including surgery, nursing, medical social work, hospice care and chaplainry.

"…the Missouri Valley Cancer Consortium accreditation," Javed continued. "Is everyone familiar with the MVCC?" he asked as he looked around the room. There were puzzled looks and head shaking, so he went on to explain.

"The Missouri Valley Cancer Consortium was formed by a group of Omaha oncologists. They have federal funding through the National Institute of Health and the National Cancer Institute. They pay for and oversee clinical trial research in our region. The federal grants support studies that look at new, experimental cancer drugs that don't have FDA approval. The studies compare the experimental drugs' effectiveness to that of FDA-approved drugs. Cathy Spelling has worked with the MVCC before and both she and I think they are top-notch," Javed concluded.

Cathy Spelling, RN, had worked at the hospital since 1990. Before that, she worked for several years at Lutheran Medical Center in Omaha. At Lutheran, she developed an interest in oncology nursing. After Cathy returned to the Fremont Area Medical Center, she earned a special certification through the Oncology

Nursing Society. She was responsible for coordination of care for any hospital patient who had been diagnosed with cancer. She was well-respected by her peers, and had a reputation for being thorough in her work.

"The hospital has been approved as a Community Clinical Oncology Program through the MVCC," Javed went on to say. "To be a fully participating member, we need to offer clinical research trials to patients. A physician must supervise these trials. The next step in accreditation is for us to identify a supervising physician and then make arrangements for a site visit of the physician's practice by MVCC."

The upside of joining the MVCC was that clinical trials would bring a lot of new patients to Fremont—patients who might not otherwise go there. Cancer patients, especially those with poor prognoses, tend to look for a "magic bullet." The term "research study" suggests cutting-edge technology that would be the "magic bullet" those patients were looking for. The MVCC had a Website that listed current cancer research trials. Once the Fremont Cancer Center and Fremont Area Medical Center were accredited, the MVCC Website would direct patients to the Fremont site for research studies. In addition, announcing their involvement in cancer research and clinical trials would be a nice story to promote in conjunction with the opening of the hospital's new building addition, the Health Park Plaza.

"I'll be glad to be the supervising physician for the patient clinical trials," offered Dr. Javed. "I did research at the Medical University of South Carolina and at Albert Einstein and I'm anxious to get back into some research."

"Cathy," a surgeon in the back of the room spoke up, "you are already in connection with the people in MVCC. How about you help Dr. Javed get ready for the site visit? I'm sure you'd have a lot of good insight to offer."

Everyone in the room nodded in agreement.

Cathy's eyes widened. She took in a sharp breath and glanced down at her notepad.

"Oh, uh, I'd be happy to," she finally stammered.

The collective gaze turned to Dr. Javed.

"Well, then, it's decided," Javed announced with some hesitation. "We will go ahead with the accreditation process. We will report back to you at the next meeting. Since there are no other issues on our agenda, this meeting is adjourned."

Cathy quickly gathered up her things and hurried out of the room so as to avoid being alone with Javed. In her heart, she rejoiced. For years, she had been trying to convince Javed that his clinic's procedures were dangerous to his patients. Now, with inspection by an independent and respected oncology group, she hoped that he would finally be forced to change his nursing practices.

Cathy's history with Dr. Javed dated back to his arrival in Fremont. She had shown interest in being his office nurse when he'd first set up his practice. Despite Cathy's experience, and Linda Prochaska's lack of experience, Javed had given Linda the job. Cathy had always wondered why Javed had elected to hire someone with no training in place of her. When the Fremont Cancer Center was short-staffed, hospital nurses would moonlight at the clinic. Cathy had worked there several times in that capacity and had been shocked by their nursing procedures. Other hospital nurses who had worked part-time filling in at the Fremont Cancer Center had made the same observations to Cathy, and had then refused to return to Dr. Javed's office altogether. Cathy had brought her concerns to Javed, but he had always turned a deaf ear.

"You just don't like Linda," he'd told her. "You're just upset because Linda got the nursing job at my clinic and you didn't," he'd told her another time.

Cathy had even been questioned by several of the patients. They had complained about Linda's unfriendly demeanor, and one had asked her about the appropriateness of reinjecting discard blood into the patient.

"They don't give chemo the way you do," one patient said to her. "They don't even wear gowns and gloves."

Once again, Cathy had brought the comments to Dr. Javed.

"Of course we don't do things the way they are done in the hospital," he explained. "We're not a hospital, we're a private clinic. If a patient has a concern, she should bring the concern to me."

The Missouri Valley Cancer Consortium Audit

On April 12, 2001, *Leslie Mayberry, RN*, and *Marissa Winke, RN*, came to the Fremont Cancer Center to make a site visit on behalf of the MVCC. The purpose of the visit was to determine if the clinic would pass inspection. If the Fremont Cancer Center practices did not follow proper protocol, any studies conducted there might be flawed. The MVCC would not fund clinical research that was potentially inaccurate.

Vice President Peg Kennedy and Cathy Spelling, RN, welcomed the MVCC officials when they first arrived at the hospital. The two hospital employees showed the MVCC nurses to a conference room near the cancer center. Peg and Cathy assured the MVCC auditors that the hospital would gladly work as a liaison between the MVCC and Dr. Javed's clinic. Everyone was excited about the prospect of Javed conducting clinical trials.

"We've had a somewhat higher incidence of port infections in the past," Peg admitted. "We believe we have that problem under control now."

"Oh, really?" Marissa asked. "Sometimes that is related to improper port procedure. We'll watch the nurses when they draw blood from the ports. Anything else we should look for?"

"Umm, is it proper procedure to reinject the discard blood into the patient?" Cathy asked innocently.

Marissa raised her eyebrows in surprise.

"No, the discard blood is to be discarded. The discard blood contains clots, fibrin, tissue, bacteria and possibly heparin. We certainly don't want that reinfused into an immunocompromised cancer patient. I can give you some references on the subject if you want more information."

"Hello, ladies," Dr. Javed interrupted the conversation as he entered the room. "Welcome, Marissa and Leslie. We're so glad you are here today and we are so anxious to get started on research trials. How do we get started?"

The group agreed that Cathy would assist the MVCC in their inspection of the Fremont Cancer Center and act as the hospital liaison. Peg Kennedy then returned to her duties at the hospital.

Javed, Marissa, Leslie and Cathy made their way down the hallway to the Fremont Cancer Center. All the chemo recliners were full, and the cancer center nurses were scurrying between patients and the chemotherapy admixing area. Dr. Javed invited the three visitors into his private office and then summoned in his staff. He made introductions and explained why Marissa and Leslie were there. Linda Prochaska's reaction made it clear that the staff of the Fremont Cancer Center had no previous knowledge of either the audit or Javed's intention to conduct clinical trials.

"As you saw, we are very busy today. I don't know that we have time to work with you," Linda said, looking pointedly at Cathy.

"We just want to observe. We don't want to take you from your patients," Marissa explained. "We promise to stay out of your way."

"We are really short of space. I don't think we can accommodate three extra people moving around the chemo room amongst the recliners," Linda insisted.

"I'll go on back to fourth floor. I'm not needed here and they need me on the floor," Cathy offered. "Leslie, you can call me later if there is any way I can help."

Over the next four hours, Marissa and Leslie took notes as they observed Linda and the rest of the cancer center staff as they worked with patients.

April 19, 2001

In the days following her inspection, Marissa compiled a five-page report. It listed numerous OSHA violations, including:

1. Lack of protective equipment (masks, gowns and gloves).
2. Chemo-contaminated supplies were discarded in the regular trash.
3. Food and food supplies were present in area where chemotherapy was mixed.
4. No spill kit, no eye wash kit, no anaphylaxis emergency kit and no extravasation kit.

The report also listed numerous violations that endangered patients:

1. No alcohol wipes were used.
2. A chemo waste bucket and used syringes were left inside the chemo hood, thus contaminating it. Needles were left in vials of sterile saline and the nurses were reusing syringes.
3. Drugs were mixed incorrectly with the wrong amount of diluent.
4. Drugs were not fully mixed before they were injected into patients.
5. Unmarked drugs were administered and stored without labeling.

Altogether, twenty-six serious violations were listed in the report. Marissa went on to write that nursing practices were poor and "do not protect the employee or patient. This is a tremendous liability for Dr. Javed as well as the hospital." She did not recommend initiating clinical trials in Dr. Javed's office.

April 23, 2001

Several days later, Marissa and Leslie returned to the Fremont Cancer Center to present their report to Dr. Javed and his staff in person. They first met with Dr. Javed and Cathy Spelling, RN, in the radiation oncology conference room.

"Dr. Javed," Marissa began. "We saw some good things in your clinic, but we also saw some serious errors that need to be corrected."

Marissa slid the five-page report across the table to him while Cathy took notes.

"Oh," Javed replied as he glanced at the findings. "We'll have these little glitches fixed in no time. When can we begin clinical trials?"

"I'm sorry," Marissa shook her head. "At this time, we are not recommending your facility for clinical trials. Let's go through this report line by line and you will see what needs to be changed. Let's start at the top. 'Food and food supplies are set up on the same cabinet space where chemotherapy is stored, mixed and set.'"

"We have very limited space and resources," Javed protested. "We just don't have any other place for food. But really, I'm back in the mixing area ten times a day and I've never seen any food there."

"Well, let's move on," Marissa continued. "'Drugs were observed being admixed incorrectly, with the wrong amount of diluent.' The drug was cloudy in the vial, so it was obviously not mixed completely. Yet it was drawn up and put into an unmarked bag. These are serious problems," she stressed. "Look, Dr. Javed, the hospital has offered you their help and your nurses could use some tutoring. I'm sure someone from the hospital would be willing to give your nurses some much-needed training."

"That is a good idea," Javed sputtered. "We could use some help around here."

His voice took on an edge.

"However," he went on. "We are a private practice, not a hospital, so we do things differently. I don't know if what you observed about admixing is true. I'm never back in that part of the clinic," he declared, apparently contradicting himself. "My nurses are knowledgeable and I think when things are going well, we need to stay on course."

"Perhaps the hospital pharmacist can help with the admixing of chemo," Marissa suggested diplomatically.

"The hospital pharmacists don't know anything," Javed spoke forcefully, and his face reddened. "I don't want any help from the hospital. There have always been riffs between my nurses and the hospital nurses. Actually, Cathy shouldn't be involved with getting us set up with the MVCC at all. She's argumentative and just gets my nurses riled up."

"Frankly, Doctor, your staff is negatively affecting patient outcomes here," Marissa insisted. "This is a serious situation. We'd be happy to enroll your nurses in some classes in Omaha. At a minimum, your nurses need to spend a day there in an oncology clinic or with a pharmacist."

Dr. Javed drew in a deep breath and let it out slowly as he tried to regain his composure.

"Ms. Winke, we want to take good care of our patients," he said earnestly. "I understand that you have some concerns and I'll do what I can to work with the staff to fix the problems. I ask that you respect my privacy and not give a copy of this report to hospital administration until I have a chance to look it over and see what needs to be corrected. Would you be willing to go over this report with my staff and perhaps work out a plan to correct these problem areas?"

"Surely," Marissa answered.

"I would really appreciate it," Javed concluded as though he had a pressing engagement somewhere else to attend. "Thank you for coming out today."

He stood up and left the room, abruptly ending the meeting.

Marissa, Leslie and Cathy found Javed's nurses, Linda, Raegene and Heather, in the chemo room. It was near the end of the day, so there weren't any patients around. Again, the three Fremont Cancer Center nurses were surprised to see the MVCC nurses. After everyone was seated, Marissa and Leslie shared the contents of the report. Linda became red in the face, crossed her arms, and then slammed her hand down on the arm of the chair. She was furious. She didn't like anyone questioning her patient care.

As Marissa continued through the report, Linda became sullen and then refused to answer altogether. Raegene seemed overwhelmed by the information and said nothing during the entire meeting. Heather asked questions about procedures and was genuinely concerned and angry that she and patients had been exposed to health risks in the Fremont Cancer Center. After forty-five minutes of uncomfortable dialogue, Marissa and Leslie offered to help in any way they could. They asked Linda to get back to them and to let them know how she would like to proceed. Again, Linda refused to respond, so they excused themselves and left.

There was a moment of uncomfortable silence. Heather and Raegene felt like they had just taken a beating, and could see that Linda was about to explode.

"My gosh, did you know we were doing *so many* things wrong?" Heather finally asked. "I'm going to find a class to take to bring my skills up."

"I've already taught you everything you need to know," Linda finally said snidely. "You don't need any classes."

Linda slapped her hand on the arm of her chair. "But the thing I want to know," she barked, "is where's Javed? Why wasn't he here to stand up for us? I'm going to call him and ask him. The coward."

Linda angrily fumbled with her cell phone as she dialed Javed.

"Why didn't you tell us the MVCC was coming today?" she snapped at him when he finally answered. "You should have prepared us. And why weren't you here to stick up for us?"

"Ask him," Heather whispered as she motioned to get Linda's attention, "to inform us of what changes are going to be made."

Linda passed the question on to Javed. A few more moments passed in silence as she listened to her cell phone. Suddenly, she snapped her cell phone closed in anger.

"He says we should consider ourselves informed," she announced in a rage. The three women sat in silence. They were overwhelmed.

"Do you think I shouldn't be mixing chemo?" Raegene finally spoke up, still in a daze. "I may not be an RN, but I know what I am doing," she insisted. "And why in the world can't I be around chemicals just because I am pregnant? Do they think being around chemo will cause me to have a two-headed baby? Give me a break. I don't want to sit at the front desk with the receptionist. I'd be bored out of my mind."

"Don't worry about it, Raegene," Linda spoke up, still upset. "I trained you how to mix chemo, and I know what I am doing. If the MVCC comes back again you just stay up front in the reception area for the day. Otherwise, you just keep doing your job the way you have been. Who are these people and why did they come in here and nose around, anyway?"

April 24, 2001

The next day, Heather went up to fourth floor of the hospital and caught Cathy Spelling as she was exiting a patient's room.

"Cathy, could I talk to you a minute?" Heather flagged her down.

"Sure," Cathy answered, slightly surprised. "Let's go into the conference room."

When they were settled in the conference room, Heather began.

"I'm very concerned about the MVCC report but I think I am the *only* one who is concerned. I'm just doing what the doctor is telling me to do. Javed seems upset at the findings but he's not interested in changing things. He did ask Linda to order an OSHA manual, but that is all. It was made very clear to me that I'm not in charge down there. But I want to do things right. I did some Internet research last night and I made copies of the information and gave it to Linda and Raegene. Do you have anything I can use?"

"I've got some books I will bring you," Cathy offered with a smile.

"Thanks, Cathy, I'll take anything I can get my hands on," Heather responded gratefully.

May 1, 2001

"Ms. Winke? This is Dr. Javed," he started the phone conversation behind the closed door of his private office.

His voice was much more controlled than it was the last time they had spoken.

"I received your official follow-up letter, which contained your written report. I have met with hospital administration about it a couple of times," he lied. "We think you are right. This is not the time to begin clinical trials. We are building a new cancer center in Fremont and when we get moved into that, we will have more space, which will be more conducive to the needs of the patients and to research."

"Oh, I see," Marissa, answered.

"Can I call you when we are all settled into our new facility, and have you reconsider us for clinical trials?"

"Sure. And in the meantime, if you need any help, as I told you before, we're here to help," Marissa responded.

May 1, 2001—Later in the Day

Cathy Spelling walked briskly down the hall in the Fremont Area Medical Center to Vice President John Hughes' office.

"Did you know that Dr. Javed has decided not to participate in the MVCC clinical trials?" she burst out the instant she stepped through the door.

"No, really? Why not?" Hughes' brow wrinkled in puzzlement.

"I'm not sure," Cathy answered. "I know there were some unfavorable findings in the report from MVCC."

"A report from MVCC?" Hughes said with surprise. "I haven't seen any report. I didn't know they sent one. We want to participate in clinical trials and we can't do that without Javed being onboard," he declared. He was not pleased with the fact that he was not told of the report.

"Actually," Cathy confessed, "I've seen the report, but Dr. Javed asked me not to disclose the results. He asked us to 'respect his privacy.'"

"All right," he said begrudgingly. "I'll call the MVCC directly. Thank you."

Cathy nodded and turned to leave. As she left his office and made her way back through the hospital, she felt uncomfortable with the whole situation. She had repeatedly tried to address the dangers in the cancer center with Javed, but to no avail. On top of that, Javed had then put her in the uncomfortable position of withholding the report results from her boss.

"Hello. This is John Hughes, vice president of the Fremont Area Medical Center," he began after dialing the MVCC. "Is Marissa Winke in?"

He was riddled with anxiety as he waited for Marissa to pick up the line. The clinical trials were important to the hospital. Now, Javed had put that all in jeopardy, and it seemed like he was the last one to know.

"Marissa. Hi. John Hughes here," he began when she finally answered. "Hey,

I just wanted to call and see how the hospital's enrollment in clinical trials is coming along."

Marissa was surprised.

"Oh." She paused in confusion. "Mr. Hughes, I just talked to Dr. Javed this morning. He said he had visited with the hospital administration and the consensus was to wait until after the new cancer center is completed. Is that different from what you understood?"

"Uh, well, I guess I didn't know the final decision had been made," he fumbled for words. "Can we still work toward getting Javed involved in clinical trials? It's very important to the hospital to provide this type of service to our community."

"No, Mr. Hughes, I'm sorry," she answered. "We simply feel that the poor nursing care there would undoubtedly affect research outcomes. As our report said in great detail, there are some serious breaches of standard patient care. We can't allow your cancer center to do trials until those issues have been resolved or improved. Frankly, your cancer program needs to make some major changes. And," she emphasized, "I'm not only talking about making changes so that you can conduct research trials. I'm talking about changes for the safety of your patients. I feel I have a moral and ethical obligation to make you aware of what I observed there. The poor practices at your cancer center are not only in breach of OSHA regulations, but they are undoubtedly affecting patient outcomes. Your patients' health is at stake. Your cancer program's reputation is at stake."

She paused for a moment, so the importance of what she had said could sink in.

"But believe me," she continued. "We would be happy to assist you in making improvements. We can provide you nursing education, literature, whatever we can do to help."

"Thank you, Ms. Winke," he said dejectedly. "Would you just put all that in a letter please? I appreciate it very much," he said as he hung up the phone.

He immediately buzzed his secretary through the intercom. "Set up a meeting with Dr. Javed here at my office," he instructed her. "Ask President Leibert to attend."

"Yes, sir," she answered. "For what day of the week?"

"Immediately," he commanded. "I need to see them this afternoon."

May 1, 2001—Late Afternoon

"Thanks for coming to meet with us," Hughes said as Javed entered his office.

"Sure," he answered as he nodded politely and sat in the chair next to Mike

Leibert, across the desk from John Hughes. "So, what's going on, gentlemen?"

"Well, Tahir," Leibert quickly responded. "John just caught me up to speed on the MVCC clinical trials. I understand you have made the decision to put them off until we have finished building the new facility."

"Well," Javed glanced from Mike to John and then back again. "I just told the MVCC that perhaps it would be better to start doing clinical research once the new facility was up and running and we had more room."

"I have to say that I don't think it was fair of you to make that decision on your own," Leibert said sharply. "These clinical trials are important to us."

"Well, I—"

"On top of that," Hughes added, cutting Javed off. "You left the MVCC with the understanding that you had conferred with us about it, and that the decision was made with the hospital's consent."

"This all just could have been handled differently," Leibert commented.

Javed leaned back into his chair.

"I know," he sighed. "I know. I'm sorry." He shook his head. "I apologize. This whole MVCC thing has just got me a little rattled. I should have talked with you first. I just didn't know what to do. Marissa put me on the spot, and I didn't know what else to say."

There was a moment of silence as Javed looked away in discouragement.

"The most important thing is fixing this problem," Hughes finally commented. "How about this? We'll set up an action plan. We can sit down together and go over the MVCC report. We can work together to get a few changes made in your nursing procedures and then we should be back on track with the MVCC."

"I think that is a good idea," Leibert added with a smile.

The tension in the room had been broken.

"Absolutely," Javed replied. "We'll get the trials up and running."

Leibert and Hughes had several trump cards that they could have played to coerce Javed into making the necessary improvements in his clinic. The lease between the hospital and Javed stated that the cancer center had to abide by all hospital policies and procedures. Arguably, the hospital could have terminated Javed's lease if he did not make the Fremont Cancer Center conform to the hospital's infection control policy. However, Leibert and Hughes interpreted the lease clause regarding abiding by hospital policies and procedures as applying to environmental issues only (e.g., handicapped accessibility or fire escape plans) and not to medical issues.

In addition, under hospital bylaws, Leibert and Hughes could have also theoretically revoked Javed's hospital privileges when he did not follow the hospital's infection control policy (2001 FAMC bylaws, Article 7). They also had an overriding executive power under hospital bylaws to immediately suspend Javed's privileges because he was endangering the public on hospital grounds. By revoking his privileges for either of these reasons, they would have effectively shut down his practice. They did not invoke the hospital bylaws because they did not believe the bylaws applied to physician behavior in private practice.

Later that day, Mr. Hughes wrote a letter to Dr. Javed reviewing the meeting. He emphasized the good future relations between Javed and the hospital.

"I appreciate your efforts and your expertise as we work together to achieve our common vision of an exceptional cancer center in our community," he wrote.

Nine days later, Mike Leibert, president and CEO of the Fremont Area Medical Center, announced a new building project estimated to cost more than $8 million. The project was to house, among other things, the Fremont Cancer Center. An article in the May 10, 2001 *Fremont Tribune* stated: "Hospital officials worked closely with the cancer center staff to identify specific growth needs of the clinic."

With Javed onboard, the new facility was going to give the hospital an opportunity to be one of the premier cancer treatment facilities in the state.

Heather Fights the Tide

After the MVCC audit, Heather was a woman on a mission. She read everything she could get her hands on about oncology nursing. She formed a working relationship with the hospital pharmacist, who taught her how to mix drugs correctly. She collected the insert information for each drug and kept them in a recipe file box. She threw away outdated drugs after everyone else left the clinic. She began labeling everything appropriately. She studied the information on universal precautions for infection control that Gerri Means gave her.

Heather began drawing up fifty individual syringes of sterile saline from the large, 500cc bag in the morning and using a different one each time it was needed. She no longer reinjected the discard blood into patients. She secured proper hazardous waste disposal items, a spill kit, gloves, gowns and an emergency kit. She moved food items and other contaminants away from the chemo mixing area. In short, Heather did her best to correct the MVCC findings. She was determined to make the improvements in spite of the fact that both Javed and Prochaska were unenthusiastic about her efforts. Eventually, Javed came around and rewarded her efforts by naming her the safety coordinator of the clinic. Linda and Raegene, however, were resistant to change, and did not improve their technique.

June 12, 2001

Once Heather finished cleaning up the cancer center procedures, it was time to contact the MVCC again. Javed hoped that this time, they would be approved for clinical trials.

On June 12, 2001, Marissa and Leslie returned. They were greeted first by Raegene Lawson. This time, she was seated at the receptionist's desk and was not on the floor, around dangerous chemicals, as before. The MVCC auditors both noticed. They didn't know that she had only been stationed there for the day. Nor did they know that once they left, she returned to her nursing duties.

Heather gave the MVCC nurses a copy of a report identifying her improvements and showed them all the changes she had made. Their visit lasted approximately one hour and they did not see Dr. Javed at this visit. Marissa and Leslie were so impressed with Heather's diligent work to improve the office conditions that Marissa wrote a letter to Dr. Javed informing him that Heather's changes had now made it possible for the MVCC to authorize clinical trials.

Dr. Javed falsified a memo to his own files, stating that he had met with the two women that day.

The Missouri Valley Cancer Consortium audit documented the procedures that led to the largest American outbreak of hepatitis C in history. The purpose of the audit was to accredit the Fremont Cancer Center for clinical trials. However, no clinical trials were ever conducted at the Fremont Cancer Center.

CHAPTER 10

Yet Another Offer to Help Javed's Clinic

"You know, you can make a rule, but bacteria, infectious agents, viruses, they do not follow [it]. They don't exclude themselves just because that space is leased to Dr. Javed."
—Dr. Thomas W. Froelich, MD
(Expert witness testimony, October 5, 2004)

Late April, 2001

Rod Koerber looked up from his laptop, stretched, and looked at the clock. It was quitting time, so he shut down the computer. As he leaned back in his chair, the phone rang.

"Koerber," he said into the receiver.

"Doctor, this is Gerri Means. We have a problem."

"What's going on?" he sighed.

"I just wanted to let you know that I've heard that a patient is convinced she contracted hepatitis C from Javed's clinic. It's not substantiated yet, but I thought I would let you know what I heard."

"Thanks, Gerri. We'll see what comes of it," Rod said and hung up.

This wasn't the first time that week that Dr. Koerber had heard rumors about Javed as they were bantered around the hospital. He had overheard a conversation in the doctor's lounge about the MVCC audit. He swiveled in his chair and reached into a file cabinet. He pulled out Gerri's memo of February 21, 2001, and quickly flipped through it, and the attached article from *Annals of Internal Medicine*. It detailed how hepatitis C could spread through an oncology clinic through reuse of syringes to access a large saline bag. He studied the memo a long time and then stared into space. A long-overdue realization dawned. If the patient report was true, Javed's assurances of proper nursing procedure could not be trusted.

The hospital's infection control plan defined Dr. Koerber's duties as the chairman of the infection control committee. It said that anytime "patients, visitors, medical staff or employees" of the hospital were in danger of contracting an infectious disease, it was his job to make sure they were protected. The plan went on to state that if he knew of a potential danger that was not prevented by current infection control policies, he was obligated to take emergency measures to protect the public. He was even given the specific authority to isolate and close off any area of the hospital where the danger existed.

Dr. Koerber believed that under the hospital's bylaws and infection control plan, he had no authority to intervene in the cancer center. In addition, he did not believe he had the ability to warn Javed's patients of their risk of exposure. He handwrote a note and attached it to Gerri's memo. He dropped it into a manila envelope and addressed it to Dr. Javed, to be sent via hospital mail. He did the only thing he thought he could do—and that was to offer to discuss the situation with Javed once again.

May 16, 2001

Dr. Javed continued to update the sticky note he had placed inside the cupboard in the chemo room. It now held the names of five patients who were infected with hepatitis C. He let the nurses know that they should be especially careful around these five patients.

Since these names were on the line log, Gerri Means asked Javed if he could shed any light on their hepatitis C diagnoses. Javed reviewed their medical charts and compiled a report denying that they contracted hepatitis C though his clinic. He then invited Gerri to come to his office and shared the report with her.

It was obvious that each of the patients had contracted the disease at his office. They all had the same virus, and most of them had no other reasonable means of contracting the disease. Still, Javed was not ready to concede anything.

"I believe this patient has a history of IV drug use," he told Gerri as they went over each patient on the list. "This patient cut her hand throwing trash into a trash can at a movie theater several years ago. It's quite possible that what actually cut her hand was a hypodermic needle. Hypodermic needles are everywhere these days. It's quite possible that the hypodermic needle had the hepatitis C virus on it."

"Oh," Gerri answered. "I wasn't aware of that."

"Yes," he continued as he pointed further down his report. "And this patient had her port flushed here, but not with saline."

Gerri accepted his explanation, although he did not explain how a port could be flushed without saline.

"Oh," she said again. "Well, I have received a number of patient complaints about the reuse of needles here in your clinic. Is it possible that—"

"I swear to God, no," he cut her off. "I can assure you that is not even a possibility. Gerri," he said sincerely, "you have to understand. I regularly watch my nurses to ensure that they are using proper protocol. The other day, I spent all afternoon observing chemotherapy infusions. There is no way these people got hepatitis here."

Gerri thanked him for the visit, went to her office and put together a memo about their meeting. *Well,* she thought to herself as she finished the memo, *he said there have been changes made in his office. I'm sure that between administration and Dr. Koerber, things will be handled through the back door. I think we have the mess at the Fremont Cancer Center cleaned up at last.*

CHAPTER 11

The Valerie Wheaton Story

Winter 1997

Valerie and John Wheaton sat drinking coffee in the Methodist Hospital cafeteria in Omaha, Nebraska. It was a cold and dreary day. Valerie had recently been diagnosed with breast cancer and they had been struggling to find an oncologist to treat her. Their family physician in Wahoo, Nebraska, had recommended one in Omaha, but they didn't like his cold, brisk demeanor. They hoped to find a cancer doctor who would be approachable and knowledgeable.

Time was of the essence, not only because of Valerie's diagnosis of advanced breast cancer, but also because John was a farmer. When springtime came, he would have to return to the fields and would not be able to drive Valerie to Omaha for her appointments. They tried to be brave for each other, but time was slipping by and desperation began to creep into their conversation.

"Let's try the University of Nebraska Medical Center," John suggested. "There must be a number of oncologists there. Surely we can find one who will take time to visit with us."

They gathered up Valerie's medical records and headed across town. After telling and retelling their story to a number of receptionists and nurses, they were finally led back to meet *Dr. Jay Everett*. He was the compassionate, qualified physician they had been searching for. He agreed to treat her and suggested that the Wheatons stop at the patient advocacy office to begin their paperwork.

Dr. Everett felt that the best way to fight Valerie's cancer was to have her undergo a procedure known as a stem cell rescue. It was a very taxing procedure with a lot of risks, and it was also very expensive. Time passed agonizingly slowly while they waited for insurance authorization. Eventually, the final ruling came. Valerie's health insurance company would not pay for the procedure. Valerie would have to settle for cancer surgery and conventional chemotherapy.

Twenty-three lymph nodes were removed during her mastectomy and all of them tested positive for cancer. Although cancer was not found anywhere else in her body, there was concern that the cancer would show up somewhere else in the future. When she finished chemotherapy, Dr. Everett recommended that her vascular access devise (port) stay in place, in case she would need more chemotherapy. As a result, even though she was done with chemotherapy, she needed to have her port flushed regularly.

When the winter was over and spring finally came, Dr. Everett recommended that Valerie undergo radiation. Since John had already begun spring planting, Valerie decided to go to the Fremont Area Medical Center for radiation. Fremont was only about twenty miles from their farm, so it was a much shorter drive. While she was there, it was convenient for her to walk across the hall to the Fremont Cancer Center for port flushes.

Valerie was happy with the service she received at the hospital's radiation clinic. The Fremont Cancer Clinic, on the other hand, was a different story. Linda was rude and her technique was worrisome. Valerie noticed at UNMC that the nurses used three different syringes when drawing blood and flushing her port whereas Linda used only two. Valerie mentioned this difference to Nurse Tilson when she had her port flushed in the outpatient department at the hospital. Nurse Tilson encouraged her to visit with Gerri Means to share her concerns.

Gerri doesn't know me, so why should she believe me? Valerie thought to herself. She decided not to call her.

Valerie's blood counts dropped during radiation. As a result, she had to take growth factor shots, but the counts continued to remain low. Her radiologist, Dr. Janet Pieck, wanted her to have a blood transfusion. Dr. Pieck knew, however, that she would have to convince Dr. Javed to order the transfusion. She had tried to persuade Dr. Javed to order a transfusion on other patients, but Javed was adamantly against the procedure.

"You know the problems with transfusions," Javed had argued. "There's too much risk of hepatitis C. Just be patient and send her over to me for the growth factor shots. The counts will get up to where we want them soon enough."

"Javed, blood transfusions raise the blood count immediately. As you know, radiation works better when the level is up to twelve grams percent. It takes a month for the growth factor shots to work. By that time, the patient will have finished radiation so the shots wouldn't have had time to be effective. We are far more likely to help a patient with a blood transfusion than to expose them to hepatitis C. I'm not worried about transmission of hepatitis C through a blood transfusion," she had argued.

"Well, maybe you should be," he'd declared. "I just don't trust transfusions. I recommend you stay the course with the growth factor shots."

Javed had a motive for promoting growth factor shots instead of transfusions. He charged hundreds of dollars for each shot. Many chemotherapy patients needed several shots per week. On the other hand, he couldn't make any money from transfusions because Dr. Koerber had not given Javed permission to give them at his clinic.

June 1, 2001

When Valerie finished radiation, she continued to go to Dr. Javed's clinic for port flushes. Her worries about the cancer center's nursing technique kept gnawing at her. Finally, she decided to ask Dr. Pieck at a radiation follow-up visit.

"Okay," Dr. Pieck said at the end of the visit. "Everything looks good."

Valerie stammered and avoided eye contact with Dr. Pieck.

"Valerie, is there something on your mind?" Dr. Pieck asked.

"Well, I'm not sure. I just don't know."

"You just don't know what? What's troubling you?"

"Dr. Pieck, is it proper procedure to flush a port with saline from a large, multi-use bag?" Valerie asked.

"Well, yes, it can be done that way, although I think more commonly now, nurses are using single-dose vials of saline. Why do you ask?" Dr. Pieck replied.

Valerie chose her words carefully. She was a hard-working farm wife and her education did not extend beyond high school. She did not want to overstep her bounds.

"Linda Prochaska uses a syringe to draw my blood and then pulls out saline from a large bag to flush my port with the same syringe. I watched her do the same thing with the patient ahead of me. If I go for a port flush in the morning, the saline in the bag is clear. If I go in the late afternoon, it is cloudy pink with bits of debris floating in it. Does that sound right to you?" Valerie asked anxiously.

This time, Dr. Pieck drew in a deep breath.

"Excuse me, Valerie, tell me this again. Linda uses the same syringe on you that she used on the previous patient?"

"No, I have my own syringe. She uses it to draw a blood sample out of my port. After she puts my blood in the specimen vials, she uses the same syringe to draw saline out of the large bag and then flushes my port with the saline in that syringe."

"One more time, Valerie. Tell me exactly what you saw."

Valerie went over the procedure again, being as specific and careful in her description as she could.

Dr. Pieck had been watching Valerie closely as she spoke. Her eyes took on a faraway look as she turned over Valerie's account in her head.

"This doesn't sound right," she finally spoke as she turned her gaze back to Valerie. "You wait here. I'm going to get someone to listen to this."

She left the room and walked quickly to the suite of administrators' offices across the hall.

The door to the exam room closed behind Dr. Pieck as Valerie closed her eyes and felt her stomach churn in anxiety. Who would be in the room next? Would it be Javed? Or Linda? Would they believe her, dismiss her as a fool or call her a liar?

"What's wrong, Valerie?" Dr. Pieck's nurse asked quietly as she put her hand on Valerie's forearm.

Valerie began to cry.

"I'm just so scared. I've been worried about this for so long—two years now. I've asked the Lord for strength to tell someone about this. I'm just afraid no one will believe me and nothing will be done."

The door finally opened and Vice President John Hughes walked in alone. He listened to Valerie's story carefully and asked a few questions. He seemed genuinely concerned. His attentiveness and respectful demeanor was encouraging.

When John Hughes was finished with his questions, he addressed Valerie gently.

"Valerie, I can tell you are uncomfortable with the port flushes at Fremont Cancer Center. I suggest that you go elsewhere for your port flushes. Experiencing cancer is enough of an emotional burden. You don't need to put yourself through any more anxiety. I wish you the best, Valerie," he said as he stood up to leave, extending his hand to her. "If there is anything we at the hospital can do for you, please do not hesitate to call."

The hospital's bylaws included an emergency clause. It stated that whenever patients were in immediate danger, members of the hospital administration had the option of immediately suspending a physician. John Hughes believed the bylaw pertained only to a physician's actions within the hospital and it had no authority within a private physician's clinic, so he did not invoke the emergency clause to suspend Javed's hospital privileges.

"Do you think anything will change?" Valerie asked the nurse after Hughes left the room.

"Oh, surely it will," she answered optimistically.

"I really hope so," Valerie replied.

It was more of a prayer than a hope—one that would go unanswered.

June 8, 2001

It was John and Valerie Wheaton's wedding anniversary. She and John were going to host all their children, in-laws and grandkids that evening for a celebration. As she sat in her family doctor's office that morning, she was mentally going through her "to do" list when her doctor walked past the open door.

"Hi, Valerie," he said with surprise. "I didn't see your chart pulled. Are you here to see me?"

"Oh, no, Doctor. I'm just here to have my port flushed," she answered.

"Port flushed? I thought you went to Javed for that?"

"I did, but not any longer. I wasn't comfortable with the procedure they used."

"Procedure? What is it about a port flush procedure that made you uncomfortable?"

Once again, Valerie explained to a professional healthcare worker the port flushing procedure used at Fremont Cancer Center. Her family doctor listened carefully and then became very concerned about her health.

"Well, Valerie, this is very worrisome. You could have contracted AIDS or hepatitis from that contaminated saline bag. I want to do some blood tests on you and make sure you are all clear. Let me take a blood sample and I'll order all the necessary tests. Let's hope that nothing shows up," her doctor offered.

Valerie tried to be upbeat and festive for the anniversary party that night but her mind was racing. AIDS? Hepatitis? She had been consumed by a cancer battle for three long years.

"Please, Lord," she prayed. "Spare me another health battle."

Days passed in a fog of worry. Finally, five long days later, her physician called her.

"Well, Valerie, I'm sorry to tell you the results show that you have hepatitis C," he began.

"Is that all? Not AIDS?" Valerie asked.

"Yes, that's all that showed up. I think we should repeat the testing just to be sure. Would you come in this afternoon for another blood draw?"

June 19, 2001

On Tuesday, Valerie's doctor called again to confirm the report. Valerie had hepatitis C. In the past few days, she had educated herself about hepatitis C and knew that it was not an insignificant disease. Her life had been turned upside down once again.

"Mom, you must call the hospital and tell them," daughter Mary Lynne insisted. "They need to know and they have a duty to do something."

"But who do I call?" Valerie asked. "Who will do anything about this?"

"Call that John Hughes you told me about. You thought he listened to you. Maybe he will get something done," Mary Lynne answered.

Valerie placed a call to Mr. Hughes. His secretary told her that he was out of the office for the rest of the week but that he would call her the following Monday. Valerie sat down at her kitchen table, put her head in her hands and wept in frustration and grief.

Within minutes, the phone rang.

"Valerie? This is John Hughes," the voice began. "How can I help you?"

"Mr. Hughes, I have hepatitis C and I got it at Fremont Cancer Center."

"Oh my God. Are you sure?"

"Yes, I got the confirmatory tests back today. Mr. Hughes, you must do something. No one else must go through what I am going through."

"Yes, I agree. Have you told your story to Dr. Javed?"

"No, I have not. I was always afraid that if I complained to Dr. Javed about Linda, she would be even meaner to me."

"Let me set up a meeting between you and Dr. Javed. Let's hope that when he hears your story, he will let Linda go. I'll call you back," John Hughes offered.

June 20, 2001

The next day, Valerie and Dr. Javed met in his clinic after hours. He listened quietly to her story and said nothing. It was a brief meeting. Valerie felt that he looked and acted like a trapped animal.

June 21, 2001

Nurse Prochaska carried out her duties as usual in the Fremont Cancer Center. Nothing appeared to have changed as a result of Valerie's visit with Dr. Javed.

June 22, 2001

Mike Leibert, John Hughes, Peg Kennedy, Dr. Rod Koerber, another physician, Deb Wohlenhaus, and Gerri Means met at nine o'clock that morning. John informed the group of his recent conversations with Valerie Wheaton and her diagnosis of hepatitis C. He also let the group know that Valerie had spoken to Javed two days prior but that Prochaska was still employed at the cancer center.

"Ms. Wheaton did not have her lab done here at the hospital. So her positive hepatitis C diagnosis wasn't noted in my line log," Gerri commented.

The group came to two conclusions. First, that Gerri would make the state aware of the "issue." Second, that Linda's behavior did not bode well for future compliance with rigorous infection control standards and that Dr. Javed needed to be informed of the group's concerns.

Gerri called the Nebraska Health and Human Services. The "issue" was taken to state epidemiologist Dr. Tom Safranek. Gerri was told that the state was only keeping count of the number of reported cases. She was told that she should talk to Bob Semerena, director of investigations.

A July 31, 2003 article in the *Fremont Tribune* said that the state "was not made aware of problems at the clinic until September 2002, two months after Javed left the country."

An investigation of the Fremont Cancer Center should have commenced immediately. It did not. No one from the Fremont Cancer Center or the hospital or Nebraska Health and Human Services warned Javed's past or present patients of the potential risk of contracting hepatitis C from the clinic. At that moment, more than ninety other Nebraska outbreak victims had hepatitis C but did not know it. Most of them wouldn't know until the outbreak finally became public knowledge—fifteen months later, in October 2002.

The group decided that John Hughes should talk to Dr. Javed. He met with Javed at ten that morning. By noon, Linda was no longer employed at the Fremont Cancer Center.

CHAPTER 12

■

Evelyn Recounts Her Second Diagnosis

December 8, 2001

"Mom, hurry up, I'll be late for basketball practice!" Alex yelled to me through the closed bathroom door. I was frozen in place in the shower, feeling a lump along my mastectomy scar.

I wondered if it was just scar tissue. Surely it was. There was no reason to even mention it to Tom. It would just worry him needlessly.

After I dropped Alex off at the gymnasium, my car found its way to Tom's office. I didn't want to burden him, but the more I thought about it, the more I fretted. It was a Saturday, and it was Tom's weekend to see patients in the office. I had finished chemo eight months earlier and I was happy that my hair was growing back. I was no longer nauseous. My blood counts were normal again. I was still very tired, though. Dr. Javed gave me the "everyone is different" explanation when I mentioned my fatigue to him. He told me that most people are tired for about a year after chemo, and that I would be feeling "peppy" soon.

I found Tom in the back hall of his office.

"Hi." He smiled. "What's up?"

"Oh, I, uh, just thought you might check out something for me," I said as casually as I could.

In the exam room, Tom's face wrinkled into a frown as he felt the lump.

"I'm going to call Javed and ask him to see you today," he declared.

"But it's Saturday," I pointed out.

79

"That's okay. He may be in town making rounds anyway."

"Oh, let's not bother him. I'll go to his office on Monday."

It was too late. Tom had already dialed the phone.

"Hello," he said. "Tahir? Tom McKnight. Would you come out and see Ev? She has a lump right on her mastectomy scar. We'd really feel better if you would take a look at it. Great. See you then," he said as he hung up.

Tom and I had become friends with Tahir during my cancer treatment. When Fouzia had returned with their children after their year-long separation, we had gotten to know her as well. During a clinic visit that May, Tahir had mentioned that she and the kids had returned.

"And I'm overjoyed," he had said, grinning broadly.

Our friendship with the Javeds had made me consider the terrorist attacks of September 11, 2001 with a broader view. As I'd gotten to know them, I'd felt empathy for them. I couldn't imagine how they must have felt living in a foreign country where many people had tied their skin color and their religion to terrorist attacks. The day after 9/11, I had baked a fresh apple pie and dropped it off at Tahir's office with a "thinking of you" card. I wanted them to know that Americans were generally open-minded, even though many were angry at the time.

Tahir had thanked me for the pie the next time I saw him.

"Oh, the 9/11 attacks were a terrible thing," he'd commented. "I only hope that those responsible will be found and punished," he had said, looking very grave.

Dr. Javed met us at the door to the Fremont Cancer Clinic two hours after Tom called. He waved away our thanks for coming to Fremont from his home in Omaha.

"We were coming anyway," he explained. "The kids and Fouzia are waiting for me in the car. The kids want a puppy so we are going to the Humane Society when we are done here. We figure the farm dogs from Fremont will be better behaved than the city dogs of Omaha," he laughed.

Javed was quiet and serious as he examined the lump.

"I'm sure that the lump is just some extra scar tissue," he said as he sat down, and took off his gloves. "But we can biopsy it if you like."

"If you're sure it's benign that's good enough for me!" Tom said.

Tom didn't weigh more than 150 pounds soaking wet, but he nearly knocked Javed off his stool with a big, happy, bear hug. I was sitting on the exam table with my gown still open in the front, watching the exchange. The most memorable thing about it was how uncomfortable Tahir looked smothered in

Tom's hug. I thought that perhaps he was unaccustomed to males showing that kind of affection to one other. Looking back, I wonder if his conscience was gnawing at him. Maybe he felt guilty because he did not deserve our complete trust.

I mentioned the lump to Dr. Javed a month later when I went to see him.

"You know, I think it is a bit larger than it was last time," he said seriously. "I'll schedule a biopsy."

January 8, 2002

It was cold, windy and snowing on the day Dr. Javed walked across the street to give Tom my biopsy results. He arrived at the clinic unannounced but the front office worker immediately showed him to Tom's private office. When Tom saw him waiting in his office, his heart sank. In the three years that Javed had been in town, he had never come to Tom's office.

"It's malignant," Javed said as tears welled up in his eyes. "Koerber and I looked at the slides together just now. I'm so sorry. Will you tell Evelyn or do you want me to?"

"I'll tell her," Tom answered as his own eyes spilled over with tears. "She'll want to talk to you, though. Can we come over later?"

"Sure." Javed stood up to leave. "I know this is a shock to you but I want you to know we will get through this together."

Tom walked across the McDonald's parking lot to see me.

"I have something to tell you," he said.

I had heard that line before. He didn't need to tell me the rest of the story. In tears, we bundled up in our coats and crossed 23rd Street to the hospital.

We met Javed in his clinic, and the three of us sat together, digesting the news. "I think you will certainly need a wide excision mastectomy and radiation," Dr. Javed said. "And, because of the positive lymph node found during the first mastectomy, I suggest a stem cell rescue. It's a very difficult and taxing procedure, but I think it is our best hope for a cure. Essentially," he explained, "we harvest stem cells from your blood. Then you check into the hospital for heavy-duty chemotherapy—six to ten times the strength of the chemotherapy you got before."

The procedure sounded horrific.

"The theory is," he continued, "that the chemo will kill fast-growing cells in your body, particularly the cancer cells. In the process, the strong chemo eliminates your white blood cells. When this happens, the stem cells we took out will be given back to you so that your body will start making white blood cells again."

Tom and I looked at one another as the full gravity of the situation weighed on us.

"One downside is that as we kill the fast-growing cancer cells, we also kill all the other fast-growing cells in your body. The cells lining your mouth and your entire digestive tract are fast-growing. Therefore, the side effects include mouth sores, nausea, diarrhea, vomiting, indigestion, fever, chills, rash, muscle and joint pain, weakness, hair loss and fatigue. You will have to stay in the hospital about three weeks. At least one of those weeks, you will be in intensive care."

The more he talked about a stem cell rescue, the less I wanted one.

"Look," Javed went on, "I think of you as a sister. I would recommend a stem cell for my sister or my mother or my wife. I think it offers the most hope for success."

"I'd like to have a complete cure," I answered softly. "But for now, I just want to see Alex graduate from high school."

I blinked back tears of despair.

"You will see Alex graduate from college," he said with conviction.

For the next six weeks, we went to one medical consultation after another. Despite Javed's confidence, I wanted all the information I could get. Chemotherapy had been miserable the first time I had taken it. The stem cell rescue would be *six to ten* times worse, and sounded more like torture than treatment. Still, no one seemed to have a clear idea of how to treat my cancer. Oncologists at the Mayo Clinic and the University of Nebraska Medical Center did not wholeheartedly agree with Javed. They were not convinced that the stem cell rescue was the best option. The procedure was extremely risky, and the research to show that it could defeat my cancer was inconclusive.

Tom and I debated it for weeks. I spent night after night staring at our bedroom ceiling, thinking about my future. I didn't want to die. I wanted to see my sons grow up and become the kind of upright and gracious father that Tom was. Even so, it was an almost impossible decision. The specter of isolation from family and friends for three weeks, as well as the nausea, vomiting, fevers, chills and pain was so frightening to me that I felt sick to my stomach whenever I considered it.

In the end, through the grace of God and the support of loved ones, I found enough courage to go ahead with the very challenging stem cell rescue. Dr. Javed's encouragement was a big factor in my decision. He thought it was the best option for fighting cancer. If I had to go through the stem cell rescue to see Alex graduate from high school in three years, then I would.

The largest part of "encouragement" is "courage." With his quiet assurances, Dr. Javed helped me find the courage I needed to go through with the procedure. He also supported Tom in the process.

"You need to be strong for Evelyn," he told Tom after one of my visits to his office. "She's really having a tough time right now, and we don't want her to back out of the procedure. Spend some time with her tonight and assure her that we will all help her get through this."

It was ironic that I turned to Tahir Javed for support—the same physician who, unbeknownst to me, gave his patients reduced doses of chemotherapy to save money. When I was diagnosed the first time, Dr. Javed told us that I had a ninety-six percent chance of cure. Instead, the cancer returned in less than one year. I have often wondered if I received less chemotherapy than I needed in the first round of treatment, which allowed the cancer to recur so quickly. There is no way to know, since Javed was also falsifying medical records.

February 8, 2002

Before I could have the stem cell rescue, I had to undergo an onslaught of blood tests, radiology tests and lab tests. One day, several weeks before the procedure, Tom let himself in through the back door of my office yet again.

"I have something to tell you," he said, looking serious.

I had heard this twice before, so I knew that whatever the news was, it was not good. I had no idea how far-reaching and how life-altering the news would be, however.

"You have hepatitis C," he said. "The lab test is positive, but I have no idea how you got it. Javed mentioned it a couple of months ago, but the test was negative then. I know that there is an incubation period before the virus becomes detectable, which may explain why your test was negative before and is positive now. But it still doesn't explain *how* you got it, since you have no risk factors. I still can't believe," he said, shaking his head. "I've got to believe the positive result is a lab error."

He could see I was overwhelmed.

"I suggest we just put this information in the back of our minds," he comforted me. "Let's not worry about it for now."

That sounded good to me. I was within a hair's breadth of refusing the stem cell rescue altogether. I was so scared of the upcoming procedure that I was happy to ignore any other diagnosis that might require more medical treatment. I promptly put it out of my mind without asking even a single question about hepatitis C.

February 18, 2002

I packed a bag with pajamas, hats and music, and said goodbye to my sons and mother. Tom and I stopped at our church, where I received the Sacrament of the Sick before we went on to Omaha. The stem cell rescue was done at the University of Nebraska Medical Center.

Before I checked into the hospital, I was examined by my UNMC oncologist.

"Evelyn," She began. "You know you have hepatitis C. I need to know more about the extent of this disease before we proceed with the stem cell rescue. It may be best not to do the stem cell rescue if the hepatitis C will complicate things. I'd like you to have a consult with our gastroenterology department. Can you go there now if they can work you in?"

It was a bolt out of the blue.

"Not do the stem cell rescue?" I asked, befuddled and a little angry.

I had agonized over it for weeks. Now there was a possibility it would be cancelled.

"I really want to go ahead with the stem cell rescue," I stated adamantly. "This has been too much emotional work for me to give up now."

Dazed, we found our way through the maze of hallways to the UNMC gastroenterology clinic. I was first seen by Dr. Richard Gilroy. In a different time and place, I would have noticed how young and handsome he was, and how engaging his Australian accent was. Today though, was strictly business. I wanted to know what hepatitis C was, and how it was going to affect my cancer treatment.

Dr. Gilroy took my history. We went over all the possible risk factors for contracting hepatitis C. He asked if I'd had any blood transfusions, drug abuse, alcoholism, multiple sex partners, or lived with anyone who had hepatitis C.

"Have I had sex with anyone who had hepatitis C?" I asked him back, aghast. "Have I ever drank to the point of passing out? *No.* And, no, I never had any 'youthful indiscretions.'"

"Well, in one out of five cases," he commented, "the cause is unknown. So I guess we will never know how you contracted hepatitis C."

When he stepped out of the room, he stopped and scanned his notes.

I wonder if she could have gotten it through chemotherapy, he thought to himself. *No, not in the United States. Not in the twenty-first century. That sort of thing only happens in third world countries now.*

Back in the room, I felt horrible.

"You do believe me, don't you, honey?" I asked Tom. I was terrified to hear his answer. "I've never cheated on you. I swear. I've never been with anyone besides you."

"Of course, sweetheart," he quickly consoled me. "I know that. Don't even *think* those things. The thought of you being unfaithful to me has never crossed my mind. I guess we'll just never know how you got hepatitis C. But I'm going to have them draw another blood test on you. I still don't even believe you have hepatitis C. We're not going to tell anyone about this diagnosis right now. We have enough on our plates without adding more challenges. For right now, I'm going to ask Vincent not to put your test results in your medical chart. It will be in your UNMC chart, and that's good enough."

Dr. Vincent Osborn was one of Tom's partners in the medical practice and he had been our family physician for years. He and Tom shared office space and some employees. Although Dr. Osborn's charts were separate from Tom's, anyone in the building could have access to my chart since Tom and Vincent often covered for each other.

Tom and I looked at each other. I was beginning to understand how embarrassing and stigmatizing a diagnosis of hepatitis C was. I didn't even want my healthcare providers to know I had the disease.

We left UNMC and returned home to Fremont to a barrage of questions from family and friends.

"Why did you come home? Why didn't you have stem cell rescue? What's going on? When are you going back?"

"Some of the tests show a slight problem with my liver enzymes," I told them. "The doctors want to do a liver biopsy first. It shouldn't be a big deal. I'll probably be back to do the stem cell rescue next week."

The Stem Cell Rescue

The second hepatitis C test continued to show the presence of the virus. A liver biopsy showed mild inflammation but no cirrhosis, so we decided to proceed. I returned to UNMC the following week for the stem cell rescue. It was even worse than I had feared. The fevers, chills, rash, nausea, diarrhea, weakness, joint pain, muscle pain and mouth sores made it a grueling experience. Fortunately, Tom or my sisters were with me every waking moment, comforting and caring for me. Even though their faces were covered in masks, I could see the concern in their eyes and feel their loving touch through their latex gloves.

Before I'd entered the hospital, I'd had my newly grown-in hair cut short. During my initial round of chemotherapy, I had hung on to my hair as long as possible. When it had fallen out, it had come out in huge handfuls. I had washed out a clump of hair about two inches thick that covered the entire drain in the shower. I had asked my son, Luke, to comb out the rest for me. We'd sobbed as he'd filled an entire wastebasket with hair.

This time would be different. I asked Tom to shave my head in the hospital a day or two before it was expected to fall out. Tom really didn't want to shave my head, but I insisted. I caught sight of him in the mirror as he was applying the clippers to my head and saw tears dampening his mask. I have never felt so loved in my life. Having lived through baldness once before, I knew that hair loss was really inconsequential. Losing my hair a second time was of no importance. Feeling Tom's love for me was all that mattered.

A bright spot in the hospital stay was a visit from Tahir and Fouzia Javed. Visitors were discouraged, so if I had been able to think clearly, I would have been surprised to see them. They were the only visitors I had other than close family. Their encouragement meant a lot. It wasn't easy for them to come to see me. They brought their three small children and had them stay in the TV lounge while they visited me in my hospital room.

Cancer made me think about time. As I lay in the hospital bed, I contemplated how much time I had left on this earth. What should I do with that time? How could I use my time to make a positive contribution to the world? I remembered the people who I'd sat with in the chemo room at Fremont Cancer Center. I knew that several of them had died. I wondered why I had been given more time than they, even though we had the same disease.

One thing the stem cell rescue taught me is that time *passes*. The time of the awful stem cell rescue passed. Although I was only in the hospital three weeks, it seemed like three years. However, the time did pass and I returned to my beloved home in Fremont. The following months of recuperation—although not as difficult as the stem cell rescue—were also difficult. As I recuperated, I was certain that the stem cell rescue would be the most physically demanding time I would ever have to face. Fortunately, I was not able to see my future and what awaited me two years down the road.

CHAPTER 13

◼

More Hepatitis C

February, 2002

Monica Weber fumbled with her keys and juggled a bag of groceries as she hurried to open her front door. She rushed to answer her phone ringing inside, but she was too late.

Without urgency, Monica carried her groceries to the kitchen before returning to close the front door. From across the room, she could see the answering machine light blinking. It had been a long day. Between work, a doctor's appointment and grocery shopping, she was nearly exhausted.

She walked to the sofa and sat down with a relaxed sigh as she reached across to the answering machine.

"Monica," the voice came on after she pushed the button. "This is Doctor Osborn. Your blood tests are in. Your liver enzymes are very elevated. I'm quite concerned about this. Please come to my office the first thing Monday morning and we will talk about what we need to do next."

Monica's heart sank.

"What does that mean?" she wondered. "God, is it something bad? It must be, since Dr. Osborn said he was 'quite concerned.' Has the cancer spread to my liver now, two years after it was first diagnosed?"

It was late Friday afternoon, and she likely wouldn't be able to reach Dr. Osborn. The thought of spending the whole weekend in uncertainty added to her anxiety.

She dialed Dr. Osborn's office number and miraculously, the receptionist answered. Monica relayed the message to her from the answering machine and pleaded to speak to him. After a few moments, Dr. Osborn picked up the line.

"Dr. Osborn, what does 'elevated liver enzymes' mean?" Monica's voice shook.

"Well, Monica, it is too early to say. We need to do more testing. But I do want to warn you. I am worried that the cancer has spread to your liver. Come in first thing Monday morning and we will begin tests that will tell us what we are facing."

Monica hung up and collapsed into a chair. She was a recent divorcée. All her children were grown. She felt all alone. It was too much to deal with by herself. One by one, she called her children for support. They rallied around her and came home for the weekend. They cried together. They reminisced together. They laughed together. They also made plans: plans for Monica's care; plans for her finances; and plans for her funeral. By the time they left, Monica felt a bit stronger and more able to face the future, however long or short that future would be.

A week after the battery of tests, Monica received the news. She did not have liver cancer—she had hepatitis C.

"What's that?" she asked. "I've never heard of it."

"It's a blood-borne virus that attacks the liver. Some people can live a very long life with it, but others have more immediate difficulty. I'm going to set you up with a gastroenterologist in Omaha, *Dr. Ted Matthews*. He can answer all your questions better than I," Dr. Osborn advised.

Well, I don't know what hepatitis C is, but it's got to be better than liver cancer, Monica thought to herself as she hung up. *The treatment can't be as bad as the treatment for breast cancer.*

She would find out differently.

April 4, 2002:
Evelyn Describes Events After Her Stem Cell Rescue

Tom accompanied me to Javed's clinic for an office visit. After Dr. Javed finished examining me, we thanked him for the Pakistani meal that Fouzia had prepared for our sons, and then asked our questions.

"What about the hepatitis C?" Tom asked pointedly. "How will it affect her life? How do you think she got it?"

"Oh, I don't think it will cause her any problems," Tahir answered unconcernedly. "I think we should concentrate on defeating the cancer right now."

Tom was not satisfied.

"But how do you think she got it?" he persisted.

"I guess we'll never know," Javed answered evasively while reaching for some papers. "By the way, would you like to see the plans for the new cancer center?"

He changed the subject. "The administration and I have been working on plans and I just got this updated set back."

It was the first time we had seen the actual plans for Health Park Plaza. It was going to be a beautiful facility, with far more room for Javed's clinic.

"I'm just very anxious for it to be done," he commented as he unrolled the blueprints. "It will be so nice to have more space. It will be much more comfortable for the patients."

June 2002

Now that I was home, Tom returned to his medical practice full-time. My hepatitis C diagnosis continued to gnaw at him. It was too much for him to deal with on his own, so he shared the news with his trusted nurse, Jean Shafersman. He was tired of hiding our secret, and it was a relief to talk about it with an old friend. She had recently watched her own son, Byron, undergo chemotherapy, so she knew what it was like to watch a loved one suffer. Byron was active, healthy and only nineteen when he was diagnosed with stage IV testicular cancer several months after I was diagnosed with breast cancer. Jean consoled Tom, and they encouraged each other in their roles as caregivers.

One day, Jean came into Tom's office and shut the door behind her.

"Doctor, I noticed that Byron's liver enzymes are elevated. And so are another patient's, Toni Heiman. Do you think they should be tested for hepatitis C?"

Tom sat back in his chair as she took a deep breath and continued.

"Here's what I am thinking. When I sat with Byron through chemo, there were some nursing practices that went on that I didn't think were right. I told Dr. Javed about it and he said he would take care of it. But I don't know if he did and I'm worried that hepatitis C may have spread through the Fremont Cancer Center, through unsafe nursing practices. Both Byron and Toni got chemo at Javed's clinic."

"Oh my God, Jean," Tom said as he put his head in his hand. "You might be right. Oh my God! Or wait," he cautioned as another grim possibility dawned on him. "Do you think it was spread through our clinic? Think about it. Byron, Toni and Evie all had blood draws here. Could it be spreading through our lab?"

It was a horrible concept. Tom had spent his entire adult life helping the ill. The thought that his clinic might have given patients hepatitis C was gut-wrenching.

"Well," Tom broke the momentary silence. "Either way, we need to know. We need to get to the bottom of this. If there is an outbreak going on here we need to report it to the state and get it under control. I'll order the hepatitis C tests on Byron and Toni. Is there anyone else we should test?"

Over the course of the next several weeks, Tom and Jean reviewed patient charts, looking for patients with elevated liver enzymes. When they were finished, Byron, Toni and Cheryl Gentry were diagnosed with hepatitis C. With my diagnosis, there were now four unexplained cases of hepatitis C. We had all had lab draws at Tom's family practice, and all had received chemotherapy at Fremont Cancer Center.

July 1, 2002

Tom saw Tahir Javed in the hallway at the hospital.

"Tahir, could I speak to you a minute?" Tom said.

"Sure, let's step into my office," Javed replied.

"You know, I have continued to wonder how Evie got hepatitis C," Tom explained. Well, I looked around my practice and discovered three others have it. None of them have any risk factors but they have all been treated at the Fremont Cancer Center and they all have had lab draws at my office. Do you think that the virus was spread through one of our clinics?"

Javed took in a sharp breath.

"Well, I don't see how, but we need to look into this. We'll have Gerri Means do a chart audit on both of our practices. I'll get together with her today or tomorrow and get the process started."

They parted company but promised to keep in contact. Javed did not tell Tom of the sticky note inside his chemo room cupboard listing the names of patients with hepatitis C. The note had been in place for more than a year.

Later in the day, July 1, 2002

Dr. Javed met with Gerri Means at his office. He gave her the names of two newly diagnosed cases of hepatitis C in his practice and the names of Dr. McKnight's four cases.

"Doctor, I do not have your names on my line log," Gerri replied. "Where did they come from?" Gerri apparently was unaware that Javed sent much of his lab work to the University of Nebraska Medical Center.

"Gerri, I swear to God I do not know," Javed answered a different question than Gerri asked. Gerri was asking about the identity of the pathology lab, but Javed answered the unspoken but all-important question of how the patients contracted the disease.

"I wonder if the virus is spreading through Dr. McKnight's lab," Javed proposed. "I think you should run a chart audit on his clinic. You can use my two names as a control," he suggested. "Are you seeing an increase in hepatitis C in the hospital?"

"Well, I didn't think so. Dr. Dinsdale asked me that same question more than a year ago and I didn't see anything then. Let me do some digging and I'll get back to you," Gerri promised.

July 10, 2002

Javed met with Gerri so she could share the results of her investigation with him. He was surprised to find that instead of running a chart audit on Tom's practice, she had compiled a timetable on his clinic. She also brought copies of medical articles discussing cross-contamination and asked questions about his use of a community saline bag for the port flush procedure.

Her presentation made it clear. Gerri had figured out what had caused the six new hepatitis C cases. In actuality, she had figured it out some sixteen months earlier, when she had authored her February 2001 memo to Dr. Koerber.

After their meeting, Dr. Javed walked out to the hospital parking lot. He had a lot to think over on his drive home that day. He had decisions to make.

July 11, 2002

Tom hadn't heard anything from either Tahir Javed or Gerri Means for days. So, he stopped by Gerri's office in the hospital.

"Gerri, have you found out anything in your chart audit of the hepatitis C cases? I'm really anxious to clear up this mystery. Especially if there are any problems that need to be fixed," he stated.

Gerri had spent a fair amount of time on the issue but was reluctant to share her findings with Tom.

"Yes, I've been talking to Dr. Javed about the situation. You need to talk to him," she stated firmly.

"Oh, has he figured out what has happened?" Tom asked.

"You just need to talk to him," Gerri said with finality. She closed her notepad to signal that their meeting was over.

Tom left Gerri's office and walked directly to the Fremont Cancer Center. He dispensed with small talk and got right to the point.

"Gerri Means told me to talk to you. What did you find out about the hepatitis C cases?" Tom demanded.

"Actually, we are working on a chart review. Don't worry, we will get to the bottom of this," he said reassuringly. "I'm sure we'll figure it out. Just give me a couple of days."

"A couple of days" was all Javed needed. Two days later, he fled the country.

CHAPTER 14

Javed Flees the Country

"I think he is a jerk. I think he's an asshole. What do you want me to say about him?"
—Michael Leibert, president of Fremont Area Medical Center,
referring to Dr. Javed during sworn testimony on May 25, 2004

July 13, 2002

"Did you hear the news, Tom? Javed is going back to Pakistan. His mother had a stroke and he's going back to see about her care," said a gray-haired surgeon over the top of the newspaper he was reading.

Tom was walking through the hospital doctor's lounge on his way to the medical records department. There were several other doctors in the lounge, and a couple of them glanced up from where they had been watching television. The old surgeon was anxious to fill them in on the latest scuttlebutt. Tom had spoken to Javed just two days earlier about the four patients with hepatitis C. Javed hadn't mentioned anything about his family then.

"No, I hadn't heard that," he said with concern for Javed's family. "When did his mother go back to Pakistan?" Tom asked.

"I don't know, but apparently, she is very ill."

"I bet he feels terrible about it." Tom sighed, shaking his head. "I know he wanted her to stay in the US In fact," he continued, "Javed said he was going to call Homeland Security and tell them that she was a terrorist so that she would not be allowed to board a plane. Can you imagine anyone believing a seventy-year-old woman is a terrorist?" he scoffed. "You know, Tahir brought his mother to live with his family in Omaha just this last year. His whole family was working on getting a visa for his father to come over, too. His father was a very accomplished physicist. The University of Nebraska at Omaha said they would give him a teaching position anytime he could get here. It hadn't been a problem for his mother to come to the United States because she arrived before September 11. But since 9/11, it has been one insurmountable hurtle after another for them."

"I heard that too," one of the younger physicians interjected from a chair near them. "Tahir said that after about eight months of futile paperwork, Mrs. Javed couldn't stand being separated from her husband any longer. That's when she returned home to Pakistan. Tahir told me that he really didn't want her to go. He said that he and his siblings did everything they could to persuade her to stay. They were confident that their dad would be allowed into the country and wanted their mother to wait for him in the comfort and safety of the United States."

"That's terrible," the older, gray-haired surgeon interjected. "But why didn't his father come over when his mother did, before 9/11?"

"Tahir said his father was attending to the hospital he underwrote along the Afghanistan/Pakistan border. The area is very remote and very poor. The Javeds come from there, and have become so successful that they wanted to give back to their native people. His parents lived at the complex and managed the day-to-day operations of their hospital. Tahir and his siblings go back there on holidays to help out. They also run a successful fundraising effort for the compound through the Internet."

"Wow," the surgeon commented. "That's an impressive story. How generous of the Javeds. You know," he continued, "it's amazing what the Internet can do. Can you imagine a rural hospital out in the middle of nowhere taking donations from all around the world through the Internet?"

They had no way to know that the Javed family would close down the Website in the next few days.

"Tahir's father was very attached to the complex and found it was hard for him to leave it, but finally, I guess he realized that he had to. Tahir said it was not a safe place. I told him that I would like to see it. But, he said the area was becoming increasingly unsafe due to clashes among local militant groups. Apparently, it's a bloodbath over there—constant fighting between the tribes," the surgeon explained.

"When peace returns to the area," Tom said, shrugging his shoulders, "maybe Evie and I will go over and help out. I don't know if I can convince her right now, though. She is in the middle of a battle with cancer—I don't think she wants to go looking for more peril," he said with a sigh.

Later That Day
When Tom got home from the hospital, he called Tahir.

"You're leaving us, Tahir?" Tom asked.

"Oh…yes. I am catching a plane at one o'clock. My mother had a stroke. She is in our hospital on the border, but there are not many services there so I want to bring her back to Sialkot. Between my dad's sketchy reports and the terrible phone connection, I can't tell how bad she is. I feel very responsible because I am the oldest son and I never should have let her leave the US," he said, choking back tears.

Tom could hear the pain in the man's voice, and it hurt him to hear his friend suffering.

"You did all you could, Tahir," he gently comforted Javed. "We'll check in on Fouzia and the kids while you are gone. Any idea how long you will be?"

"Unfortunately, I'm afraid it might be as long as two weeks. They are in a very remote and mountainous area with very poor roads. It takes some time to get there. If she is not in stable condition, we'll have to stabilize her before we can head to the city. I'd appreciate it so much if you would look in on Fouzia and the kids. We'll talk when I get back," he said. Tom could hear that he was barely able to keep from sobbing.

"Goodbye, Tahir. Godspeed. We'll pray for you and your family," Tom finished.

"Thank you. We need your prayers."

Evelyn Describes the Following Weeks

Over the next several weeks, Tom and I spoke to Fouzia and the kids weekly. We took them to the Durham Western Heritage Museum in Omaha to see a dinosaur exhibit one day.

"How is Tahir's mother? Any news?" we asked her anxiously.

"We just can't seem to make a phone connection. I've tried and tried but I can't reach them. I think that means that they are driving to Sialkot now. The last time I spoke to him was about a week ago. He said she was very bad. All we can do is pray," Fouzia replied, wiping tears from her eyes.

Over the weeks that we called Fouzia, the report was always the same. She had a hard time reaching him. When she did, the connection was poor. From what she understood, her mother-in-law was very ill and Tahir could not leave her. The possible two-week absence stretched into three weeks, five weeks, and then seven weeks.

Before he'd left, Dr. Javed had sent letters to his patients, explaining his absence and informing them whom to contact for medical care while he was gone. He listed Dr. Janet Pieck, the radiation oncologist at the hospital, and Dr. M. Salman

Haroon, his soon-to-be-partner, as the physicians covering for him "during his absence." None of us imagined that his absence would be permanent.

A Visit to the Cancer Center

When Javed left, I was still suffering the effects of the radiation treatment. In early August, I stopped into the Fremont Cancer Center. I had developed radiation pneumonitis from damage to my upper right lung during radiation therapy. I was weak, wracked by suffocating coughing spells, and short of breath. My newly sprouted hair made my scalp itchy under my scarf. I was dead tired, but couldn't sleep because the steroids prescribed to treat the pnuemonitis made me agitated. The skin on my right chest was broken and weeping from the radiation, which made using a breast prosthesis impossible. I was wearing a poncho over my clothes to camouflage my missing breast even though it was ninety-five degrees outside. I was so hot that that my penciled-on eyebrows and eyelashes melted off, leaving lines of brown perspiration down my cheeks. I was truly miserable.

Although I was receiving quality medical care, I wanted to be cared for by Dr. Javed. I had become attached to him through the long months of cancer treatment. I hoped there would be word from Tahir that he was coming home soon.

"Hello, June," I said to the receptionist. "Any word from Dr. Javed?"

"No, not lately. I'm sure we will hear from him soon, though. I think he will be coming home next week," she offered optimistically. "We're looking forward to Dr. Haroon joining us. Have you heard about him? Here is his picture."

She offered me a laminated newspaper clipping that was on display on the counter. It was an article paid for by the hospital and published in the Fremont Tribune. It said, "Welcome to the hospital cancer team, Dr. Haroon." It described Dr. Haroon's qualifications and went on to say that "Dr. Javed is currently attending to a family emergency and asks for prayers for his mother's recovery."

"Yes, I know about him. I hope he likes it here and I hope Dr. Javed comes back soon. Well, here are my latest lab reports. We'll just hope for the best for Dr. Javed and his family," I said as I left the Fremont Cancer Center.

As I walked down the hallway of the hospital, I thought of the many times I'd sat with Javed in his private office. I pictured him sitting at his desk with his dark, handsome face wrinkled in concern. I had shared my deepest fears with him there and in return, he had offered unwavering encouragement. Remembering these times, I felt comforted in the belief that he cared.

I didn't know it at the time, but Javed's private office had undergone a transformation a few weeks previous. The wall opposite his desk was nearly empty. All his many framed diplomas and citations were gone except one—his license to practice medicine in the state of Nebraska.

■

CHAPTER 15

Some Upsetting Conversations

September 10, 2002

"Dr. McKnight, Dr. Matthews is on line two," a voice interrupted Tom's examination of a patient.

"Excuse me, Toni, I'll be right back," he said as he exited the exam room.

Tom went into his office and picked up the phone.

"McKnight," he said into the receiver.

"Tom, this is Ted Matthews. I think we have talked before. I'm a gastroenterologist in Omaha."

"Sure, Ted. What can I do for you?"

"Well, I spoke to Gerri Means and she suggested I call you. I have two Fremont patients now who have no risk factors but have recently been diagnosed with hepatitis C type 3a, which is a relatively rare type. Can you shed any light on this?"

"Am I their physician?" Tom asked with anxiety as his stomach knotted. His instant reaction was to worry if his lab was the cause of the infection. He had not heard anything from Gerri Means about a chart audit since Javed had left seven weeks earlier.

"No, Dr. Javed is."

"But am I their primary care physician?" Tom persisted.

"Let's see. I'm looking at their info sheet in their charts. Uh—no."

"Is their physician *Andrews*, Beacom, Osborn or *Smits*?" Tom asked, listing his partners, who shared lab services with him in their clinic.

"Umm…who did you say? Andrews, Beacom, Osborn, Smits… No. None of them are listed as the primary care physician. Do you want me to call their primary physician? I called you because Gerri Means told me to. She indicated that you might have some information about these hepatitis C cases. I know this is odd," he confessed. "I don't really understand it myself. But if you'd rather I call their primary physician—"

"No, no." Tom took a deep breath and sat down. "Go on."

Even though it was now clear that hepatitis C had not been spread through Tom's lab, he still felt anxious. How *many* hepatitis C cases were there? He knew of his own four and now, Matthews was telling him of two more. He didn't yet know of Dr. Dinsdale's cases or the several others that had been found a year earlier. He didn't know about the two recent cases that Javed offered to Gerri Means to use as "controls." But he did know that even one case of hepatitis C was one too many.

"Well, like I said, I have these two cases and it doesn't make sense. Their hepatitis C is genotype 3a. That is an extremely rare type of hepatitis C here in the Midwest. It's more common in third world countries. But here, it is nearly unheard of. To have two cases at once perplexes me."

"I know," Tom replied. "I have four cases myself. I don't know where they are coming from. But we need to find out."

"Oh my God," Matthews muttered.

"The common factor among my four patients is that they all went to Javed for chemo," Tom continued. "I've been waiting for him to come back from Pakistan and then I'm going to insist on a full-scale audit on the cancer clinic's charts."

"How long has he been gone?"

"Seven weeks." Tom shook his head. "But with your two new cases, we really cannot wait any longer. I think we should call in the state to investigate this."

"I agree," Matthews answered.

"Since you've done genotyping on your patients, maybe you should be the one to call. Talk to the state epidemiologist, Dr. Safranek."

"I'll be glad to. We'll get to the bottom of this," said Dr. Matthews, unknowingly echoing Javed's words of nearly two months previous. "I'll call Safranek right away."

When the two men hung up the phone, Dr. Matthews did as he promised and called Dr. Safranek. Dr. Safranek was jolted by the news. If the report was true, this was a very serious matter.

September 11, 2002

Dr. Tom Safranek called Tom McKnight the next day. Dr. Safranek asked if he could come to Fremont and discuss the hepatitis C situation. At their meeting, Safranek introduced Dr. Alexandre Macedo de Oliveira from the national Centers for Disease Control and Prevention (CDC). Dr. Macedo was a medical epidemiologist who was originally from Brazil. He had been sent to the Nebraska office for a two-year fellowship and would be conducting the investigation.

"Well, this is something interesting for Alex to investigate," Safranek said. "When the CDC told me he was coming, I was afraid he would have a rather dull time here in Nebraska."

It was an ironic comment to make. Dr. Safranek didn't know it at that time, but the "something interesting" turned out to be the largest American outbreak of hepatitis C in history.

"I understand," Safranek paused as he glanced at his notes, "that a Dr. Haroon joined Javed's practice and is seeing patients in his clinic. Tom, would you be willing to call Dr. Haroon and ask him if we can come into the cancer center and run an investigation? It might be easier for him to hear the news from you rather than from me. We can subpoena the records but it would be easier if we could just go in and look at them."

"Oh, certainly," Tom agreed. "I've met him and he seems easy to get along with. I'll call him right away. When do you want to start?"

"As soon as we can. Say, five minutes?"

Safranek was serious. Tom immediately reached for the phone.

"May I speak to Dr. Haroon?" he said into the receiver. "Hello, Dr. Haroon? Dr. McKnight. There are some investigators from the state here. They want to know if they can come over and look through your charts. There are a number of cases of hepatitis C coming from the cancer center and they want to see if they can figure out what's going on."

"Uh, excuse me?" Dr. Haroon asked, puzzled. "Hepatitis C? What do you mean?"

Tom took in a breath and tried to slow down.

"There are at least six cases of hepatitis C diagnosed recently. The only commonality is that they all received chemotherapy at Fremont Cancer Center. The state epidemiologist is here in my office along with an investigator from the CDC. They want to come over and look at charts. I think it would be best if you let them come in. You have nothing to hide."

"Well, certainly they can come in. But I can't believe it would be spread through the clinic. I'm sure they won't find anything."

Dr. Haroon was just as incredulous as anyone else would have been. It was obvious that Dr. Javed had kept him in the dark.

September 16, 2002

Tom walked quickly down the hospital hallway. His hospital rounds had taken longer than expected that day, and he had patients waiting at his clinic.

"Tom," a voice interrupted his quick stride. "Could I talk to you a minute?"

It was the president of the hospital, Mike Leibert.

"Um..." Tom glanced down at his wristwatch. "Sure, Mike."

"Thanks, Tom. Let's step into my office," Mike said, opening the door. "Have you heard anything from Javed? What do you think the state investigation will find?" he asked as he closed the door behind them.

"I don't know but I'm afraid it won't be good. I know of six cases of hepatitis C that may be linked to the cancer center. Even if the cases aren't linked to the cancer center, I pity those poor six patients," Tom replied.

"Yeah, well, I just wish Javed would get back here and clean up this mess. He told me he had everything straightened out after that site visit last year," Mike replied intensely.

"What site visit?" Tom had no idea.

"The Missouri Valley Cancer Consortium came out and inspected Javed's clinic because he wanted to get into their research group. They came down pretty hard on his nursing staff—cited numerous breaches of sterile technique. Hell, Dr. Koerber told him he had problems years before. But Javed wouldn't do anything about it."

Tom was in shock.

"Problems? He had problems with sterile technique? Was he reported to the medical staff or state licensure?"

"No, he said he had everything cleaned up," Mike spat out bitterly. "Well, I'm supposed to meet with some members of the board, so I gotta go. Call me if you hear anything, will you?"

Tom mulled the conversation over as he drove from the hospital back to his clinic. He would usually call me on the drive to his clinic. But that day, he didn't. I was still feeling poorly and he knew this news would upset me. He also knew that if he heard my voice he wouldn't be able to keep the startling news to himself. So he took some deep breaths and tried to clear his mind.

"I must have heard him wrong," he told himself. "Or there's more to the story that I don't know."

September 17, 2002

On Tuesday, Tom chose to walk past the hospital lab on his way out to his car. He saw Dr. Koerber entering the lab and hurried to catch up with him.

"Morning, Rod. Any word from Javed? How's his mother doing?" Tom tried to act nonchalant.

"I don't think so. Not a word. I wish he'd hurry up and get back, though."

"Did you know he had problems with infection control?" Tom probed.

"He told me he had everything cleaned up every time I called him about the problems in his clinic. I even went over every infraction in the Missouri Valley Cancer Consortium report with him line by line."

Tom had never seen Rod agitated before, but he could see that Rod was uncomfortable.

"Every time?" Tom questioned. "You talked to him about problems in his clinic more than once?"

"Oh sure, two, three times a week for several years," he admitted. "Finally, he got rid of Nurse Prochaska after that MVCC report last July. I thought everything was taken care of then."

"Did you report him to the state or bring this information to the infection control committee?"

"Gerri reported the hepatitis C cases to the state in her line log. He already had a complaint against him for personal misconduct. I don't know why he didn't lose his license for that," Rod retorted, referring to the charges against his license for personal misconduct. "And we couldn't bring him up to the infection control committee because the problems were in his private clinic, not in his care of patients admitted to the hospital."

Personal misconduct? Tom thought to himself as he walked out to his car. It wasn't what he wanted to hear. Just like most of Javed's cancer patients, Tom was hoping to find a "magic bullet" that would fix everything. He hoped there was some explanation that would exonerate Javed. He was beginning to realize there was no magic bullet, though, and that the mess wasn't going to be explained away. Still, he couldn't believe it. He wanted to hear the story one more time from Leibert.

September 18, 2002

On Wednesday, Tom saw Mike Leibert in the hall and walked with him to his office.

"Any news?" Tom asked.

"Yes, I finally got through to Javed. I told him he needed to be back here within two weeks. He said his mother is very ill and he didn't know if he could leave her."

It was the same story that Fouzia had been telling us for nearly two months.

"I'm going to send him a certified letter and make it clear that if he's not back within two weeks we will consider his practice abandoned," Mike added emphatically.

"Really? Don't you think he'll come back?"

"I'm beginning to wonder. He must realize the seriousness of the situation. I talked to his lawyer yesterday and he indicated that Javed had called him before he'd left and told him of the hepatitis C cases. Now, why would he do that if he planned on being back to take care of this mess?"

That Evening

When Tom arrived home, he found me on the couch. He sat down, pulled my legs across his lap and began to massage my aching feet. It was his usual end-of-the-day ritual while I was recovering from cancer treatment.

"I want to tell you about some conversations I had this week," he began.

Most people of my generation remember exactly where they were when they heard the news that President Kennedy had been shot. People in my parents' generation remember where they were when they heard that Pearl Harbor had been attacked. Members of my sons' generation can tell you where they were when they heard of the terrorist attacks of 9/11/01.

On September 18, 2002, at 6:36 p.m., Tom told me about the substandard nursing practices in the Fremont Cancer Clinic. It was my personal unforgettable moment in history. I remember the exact suit and tie Tom was wearing. I remember how the sunlight through the window made reflections against his profile. I remember how he counted off warning signs on his fingers until he ran out of fingers and had to start over again.

My gosh, my illness has been harder on Tom than I ever imagined, I thought to myself. *He is delusional. This is crazy talk.*

I was glad that no one else was in the room to hear him.

When he finished, I still couldn't believe it. So I asked him questions, and then more questions. Then, I rephrased the questions and asked them again. His answers were always the same. He had learned of the substandard nursing practices, which had gone on for years at the Fremont Cancer Center. At least six patients had contracted a potentially deadly disease because of those substandard practices. When the gravity of the situation finally sunk in, I became sick to my stomach.

I got up from the couch and started a new document on my computer. I titled it "Tom's notes about Hepatitis C." I typed out everything he remembered. As more information surfaced over the next month, I continued to keep notes as accurately as I could. Sadly, we would come to learn that the recorded information was just the tip of the iceberg.

September 24, 2002

Mike Leibert asked Tom to meet with him at Tom's office after clinic hours.

"What's up, Mike? Any news?" Tom asked as Mike entered the room.

"No news about Javed, if that's what you mean. But I'm worried Haroon will leave. He's pretty overwhelmed with the state investigators crawling all over the cancer center. He may bolt and I can't say I would blame him. But we need him here." Leibert shook his head slightly. "Would you talk to him and encourage him to stay? As the busiest family physician in town, you've got the leverage to reassure him that he will be busy enough here to make it worth his while. And with your wife having cancer, he has a personal connection to you."

Tom realized that it was important for the community to have an oncologist. On top of that, Haroon seemed like a good man, and a good doctor.

"Sure, we need him here to take care of our cancer patients," Tom acknowledged. "I'll talk to him."

"I just don't know how all of this will shake out. The hospital has some liability here," Tom heard Leibert say. Liebert's concerns were warranted because, even though the allegations of substandard practices involved the clinic, the clinic and Javed were generally perceived as being associated with the hospital, whatever legal distinctions the hospital would claim as between the two entities. Leibert left and Tom sat at his desk for a long moment.

This is a nightmare, Tom thought to himself as he watched the retreating hospital president. *I just can't believe everything I am hearing.*

September 25, 2002

Although I felt poorly, I still tried to work twenty hours per week. It was important for my staff, my patients and my own spirit. I needed to be there to encourage and direct the staff and to have a consistent presence for my patients. It was also important for my own sanity to go to work. When I was there, I was given peace of mind while focusing on something other than my own woes.

"You just received a beautiful bouquet of flowers," the receptionist said to me one day over the telephone intercom. "Come out to the front desk and see them."

My first thought was that Tom had sent them. I felt a twinge of guilt. I should have sent flowers to *him*. All this information about the hepatitis C fiasco was hard on him.

"Thinking of you, Mike and Shirley Leibert," the card read.

Tom and I had not told anyone, even our parents and our sons, of my diagnosis. With the intense scrutiny of patient records and lab reports at the hospital, someone had found that I was infected with hepatitis C. The news had obviously been passed on to the president of the hospital that day. Leibert did not appear to know that I had hepatitis C when he repeatedly confided in Tom in the previous days.

At that point in time, what I wanted from the president of the hospital was not a bouquet of flowers. I wanted what every maltreated patient wants. I wanted a pledge that the hospital would investigate the outbreak. I wanted a promise that the hospital would do everything in its power to insure that such an outbreak would not happen again on the campus of Fremont Area Medical Center. And finally, I wanted an offer of compassion and support in my upcoming health issues with hepatitis C.

September 27, 2002

"Thanks for meeting with me," Tom said while shaking hands with Dr. Haroon in his clinic after hours. "How is everything going here?"

"Well, the patients are very nice and the staff is friendly and helpful," Dr. Haroon answered. "But I don't like having the investigators here. I keep thinking every day that they will be finished and will leave. Do you think they will find anything?"

"I think you should be prepared for that, yes. We are finding that Javed didn't run a very tight ship. He let some bad nursing practices go on for very long time. I think it is very likely that hepatitis C was spread through the cancer center."

"What do you mean, 'spread through the cancer center'?" Haroon staggered back a bit in shock. "You mean there may be more than one case?"

"I don't have all the information, but yes. There are six cases that we know of. There could be more."

"More than six cases?" Haroon was overwhelmed. The news was crushing. When he had come out to Fremont at Javed's request, he had never anticipated anything like this. "I can't believe this. Javed was a good doctor. He was a long-time acquaintance of mine. I can't believe that he would allow this to happen. Do you think he knew of the hepatitis C before he left?"

"Yes, he knew," Tom explained. "But he is gone now and you were unfairly stuck with this mess." Tom took a deep breath. "You have nothing to hide," he spoke earnestly. "You did nothing wrong. Yes, this is a terrible mess, but the community needs you to stay and practice medicine in Fremont. The doctors of this town realize that you had nothing to do with this. So we will all continue to refer patients to you. We need you here. You can have a good practice here. Please stay," Tom pleaded.

"Stay? Well, it is getting uncomfortable here. I've still been expecting Javed to come back. I didn't know any of this. I've never been so betrayed by anyone in all of my life. And the potential legal consequences make me shiver. I'll have to think about it," Haroon answered.

"If you stay, you need to divorce yourself from the Fremont Cancer Center. Close down Fremont Cancer Center and open up your own clinic," Tom urged.

"But what if the same thing happens again? What if I hire a nurse who, unbeknownst to me, has a sloppy technique? I would be held responsible for her carelessness," Dr. Haroon protested. "In healthcare, we are all vulnerable— patients, doctors, nurses. We are all so intimately intertwined. There is such a huge risk of exposure."

"This outbreak was not caused by one nurse who had a sloppy technique. It was caused by Javed and his nursing staff, and continued for years even though other people knew about it. I'm not going to minimize the situation. If you stay, there is risk. But there is also huge potential for doing good. You can provide great comfort and healing for the cancer patients in this town. And that is the bottom line. We continue to do what we do despite the risks because of the good that we do. I know it is a lot to think about but we need you here in Fremont," Tom reiterated.

They parted company. Dr. Haroon sat at his desk with his head in his hands.

I can't believe this, Haroon thought to himself. He sat at his desk for a long time, pondering the situation.

September 30, 2002

Three days later, Tom once again ran into Mike Leibert in the halls of the hospital. Neither Tom nor Mike mentioned the flowers or my diagnosis of hepatitis C.

"I guess Javed won't be coming back for good now," Mike said.

"What do you mean?" Tom asked.

"John Hughes looked him up on the Internet. He is running for political office in Pakistan."

Tom walked away shaking his head in disbelief.

October 2, 2002

Tom was finishing his rounds on the medicine floor of the hospital when Cathy Spelling, RN, drew him into an empty room. They had worked together for years on the fourth floor.

"What's going on? Any news on Javed?" she asked anxiously.

Tom relayed the news that Javed was running for public office. Cathy was disgusted with the situation.

"I told him and told him there were problems in his clinic," she confessed. "I've told administration repeatedly through the years. Javed told me I was being too hard on Prochaska. He said I was 'sour grapes' because I didn't get her job when he first came to town. I'm telling you, there were real problems in that clinic. That's why I wanted the Missouri Valley Cancer Consortium to come in and do an audit in April 2001."

"I've heard about the MVCC report. I never have heard the details, though," Tom replied curiously.

"I knew there were terrible nursing procedures going on in that place. I figured it out when I worked there, when Fremont Cancer Center was short-handed. Other nurses knew also. Some of them were so appalled by it that they refused to go back," Cathy explained. "I knew that Javed wanted to get involved in research trials. I also knew the MVCC would come out and do an inspection of his clinic before his practice would be approved for inclusion in clinical trials. I was pretty sure the MVCC would be appalled, too. I was hoping that Javed and the administration would believe the MVCC even though they had discounted everything I said," Cathy explained.

"Some of the hospital nurses refused to work there because of the dangerous procedures?" Tom was stunned.

"Yes, some of the hospital nurses worked at his clinic when it was short-staffed. After a while, I was the only one who would go back there. But I kept going back, hoping that I could clean up the poor practices. At minimum, I knew the patients were being properly cared for when I was there. But no matter what I said, Javed insisted that his nurses could do no wrong," Cathy replied.

Tom and Cathy parted company, each sickened by the unfolding drama.

CHAPTER 16

Nebraska Health and Human Services Investigates

September 2002

When the state epidemiologist and the CDC officer first began investigating the Nebraska outbreak, they did not know of the Missouri Valley Cancer Consortium report of April 2001. Even though they interviewed hospital administration, they did not have a copy of the report. As a result, they had to unravel the mystery of the outbreak themselves.

The investigators carefully inspected the charts of the known hepatitis C cases, looking for a common thread among them. The only common link was that all the patients had been treated at the cancer center. They interviewed patients to determine what treatments they received, and who had performed them.

Several of the patients told them that the nurses did not change the syringe between accessing the patient's port and drawing saline from the community flush bag. Several patients even told the investigators that when they had chemo in the morning, the community saline bag would be crystal clear. When they had chemo in the afternoon, however, the saline would be cloudy, with bits of pink sediment floating around in it. It didn't take long for the investigators to figure out that the community saline bag had been cross-contaminated. At that point, they hoped that the outbreak was limited to the six identified patients, but they knew that there was the potential for many more cases.

The investigators began reviewing all the cancer center patient charts. They found one patient who appeared to have had hepatitis C, genotype 3a, before he or she was treated at the Fremont Cancer Center. Since they couldn't find any patients with hepatitis C3a who had been in the clinic in the six months preceding, they labeled the patient as the index (or initial) case.

Again, through patient interviews, they discovered that after Nurse Prochaska left the Fremont Cancer Center, the technique for flushing ports changed for the better. The investigators decided to set the time frame of at-risk patients starting with the index case's first visit to the clinic and ending six months after Nurse Prochaska left. The extra six months was added in an abundance of caution. Therefore, the time frame for risk of infections was from approximately March 1, 2000 through December 31, 2001. During that time, 857 patients were seen at Fremont Cancer Center. However, only 613 of them were still living at the time of the investigation.

On October 11, 2002, state epidemiologist Dr. Tom Safranek sent a letter to the 613 patients, notifying them of their possible exposure to the disease. His letter offered them free testing at a neutral site in Fremont. Nebraska Health and Human Services and Fremont Area Medical Center personnel conducted the screening. Of the 613 patients, only 486 actually participated. Patients were interviewed privately to assess their medical history and risk factors for hepatitis infection. A blood sample was drawn and tested for hepatitis B, hepatitis C and HIV. None of the patients had hepatitis B or HIV. Eighty-two of them were found to have hepatitis C3a in October 2002.

When the Nebraska outbreak became public on October 8, 2002, Dr. Javed's malpractice attorneys closed the Fremont Cancer Clinic. His patient records were sequestered in a storage facility adjacent to a cornfield near Lincoln, Nebraska. After the mass screening was completed, Dr. Alexandre Macedo de Oliveira of the CDC and Kathryn White, RN, (the hepatitis coordinator for the state of Nebraska) tackled the job of reviewing all of the 857 charts.

Their review was very comprehensive and looked at many variables: types of drugs; when the drugs were made; the surgical implants of ports; the dates patients were seen in the clinic; the dates and number of port flushes each patient received; the locations of the patients' ports; the person who performed the patient flushes; the complete history of all lab data; the patients' genders and ages; all invasive procedures performed on each patient; and the types of the patients' cancer. After their extensive review, they found that the improper port flush procedure was the only route of transmission.

Reviewing 857 charts in a brief, two-week time period was a tedious task. It was December, and it was very cold in Nebraska. The wind chill was -20° F and the aluminum metal building was unheated and drafty. It was a baptism by ice for Brazilian Alex Macedo, and he fought the cold by buying his first set of long underwear. Kathy and Alex could see their breath as they toiled in the metal building and became adept at thumbing through charts and recording data on a computer with gloved fingers.

Alex and Kathy completed their work reviewing the charts, exposing the details of the largest American outbreak of hepatitis C in history. The investigation took hundreds of man-hours, 857 chart reviews, 486 patient interviews and more that 500 blood tests. Nebraska taxpayers footed the bill, which was in the tens of thousands of dollars.

BOOK II

∎

The Aftermath
of the Nebraska Outbreak

■

CHAPTER 17

Travis Files Dorothea's Lawsuit

October 2002

"Travis," my secretary said as I walked through my law office door. "Did you hear about the cancer patients who got hepatitis C at the hospital?"

"No," I answered politely.

"My neighbor told me all about it at lunch," she added.

My secretary was well-known as a local gossip, and it was not uncommon for her to spend time after lunch bantering about "he said *this*," or "I can't believe she did *that*." So, as usual, I simply smiled and nodded as I passed her station and headed back to my private office.

I had moved to Fremont, Nebraska, from Omaha in 1999, when I'd formed a partnership with another attorney who had been in practice since 1990. We had a small, two-man firm. I liked the small-town atmosphere. It seemed like everyone knew everyone else, and contrary to the local gossip hounds' beliefs, nothing of major significance ever happened in Fremont. Moreover, I liked it that way. Then, a couple days after my secretary tipped me off, the Nebraska outbreak hit the newspapers and Fremont suddenly changed.

About two years earlier, I had become friends with Fremonters *Louise* and *Brent Mynard*. Just before I'd met Louise, her mother, Dorothea, had passed away. I had never asked Louise the specifics of her mother's death. All I knew was that Louise had been extremely shaken by her mother's passing. When the Nebraska outbreak first made the newspapers in the fall of 2002, Louise told me Dorothea's story.

In August of 2000, Dorothea had begun to experience shortness of breath, fatigue and a chronic cough. She had been a smoker for years. In late August 2000, a CT scan had revealed a malignant tumor in her left lung, and she was diagnosed with lung cancer. In September 2000, Dorothea had undergone a left lower lung lobotomy to remove the cancer. Two months later, she had been told by her treating physician that the surgery had been a success, and that she had no evidence of remaining cancer. She had been recovering well from her surgery, and Louise and the rest of her family were elated.

Shortly after this, in late 2000, Dorothea's primary physician had referred her to Dr. Tahir Ali Javed for preventative oncology treatment following recovery from her surgery. The idea was that by giving her several treatments of chemotherapy, her chances of developing cancer in the future would be greatly reduced.

Within two months of receiving oncology treatment from Dr. Javed, Dorothea had contracted a sudden, unknown infection in her blood that caused her to go into septic shock on February 18, 2001. She had been rushed to the Fremont Area Medical Center, where, with the family's consent, Dr. Javed had issued an order that if she was to go into cardiac arrest, she should not be resuscitated. Several hours later, Dorothea had passed away.

The family had a very difficult time accepting their mother's passing. Louise had taken it exceptionally hard, and upon the news of the hepatitis C outbreak at Dr. Javed's clinic in October 2002, she immediately came to see me. She was convinced that Dr. Javed had played a part in her mother's death.

My initial reaction was one of skepticism. It was hard for me to believe that a doctor would have endangered his own patients to the extent that was being speculated. At that point, I—like the rest of Fremont—was still in denial that such an outbreak could actually happen. The Nebraska outbreak was still only rumor, and no lawsuits had yet been filed. Still, Louise insisted that she wanted to get to the bottom of the matter for her family's peace of mind.

I advised her to go to the Fremont Area Medical Center and ask for a copy of Dorothea's Fremont Cancer Center records from the hospital and Dr. Javed's office. Once I secured Dorothea's medical records, I promised to have a physician look them over and meet with her family to explain why her mother had died so suddenly.

Days went by and Louise finally returned to my office, even more frustrated and upset than before. After repeatedly being sent from one department to another within the hospital, she and her family had been told that they could not have her deceased mother's medical records. I was sure that this was just a misunderstanding due to improper completion of paperwork. Louise was not used to working with hospitals or retrieving medical records, so I helped her fill out the proper medical release forms and sent her back to the hospital with them in hand. Once again, she was told she could not have her mother's records. No legal reason was given to the family.

Frustrated with the way Louise was being treated, and seeing the emotional toll this entire records fiasco was taking on her, I had a subpoena issued, which demanded that the hospital and the clinic release Dorthea's records to the family. I was shocked when the hospital and Javed's clinic refused to comply with the subpoena without explanation.

The simple task of collecting Dorothea's medical records of her last days of life was becoming absurdly difficult. It appeared that something was seriously wrong. I had never seen a situation wherein a medical provider would not provide a patient's medical records. Furthermore, the continued, unexplained refusal to provide the medical records only seemed to further Louise's suspicions that her mother had been subjected to foul play.

As Louise sat crying in my conference room, I knew there was nothing left to do but file a lawsuit to get the medical records she was entitled to by law. Our backs were against the wall and I felt we had no other choice.

The following day, November 4, 2002, I filed a lawsuit against the Fremont Area Medical Center and the Fremont Cancer Center in the Dodge County District Court. I did not allege that the hospital or Dr. Javed had played any role in Dorothea's death. The lawsuit was only asking the Court to require the hospital and Fremont Cancer Center to release her records to my office, so that I could have a physician review them as I had promised Louise weeks before. I didn't realize it at the time, but the simple little lawsuit over medical records was a spark that set off a media powder keg. The lawsuit caught the eye of a local television news station from Omaha, and before I knew it, they were at my office, asking questions about Dorothea's death. Dorothea's lawsuit was the first hepatitis-C-related lawsuit filed against Dr. Javed, and it started a media frenzy. Before I knew it, Louise was on the Omaha evening news with tears in her eyes, telling her story to all of eastern Nebraska.

The next day, I received a telephone call from Dr. Javed's attorney. The clinic had, "after careful consideration," and "of its own volition," decided to release Dorothea's records to her family. I dismissed the lawsuit without making an appearance in court.

Upon receiving Dorothea's medical records from the Fremont Cancer Center, I immediately had them reviewed by a physician to determine whether or not hepatitis C had played a part in her death. It had not. She had died of natural causes, and the entire debacle of denying her family access to her records had been for naught.

CHAPTER 18

Travis Recounts the Hepatitis Hysteria

When I filed Dorothea's lawsuit, I had no idea what it would bring. It was a simple lawsuit, filed to fix a simple problem. I could never have predicted the aftermath of that short-lived legal action. My office was swamped with media coverage, and an overwhelming number of victims and their families flocked to my office, looking for help. Over the next few months, I worked virtually every waking hour, meeting with people and trying to answer their questions.

Hepatitis Becomes Big Business

As I was in the midst of meeting with victims and their families, the legal community exploded in frenzy. Hepatitis C suddenly became "big business." I have learned that there are many minor tragedies that follow a large-scale disaster like the Nebraska outbreak. One of them is simple greed. When the Nebraska outbreak went public, some lawyers saw it as an opportunity to get rich. In the end, I don't know many who did. At the outset, though, greed added to the mass confusion.

One of the biggest misunderstandings that people had about the Nebraska outbreak was that the victims were part of a class action lawsuit. This was never the case, but it was widely accepted as the truth. As a result, many of the people who came to my office following the Nebraska outbreak thought that they did not need to file their claims for damages individually. They thought that all they had to do was wait a few years until the class action was settled, and that they would then get a check in the mail for their damages.

The belief in this class action couldn't have been further from the truth, and it couldn't have come at a worse time. Under Nebraska law, the victims of the Nebraska outbreak were already nearing their statute of limitations (a law limiting the time a plaintiff can file a lawsuit after the malpractice occurs.) Those who did not file their individual claims within a short time period would be forever barred from any recovery. This meant that those who had waited around for the class action to settle would someday find out that if they needed a liver transplant, they would not receive a dime from the defendants who had hurt them.

Unfortunately, the common misunderstanding about a class action largely came from a member of my own profession. After I filed and dismissed Dorothea's lawsuit, the first lawsuit was filed on behalf of an infected victim. The attorney who filed it included language identifying it as a class action. He alleged claims on behalf of all the victims, and the local media picked up on it. He even advertised his "class action" in the local newspaper.

Under Nebraska law, there was no way in the world that the class claim was effective. Procedurally, the filing was incorrect, because he did not first obtain permission of the Court to file a class action lawsuit. Even if he had, the Court would have denied it. To file as a class action, by definition, all the plaintiffs must have the same damages. All the plaintiffs of the Nebraska outbreak had different damages. Some of the victims had died from the disease. Others lived out their lives with fewer effects of the disease. Still others fought the disease with thousands of dollars spent on grueling treatment. The reality of the situation was, however, that many people believed that they did not have to file an individual suit themselves, but merely had to wait until the conclusion of the class action.

I did everything in my power to let people know that there was in fact no such class action lawsuit, and that they had to act before it was too late. I told anyone who would listen, and even took money out of my own pocket to host public seminars on the subject. When the statute of limitations for the victims finally came and passed, ten percent of the victims had not filed their individual claims. To this day, I do not know if they simply elected not to, or if they are still awaiting settlement of the class action.

Suing the Innocent

Over the next five months, I met with hundreds of people who had questions about the Nebraska outbreak. I was hounded by the media, and eventually filed lawsuits on behalf of nineteen of the ninety Nebraska outbreak victims who filed claims. As I was preparing to file the lawsuits, I needed to identify who should be named as defendants. The last thing I wanted to do was to omit the name of someone who had caused the Nebraska outbreak. If I did, the statute of limitations against them would run and the plaintiff would possibly go without recovery.

The other thing I wanted to avoid was naming someone who had not participated in the Nebraska outbreak. I did not want to sue any innocent nurses or doctors. Filing a lawsuit is a serious endeavor. When a medical provider is named and served with a summons, their entire world changes. They have endless hours of meetings with their lawyers, and they often spend sleepless nights with the ever-present fear—albeit unfounded—that they could end up losing everything they owned if a judgment was entered against them. In reality, the medical provider's liability is safeguarded through malpractice insurance, but nonetheless, I did not want to unjustly place the burdens of a lawsuit on anyone.

As I was trying to figure out who should be listed as a defendant, I came upon a complete list of all the former employees of the Fremont Cancer Center. It was a blessing because it eliminated my first fear of mistakenly failing to name one of the proper defendants. The problem was that I was fairly certain that some of the names on the list were not the names of doctors or nurses. Some of the names had to have been Javed's receptionists and secretaries. In addition, I was fairly certain that some of the names belonged to nurses who probably had nothing to do with the Nebraska outbreak because they were not employed during the time the infections took place.

To narrow the list of names, I called the attorney who had been appointed by Javed's insurance company to defend him. I asked him if he could identify the nurses who had been working for Javed from March 2000 to December 2001. He refused. I told him I already had the names of all employees, but simply needed to remove the names that were not complicit in the Nebraska outbreak. Again, he refused to answer my question.

When I hung up the phone, I was in an awkward position. At the time, I did not even have a good understanding of how the Nebraska outbreak occurred. I did not know which of the people on the list had caused it, or who on the list could have prevented it but didn't. If I left the wrong name off the list, my plaintiffs might have to go without recovery from their lawsuit. It could mean that they would have to go without the medication they needed, or the liver transplant they may need to someday save their life. It was a life-or-death decision, so I had no choice. I had to sue everyone on the list.

Years later, I met one of the nurses who I'd mistakenly sued. She had worked at the Fremont Cancer Center, but only after Javed had abandoned his patients and absconded to Pakistan. She obviously had no liability in the Nebraska outbreak. I told her of my dilemma, and how I had no choice but to do as I had done—sue her nineteen times (once for each victim I represented.) She said she understood, and that she forgave me. I was sad to hear that the stress of the lawsuits I had filed caused her to indulge in drinking and smoking to excess. It was hard for me to hear. It was heartbreaking to know that I had caused her pain when she obviously had not deserved it, especially when she was already anguished from simply being affiliated with Javed's infamous clinic.

The Mother's Day Gift

In Nebraska, when a lawsuit is filed, it must be "served" within six months of the date of filing. Just like in the movies, to serve a lawsuit, a sheriff or process server usually personally hands the lawsuit to the defendant. The process server then sends a letter back to the Court, swearing under oath that he gave it to defendant.

Under Nebraska law, if a lawsuit is not served on a defendant within six months of the date it is filed, the lawsuit is dismissed against that defendant. If the statute of limitations happens to have run in the interim, the lawsuit cannot be refiled. The fear of not serving a defendant within the statute of limitations or six months of the filing kept me awake at night. I had nineteen victims who were relying on me to serve their suits, and one of the chief culprits in the entire Nebraska outbreak—Nurse Linda Prochaska—was avoiding service. Dr. Javed's insurance carrier had already entered his appearance in the lawsuits, so I was not concerned with serving him, even though he was still hiding in Pakistan.

Prochaska was another issue altogether. Several times, I attempted to serve her, but she seemed to be wise to the service process and avoided it at all costs. She refused to come to her front door several times, and on one occasion, refused to leave her workplace when she saw my process server waiting by her car. By the time Mother's Day 2003 arrived, she was nearing the end of the six-month period. If she could simply avoid the sheriff for another few weeks, she would get away scot-free. I was becoming desperate.

In the beginning of May 2003, I hired a private process server. We bundled the nineteen lawsuits into a box and he went to her house on Mother's Day. While she had continued to avoid service of process by "not being home" for months, she was willing to come to the door when she believed someone had sent her a Mother's Day gift. I was not there myself, but I heard that she smiled as she signed for the package.

Going Broke

Medical malpractice litigation is an expensive and risky area of law for attorneys. Typically, medical malpractice cases are done on a contingency basis. The attorney gets paid a percentage of the award received by the plaintiff. That means that if the plaintiff doesn't win, the attorney doesn't get paid. Usually, smaller law firms like mine only take on a small number of contingency cases at once. This way, they can focus most of their time on working for clients who pay by the hour (such as divorces and wills.) This enables small law offices to keep the firm afloat while they are working on the contingency cases.

I didn't know it at the time, but the media coverage of Dorothea's lawsuit would change my life. The day after the news story aired, my phone lines were jammed with calls. My small firm was suddenly swamped with Javed's patients and their families. My partner and I met with potential clients every half hour during virtually every waking hour for the better part of three months. We met with hundreds upon hundreds of people who were all in the same situation— wondering if Dr. Javed had infected them or someone they loved.

For the most part, our regular office caseload shut down. As a result, our regular income shut down, and we had to take out massive, six-figure bank loans simply to keep the firm in operation while we tried to keep up with the overload. Soon, the firm was broke. In no time at all, I was broke—pledging everything I owned to secure loans to float the failing law firm. As the cases continued for one year, then two, then three and finally four, I took on over a quarter of a million dollars in personal debt. My partner and I mortgaged everything we owned to pay the costs (medical records, expert witness fees, travel expenses, deposition fees, etc.) on our cases. I used the money to pay my share of office overhead, and to keep my own household running.

I went to lunch one day with several other lawyers from town. None of them represented victims of the Nebraska outbreak. I held my tongue as they made envious jabs at my seemingly good fortune. It wasn't any of their business to know the truth. I had already had enough grief defending my financial condition at home.

"So," one said, "I hope you remember us little people now that you are rich and famous."

"I wish I got to be on TV," another said sarcastically.

When the lunch was over, they got up and left, leaving me behind with the lunch bill. I was the "rich" one in the crowd and so I was the one stuck with the bill. With a sinking feeling, I sorted through the credit cards in my wallet to find one that wasn't maxed out.

On January 1, 2005, I took a phone call from the law firm's banker. Our line of credit was maxed out and had come due. We had barely been able to keep up with the $2,300 interest payments on our main loan, much less with paying on the loan principle. Our banker said it was imperative that we meet that morning. I told him it was New Year's Day.

"Can't we meet on the next workday?" I asked.

No. We had to meet right away. If not, the bank was going to take my house. The loan was due. Either we met or they foreclosed. I had secured the loan with my home, my car, my personal property, everything I owned. For two years, I had barely taken a paycheck, pouring every dime I had back into the cases. For the most part, my clients didn't have the money to pay the costs of their lawsuits. So I met with the banker, and we re-signed a new loan under terms that I was in no position to contest.

One month later, the first hepatitis C case settled. Soon, seventeen of my nineteen clients settled their cases. I had essentially gone without receiving a paycheck for the previous four years. I wrote a check to pay off the loans in full the next day. It was the largest check I had ever written. When the fiscal year was said and done, after paying off the loans, going through a divorce and paying taxes, I took home nearly $40,000 from the hepatitis C cases. It took me four years to earn that $40,000. For all my work and time, I earned nearly $10,000 per year for my sixty-hours-a-week employment. To this day, if you ask around Fremont, I am still the "rich guy" who claimed his prize from the hepatitis C lawsuits. Despite overwhelming public opinion to the contrary, very few plaintiffs' attorneys got rich from the hepatitis C lawsuits. I certainly did not.

CHAPTER 19

The Federal Investigation, As Told by Travis

It was another long day at the office. As had become the custom, I was spending the morning in meeting after meeting with outbreak victims.

"Travis," my receptionist buzzed me over the intercom. "Someone is here to see you."

I was far from surprised. "Someone" had been to see me every hour on the hour for the better part of the past few months.

"I'm in a meeting," I held my tongue as I answered back politely. Why was she bothering me? She knew I was busy.

"Ummm," she buzzed back. "I really think you need to come out here."

I could tell in her voice that something was amiss, so I stepped away from my office with a promise to be right back, and quickly found my way to the lobby.

With one look, I could tell what flustered her. Two men in dark blue suits with dark ties stood in the lobby. They were perfect stereotypes of every movie government agent I'd ever seen. Everything from their clean-shaven faces to their bravado postures with their fully inflated chests screamed "federal law enforcement."

"Good morning," I said, reaching out my hand.

As the first one shook my hand, I caught a glimpse of the semiautomatic handgun in a holster strapped under his arm.

Just like in the movies, they simultaneously flipped open their badges.

"I am *Agent Baker*, this is *Agent Walsh*. I am with the FBI," the more talkative one began. "He's with the criminal division of the FDA. Is there some place we can talk in private?"

"I had no idea the Food and Drug Administration even had a criminal division," I mumbled as I gestured to my conference room.

"Well, we do," the second one answered flatly.

I closed the door and sat down across the conference table from them.

"Can I get you some coffee?" I asked.

At that moment, I didn't really know what else to say.

"We are here to talk about the Fremont Cancer Center," the first one answered a different question than I had asked.

By this time, my office staff had found my law partner and interrupted him from his meetings so he could join us.

"We are here about the Fremont Cancer Center," the FBI agent repeated once introductions were done.

"First of all, let me tell you that we are not here today," he continued.

It was a cheesy, grade-B-movie thing to say, but I did not even smile. He was serious.

"No one knows we are here, and we don't want anyone to know we are here. If either of you tell anyone that we have been here, you could be charged with interfering with an ongoing federal investigation."

"Yes, sir." I nodded my head to show I understood. I didn't want to cross him. He was cold and his demeanor was that of a man who had had his badge and gun long enough to be accustomed to people following his directives.

"We understand that you two have subpoenaed medical records and other documents from the Fremont Cancer Center. We are here to review them."

At this point, everyone within a hundred-mile radius knew that we had Fremont Cancer Center records. Obviously, they too had been watching the local evening news.

"What exactly do you want with them?" my partner asked.

"I am conducting an investigation," the FBI agent said shortly. "I can't say anything else."

"You're concerned this was a terrorist attack," I said, pointing out the elephant in the room that everyone was ignoring.

"I can't say," he repeated.

"I'm investigating whether or not Dr. Javed committed insurance fraud with regard to prescription drugs. I'm trying to find out if he billed patients' insurance for treatments and tests the patients didn't know about or didn't receive," the FDA agent finally spoke up.

I could have told him what his investigation would find, if he had just asked.

I was no FDA agent, but I had already reviewed half a dozen cases wherein Javed had tested his patients for hepatitis C without their knowledge. On a couple of occasions, I had even seen cases where he had billed their insurance for "treatments" that they had never received.

"I'm just conducting an investigation," Mr. FBI repeated. "That's all you need to know. We need to see your clients' medical records. We want to see everything that you have received through your subpoenas."

My partner and I looked at one another. We were both uncomfortable with showing clients' records to anyone. Nor did we want to show them the other documents we had subpoenaed from the hospital. Our clients expected us to keep their matters private. We had a moral duty to protect them, even if we did not have a legal one.

"Gentlemen," the agent broke our pause. "You can either let us see the documents, or we can be back here within the hour with a federal warrant."

"Why don't you just get a warrant and get them from the hospital?" I asked politely. "They have more records than we do."

"Because no one knows we are here, and that is how we want to keep it," one of them replied.

The thought of letting them go through our documents did not sit well with either my partner or me. We had the medical records of dozens of former patients from the Fremont Cancer Center who trusted us to represent them as victims of the Nebraska outbreak. In addition, those metal filing cabinets in the other room contained hundreds of other client records of people who had nothing to do with this. Divorce clients, business clients, wills, trusts and dozen of other types of clients also trusted us. They had a right to privacy, too. It was an intimidating situation.

"I'll go get the documents," I muttered.

Within a few minutes, I reluctantly returned with a stack of records at least two feet tall. In an abundance of caution, I brought out only generic documents that did not specify a particular client.

One by one, we went through the documents.

"Do you have this document?" I asked, holding out the top page.

"We cannot answer that question," one of them would answer after they both inspected it closely and made notes in their little black books.

"Do you have this document?" I asked, holding out the next page.

"We cannot answer that question," he answered again. "But we would like to get a copy of it."

And so it went. For the next two hours, I let outbreak victims wait while I spent time showing documents to the government agents. I made two piles of documents—documents they couldn't tell me if they had seen, and documents they couldn't tell me if they had seen but of which they needed copies.

After they finished, they stood to leave. As they shook my hand, I wondered where all this would lead.

"Are you going to catch Javed and bring him back from Pakistan?" I asked.

It was one of those moments in life that seemed like I was in a movie.

"We always get our man," the FBI agent answered with confidence.

Several months passed and I never heard a word from either of the federal agents who had unexpectedly visited my office. As time went on, I finally saw an article in the local newspaper identifying that they had indeed been seen around town, conducting their investigation. It wasn't news to me, but I had been instructed to keep quiet about their presence, and since I didn't want an untimely vacation in federal prison, I had done so. It wasn't until the *Fremont Tribune* article came out that I figured it was alright to discuss their visit with my own family.

Finally, a year later, in the fall of 2003, my phone rang. It was one of the agents who had been out to see me months earlier.

"I just wanted to call and find out if you had any more information on the outbreak that should be included in my final investigation report," he asked.

"What's going on?" I answered his question with one of my own. "I haven't heard from you in a long time. Are you going to federally prosecute Javed?"

"Well…" He paused. He was obviously still uncomfortable talking about the status of the case. "You know I cannot confirm or deny anything about the ongoing investigation."

There was an awkward silence.

"But," he continued after the pause, "I want you to know you were very helpful to us in putting together our case. And, again, I cannot tell you why, but I've been told that we are dropping the case against Javed. I'm just writing out my final investigation report before I close the case officially. I'm being reassigned to another case."

"What?" I was shocked. "It's pretty obvious that this guy has hurt a lot of people and committed federal insurance fraud. Why are you going to close the investigation?"

I could tell by the tone of his voice that he was not happy about dropping the case.

"I can't really say, but the order came from up above." He sighed.

Suddenly, my long-held suspicions were stirred.

"We are at war in Iraq," I pointed out. "Pakistan is an ally in that war. Javed is the newly elected minister of health for Punjab Province. And no matter what he did, the United States is not going to ask a wartime ally to extradite a national official. Is that it?"

"I can't say anything," he repeated, "other than the case is closed. But if he ever steps foot back on US, soil it will be a different story."

For the next couple weeks, it was hard for me to concentrate on anything other than a feeling of betrayal for the victims of the Nebraska outbreak.

◼

CHAPTER 20

Media Coverage, As Explained by Travis

Most law schools teach their students that the value of a medical malpractice case is based on a number of factors including the plaintiff's 1) pain and suffering; 2) lost wages; 3) medical bills; 4) loss of consortium; and 5) any other damages that are special to the case. I have learned that *none* of these factors can be used to put an accurate monetary value on a medical malpractice case. The *only* value that has *any* importance is the value assigned by a jury. Every law professor in the country could review a medical malpractice case and each set a value to it, but if the jury says it is worth more, it is worth more. If the jury says it has no value at all, it is valueless.

The local media swarmed around the Nebraska outbreak. Both sides of the litigation knew that the media would have an influence on the way the public viewed the Nebraska outbreak. The media would tell every potential juror in the county what to think about the outbreak before any of the lawyers in the cases did. The media got to spend four years telling the jurors who was to blame before we got to spend our two weeks with them. Both sides knew it, and both sides, intentionally or unintentionally, influenced the way the media reported the facts. Unfortunately, it seemed that the Outbreak Victims did not get the benefit of most local media coverage.

The media portrayal of Dr. Javed was both an advantage and a disadvantage for the plaintiffs. In every other medical malpractice case I have ever seen, the accused doctor stays in the area and defends him/herself. It is often impossible for the plaintiffs' attorney to convince a jury that the doctor was negligent.

As long as the doctor looks the jury in the eyes, and tells them he tried his best, they are often unwilling to hold him liable. People like doctors. Even if they did commit malpractice, a jury will often feel that the doctor was trying to help, even if the end result did not turn out well. The fact that Javed absconded to Pakistan made him a perfect target for blame. It was going to be easy for us to convince a jury that he was a bad guy. The problem was that he was such a bad guy that the other defendants could easily jump onboard and blame him as well.

The Fremont Area Medical Center wanted to use the media to persuade the public that the hospital was not involved in the Nebraska outbreak at all. Before the Nebraska outbreak, the hospital had spent thousands of dollars on advertisement after advertisement promoting Javed. Prior to the Nebraska outbreak he had been the hospital's director of oncology and hematology. An article in the hospital newsletter entitled "The Physician's Profile: Dr. Tahir Javed makes cancer center flower," stated that when Dr. Javed had become "Medical Director of Medical Oncology at Fremont Area Medical Center, it was like putting fertilizer on a flower bed."

Once the Nebraska outbreak occurred, the hospital press releases immediately changed. Suddenly, Javed was just a tenant who had only leased space in the hospital. An article in the *Fremont Tribune* on October 18, 2002 said, "Javed leased space from the hospital for the clinic. 'He leases space from us,' Leibert said."

Time and time again, articles were run by local media that stressed the fact that in many situations, hepatitis C was a disease that usually took fifteen to twenty years to cause serious liver damage. The news articles were published so frequently that the common man on the street believed that the Nebraska outbreak was "no big deal." An October 16, 2002 article in the Fremont Tribune de-emphasized the potential dangers of the disease by quoting state epidemiologist Dr. Tom Safranek, who said, "Many people will live a perfectly normal life without ever being aware they have a Hepatitis C infection."

While a slow development of the disease may be the case for many people, it was not the case for many victims of the Nebraska outbreak because they were immunocompromised at the time they were infected. Regrettably, minimization of the seriousness of the disease was still being published after some victims of the Nebraska outbreak had died from the disease.

In some instances local newspapers seemed to be biased against the Nebraska outbreak victims when they failed to report the victim's side of issues. In June 2005, the *Annals of Internal Medicine*, a respected, refereed medical journal, released a medical article entitled "An Outbreak of Hepatitis C Virus Infections among Outpatients at Hematology/Oncology Clinic" (Ann Intern

Med. 2005; 142: 898-902.) It was written by Dr. Alexandre Macedo de Oliveria, the chief investigator of the Nebraska outbreak, among others. A companion editorial entitled "Patient to patient Transmission of Hepatitis C Virus" opined that the hospital administration had "unconscionably" failed to act on patient complaints and instead had only referred them back to Dr. Javed. The editorial went on to say that "the hospital would have served the public interest far better had the administrators immediately reported the patients' concerns" to the proper authorities.

The *Fremont Tribune* contacted the hospital attorney about the article, and then ran an article on July 20, 2005 entitled, "Report has inaccuracies." Nowhere in the article did it mention the actual findings of the medical journal's study. Instead, the article quoted the hospital attorney, who criticized the study. No plaintiffs' attorney was interviewed at all.

Another example of what I consider unfair media coverage came from the *Omaha World Herald* on February 24, 2005. In an article entitled "Taxpayers Largely Stuck With Hepatitis C Payouts," the paper said that taxpayers (our future jurors) would end up paying the "millions of dollars" asked for by plaintiffs. The article began: "Who ultimately will pay for the largest hepatitis C outbreak…in the United States? …it may be you." The paper went on to bias readers by insinuating that the Nebraska outbreak victims would likely cost taxpayers $86.1 million. The statement was completely inaccurate and absolutely ludicrous. Nebraska is a conservative state. I knew, as did all the other malpractice attorneys I worked with knew, that there was no way the victims would collect jury verdicts totaling $86 million. At the time, most of my colleagues and I would have been shocked if we ended up collecting even a quarter of that amount in total. It was a claim that focused on the theoretical rather than the reality of the situation. As a result, it served to potentially bias future jurors against Outbreak Victims. Evelyn and I, as well as other plaintiff attorneys and several members of the board of the Nebraska Medical Association, wrote letters to the editor and/or the reporter. We never saw a follow-up to the article pointing out our concerns.

Two reporters who actually stood up for Nebraska outbreak victims, in spite of propaganda, were local radio broadcaster Travis Justice and *Omaha World Herald* reporter Jeremy Olsen. Both of them spent a considerable amount of time reminding the public who the actual victims were.

My biggest frustration during the continued media blitz against the Nebraska outbreak victims was that none of the plaintiffs could respond. Early on in the cases, District Judge Samson placed a gag order on all the parties and their attorneys. The defense hoped to move venue further west, where there is a far lower per capita income than in Dodge County. At the time, Dodge County's per capita income was around $27,000. The defense knew that if the court moved venue out of Dodge County because local media coverage had contaminated the local jury pool, there was a good chance we would end up trying our cases to a poorer jury, resulting in lower verdicts.

I believe their ultimate hope was that a rural jury would be selected with a per capita income far lower than that of Dodge County. For example, if the cases were sent to a county with half the per capita income of Dodge County (like Loup County, where the per capita income was $13,372 per year), the jury could conceivably award the plaintiffs a "massive" verdict of around $20,000—thinking they were awarding the plaintiff a lifetime of savings.

The problem, of course, was that most plaintiffs had medical bills in excess of that. Nevertheless, it was the defense's greatest hope, and our greatest fear. So, as article after article was released, I told my clients to bite their tongues. In the end, it paid off because the defense's motion for change of venue was denied, and the cases stayed in Dodge County, where they belonged. The lasting downside to it all was that most people I talk to in Dodge County still believe that the Nebraska outbreak and Hepatitis C are "no big deal."

CHAPTER 21

The Jill Watson Story, As Told by Travis

"I probably shouldn't have said that, I overstated it."
—Dr. Thomas Safranek referring to his
October 31, 2002 letter to patients who had tested negative

Jill Watson was the most outspoken, determined person I represented in the Nebraska outbreak lawsuits. Most of the outbreak victims did not want anyone to know that they had contracted a disease that is associated with drug addicts and prostitutes. In addition, they didn't want their neighbors or families to know that they had filed lawsuits.

This was not the case with Jill. While most victims were hiding their disease, Jill was acting as an advocate for all the victims of the Nebraska outbreak. She may have been a stay-at-home mother of four from a small town in the Midwest, but from the outset, she spoke out about the injustices that had taken place as though she were a seasoned news anchor. The local press loved her. The defendants hated her outspoken nature, and the District Court eventually entered its gag order largely to keep her quiet. Like all the other victims of the outbreak, her life was anything but normal after she contracted hepatitis C.

The first time I met Jill Waston, I didn't understand her. She had just been tested for hepatitis C by the state of Nebraska, and she'd tested negative. It was wonderful news that many people would have loved to have heard. Yet, even with the state's letter in hand—signed by the state epidemiologist, Dr. Tom Safranek—which stated, "…you are not infected…" and that "…no further testing or medical care is necessary," Jill was still fearful that she had contracted hepatitis C.

"The state says you don't have the virus," I said, after instantly recognizing the letter.

"I know," she logically agreed. "But they're wrong. A newspaper writer already wrote an article on how I don't have it. But he was wrong, too. Something is not right. I know it."

I was baffled. Dr. Tom Safranek was the state's epidemiologist and the highest-ranking virus specialist in the state. He didn't leave any doubt in his letter.

She had already spoken to another attorney, who had reviewed the letter and explained that she didn't have a case; she didn't even have reason to be concerned. Still, she was so calm and certain of herself.

"I guess I don't understand." I looked at her skeptically.

"What don't you understand? When I found a lump in my breast, doctors told me that it was one in a million chances that I had cancer," she explained. "Then they told me I had cancer. Doctors told me that I would have a one-percent chance of getting radiation pneumonia during treatment. I got pneumonia. Anytime something happens to 'one person in a million,' I am that one person."

It was illogical, but she was so adamant that I felt I had no choice but to look into it further. Every logical part of me was saying that she couldn't have the virus, but in spite of that I couldn't tell her she was wrong. To take on her case, though, I would need to be able to prove that she was right. I didn't quite know how to begin.

Jill had walked into my office at the height of the mass hepatitis C hysteria. My law partner and I were swamped with walk-in appointments, all interested in hepatitis C litigation. He was in the other room in a meeting, but I interrupted him and brought him to my office to meet Jill.

I introduced him and explained the odd situation.

"What do you think?" I asked him.

We had worked a number of medical malpractice cases together in the past, but neither of us had ever been in a situation like this.

"Well," he answered as he pondered the problem. "I know this isn't exactly the same, but I did a case once about cows."

I remembered him working on the case. Everyone remembered him working on it. Furthermore, if anyone ever forgot, he was always quick to remind them. It had been the highlight of his legal career.

Jill looked skeptical. I could tell she had a hard time seeing a connection between hepatitis C and a case about a cow.

"In that case," he continued, "a rancher used a defective cattle vaccine and I sued the drug company that made it. After the rancher used the vaccine on his cattle, they all caught the virus and died. There were two kinds of tests that the veterinarians used to test the cattle for the virus that killed them. One was called an 'antibody' test and one was called an 'antigen' test."

"What's the difference?" I asked.

"The antigen test looks at the blood to see if the virus is present. The antibody test looks at the blood to determine whether or not the body is producing antibodies to fight the virus."

It took a moment for the difference to sink in.

"It's kind of like this," he explained. "If you want to know if a coyote is in your chicken coop, you can do one of two things. You can look for coyote tracks or you can look for the coyote. An antibody test looks for the coyote tracks. An antigen test looks for the actual coyote."

"So, when the state did the antibody test, they may have missed some people?" Jill asked.

The notion seemed far-fetched.

"Well…" My partner thought about it. "You know, antibodies are only produced by the body when the person's immune system is fighting the virus."

We all paused for a moment as we looked at each other. The same thought was on all three of our faces.

"Chemotherapy suppresses the immune system," I said.

"So," he concluded the thought, "since all these people were undergoing chemotherapy, it is very likely that their immune systems were suppressed, and that they didn't produce antibodies to fight the hepatitis C virus."

"And," I added, looking at Jill, "there may be a bunch of people out there who just got letters from the state with false negative test results."

"I'm going to get an antigen test," Jill hurried to declare.

Nebraska Health and Human Services and the CDC had tested the potential outbreak victims with an antibody test based on cost and effectiveness factors. At that time, it was not well-documented that cancer patients were not good candidates for the antibody test because of their weakened immune systems.

State epidemiologist Dr. Safranek had been on a media campaign to reassure the public that the Nebraska outbreak had been contained. If there were people who had the disease who received false negative test results, however, they could suffer horrible results. Their suppressed immune systems did not produce antibodies in response to the virus and showed that they were hepatitis-C-free.

However, their suppressed immune systems would not fight the virus. They wouldn't be going in for further testing, and by the time they had symptoms, the disease could be very advanced. Furthermore, if they did get hepatitis C from the Nebraska outbreak, their statute of limitations was nearly run. They could end up finding out that they needed a quarter-of-a-million-dollar liver transplant in a couple years and not have any recourse to require the defendants to pay for it. The state of Nebraska and the CDC had created an unintentional hazard to public health with the testing method and their proclamation of "no further testing necessary."

The following day, my law partner contacted Dr. Tom Safranek. Dr. Safranek's response to our concern was brief. In his estimation, the test Jill and the others had been given was correct 99.9 percent of the time. Furthermore, if my partner and I were to make our concerns public, Safranek felt we would be scaring the public unnecessarily. When we got his response, we questioned the validity of our theory. After all, he was the highest-ranking disease specialist in the state and we were basing our theory on a case my partner had done years earlier on cows. So, we kept our theory quiet and didn't discuss it anymore.

Several weeks later, Jill showed up at my office again.

"I told you so," she said, handing me medical test results from her new oncology doctor.

My heart almost stopped when I read the results. It was an antigen test. Her new oncologist was looking for the coyote instead of just looking for his footprints. To my disappointment, Jill's hunch had been correct. She was indeed a victim of the Nebraska outbreak. My law partner and I had also been correct about the testing method. Her immune system wasn't fighting the virus. We immediately contacted Dr. Safranek. To my amazement, he was skeptical. The CDC recommended the screening test, and he was not convinced it was inaccurate.

The following day, I filed Jill's lawsuit. The same reporter who had written an article on her first negative test result picked up on it immediately. Suddenly, the cat was out of the bag. In the meantime, Jill's oncologist had contacted Safranek to support our immunocompromised patient theory. Within a day or so, Safranek held a press conference to make another announcement. As a result of Jill Watson's test results, the state was going to retest all those people who had tested negative the first time—this time with the more accurate antigen test.

When the test results came back, seventeen more people were found to be hepatitis C positive, despite the initial letters they'd received from the state. Without Jill's unyielding belief that she was infected, Jill and the additional seventeen victims would have missed their statute of limitations, had no financial recourse and probably not have known about their disease until it was very advanced.

CHAPTER 22

The Cheryl Gentry Story

Hepatitis C can lead to liver failure. Liver failure is a slow and horrible way to die. As the virus flows through the blood stream it causes scar tissue to form in the liver. Physicians call the scar tissue "fibrosis" or "cirrhosis." Over time, the scar tissue prevents the liver from working properly.

With cirrhosis, the liver is unable to filter harmful toxins from the blood. A person suffering from liver failure will get a yellow hue to their skin called "jaundice." Liver failure affects almost everything in the body including digestion, hormones, the circulatory system and many organs. It causes osteoporosis in the bones and often leads to liver cancer. Those with liver failure become fatigued and weak, and suffer nausea and loss of appetite. Often, they become very susceptible to infections of all types, and have internal bleeding and fluid buildup. Over time, they will have cognitive and memory loss and confusion. As the toxins in the blood continue to build, the person will eventually fall into a coma and finally die. Liver failure is a medical condition that leaves the patient with two options: 1) liver transplantation or 2) death.

A hepatitis C patient with a failing liver often finds it more difficult to be accepted onto a liver transplant list than non-hepatitis C counterparts. Even with a new liver, the hepatitis C sufferer still carries the virus. Once transplanted, the process of liver cirrhosis will start over. Because the liver will scar and become damaged again in patients with hepatitis C, these patients have a difficult time qualifying for a liver transplant. In addition, many hepatitis C patients who do make it onto the transplant list die from their liver failure before a liver becomes available.

The family of Terry and Cheryl Gentry lived in Dodge County. Terry Gentry was a good man. He was quiet, humble and soft-spoken, but when he did speak, everyone in the room believed what he said. In many ways, he was a typical of hard-working, blue-collar, Midwestern men. His first priority in life was his family. He and Cheryl had been happily married for many years. Over time, their daughter had grown into a beautiful young woman on her way to college. The Gentrys' household was modest, stable and full of love.

Tragedy struck in the spring of 2000, when Cheryl was diagnosed with cancer. Since there was a new cancer doctor in town, she went to him for treatment. His clinic was touted by the hospital to be every bit as good as the Omaha and Lincoln cancer facilities, and it was much more convenient. So, Cheryl became a patient of Dr. Javed.

By Christmas of 2000, Cheryl was very close to death from her cancer. She was not ready to give up on life, however, and with Terry's and Tina's support, she fought back.

Following treatment, Cheryl's cancer went into remission. It was as though her life had been given back to her. A tremendous weight had been lifted from the Gentry household.

Time passed and all seemed well. The Gentry family did not know that she had contracted hepatitis C while receiving her cancer treatments. She and the other victims were not notified of their risk of hepatitis C in June 2001, when Javed and others recognized the risk of exposure. She had no idea that the virus was running unchecked in her body and destroying her liver. Ironically, the same cancer treatment that had put her cancer in remission had left her immune system too weak to fight the hepatitis C virus. Instead, like the other unsuspecting Nebraska outbreak victims, the virus was running wild through her body.

Within a year of her successful cancer treatment, Cheryl began feeling tired all the time. She immediately feared the cancer had returned. After some medical tests were run, she found out that it was not the cancer this time. She consulted Dr. Tom McKnight in the summer of 2002, and medical tests showed that she was suffering from the early stages of liver failure caused by hepatitis C. She was put on the liver transplant list, but it was too late. A suitable liver could not be found. With her family mourning, she passed away on March 7, 2003. It was just two years after she had contracted the virus at Javed's clinic. Her autopsy listed the cause of death as "cirrhosis with complications, secondary to hepatitis C virus infection."

If Cheryl had known about her disease at any time during the two-year period before the Nebraska outbreak became public, she could have received treatment before the virus led to her death. Cheryl was only forty-nine years old at the time she expired.

At the time, Cheryl was thought to be the first outbreak victim to die from the virus. It was later discovered that she was likely the second or third.

At her funeral mass, the priest spoke before the gathered mourners and family members. His prayers were heartfelt, and his statements were strong:

> "…Death is a thief. And, when we sense an added injustice we want to right the balance… The peace she [Cheryl] understands is what she wants for us—for you, Terry, Tina and Dennis; her sisters and the whole family and all her friends; and for all of those who carry within themselves the same infection that she carried. She would want peace for you as well… True forgiveness lies in our own heart and affects the one forgiving as much as the ones forgiven. Forgiveness, however, is different than justice. Justice seeks to right a wrong, and this is anyone's right! But forgiveness is when we choose to not let the injustice turn us bitter and angry… What will we do? How will we change? How will Cheryl's life and death affect us?"

CHAPTER 23

Healthcare Licensure Complaints, As Explained by Travis

"Do I feel bad about it [the Nebraska outbreak]? Do I feel horrific? Absolutely… It's impacted the entire hospital. But does anybody feel responsibility for what happened…? No."

—Michael Leibert, president, FAMC,
May 25, 2004

Tahir Javed, MD, and Linda Prochaska, RN

One afternoon in the early summer of 2003, I (Travis) was sitting in my law office, preparing for hearings when my friend and client, Jill Watson, came to see me. She was very upset.

Earlier that day, she had been to see her new oncologist for a follow-up visit. Although her cancer treatment was at an end and she had been declared cancer-free, she was having pain around the site of her malignancy. It was information that she had passed on to me, but that she had hidden even from her husband. She was terrified of the worst, and did not want anyone else to have to bear the fear of a reoccurrence until she knew for sure. I tried to be optimistic when she first mentioned the pain to me. I told her to pick a new oncologist and see him immediately.

"Although," I lied for her peace of mind, "I am sure it is nothing."

Jill chose to see an oncologist in Omaha. She was still so traumatized by her contraction of hepatitis C that the thought of receiving cancer services in Fremont was unbearable to her. Every day, she had to live with the fact that the hepatitis C might kill her. Her plight was now complicated by the fact that she was also fearful of a cancer reoccurrence. Adding to this, she was involved in one of the most cumbersome lawsuits in state history. Naturally, she was under a tremendous amount of stress, so it didn't surprise me when she came to my office the next day in tears.

"What's wrong?" I asked.

She was so upset that she was nearly hyperventilating.

"I went to go see my new oncologist. I picked him out of the Omaha phone book to be my new oncologist. I thought that his nurse looked familiar! I thought so!"

She was ranting, and I sat her down in my office chair to try and calm her.

"What are you talking about? Who looked familiar?"

"The medical technician who took my blood pressure. She looked a lot like Heather Schumacher, from Javed's clinic. She was Heather's sister!"

I pulled a chair next to hers and sat down for a moment as the news sunk in. It was not particularly relevant to her lawsuit, but it was interesting nonetheless. It was an unbelievable coincidence, and it was too bad that even by going all the way to Omaha, she couldn't seem to get away from thoughts of Javed's clinic.

"They took tests to see if the cancer is back. When I was sitting in the patient room waiting for my new cancer doctor to come in and tell me the test results, *she* walked in!"

"Schumacher's sister?" I asked.

"No! Heather Schumacher! She walked right in and sat down across from me!"

I was speechless.

"She is working as a nurse at his office!"

It was a terrible coincidence, and it couldn't have happened at a more stressful time in Jill's life.

"Heather walked up to me and said she wanted me to know she was sorry about what happened at Javed's office. I was just sitting there and—"

As the words fell from her tongue, I had to cut her off.

"Whoa! Whoa! Whoa!" I shook my head slightly, still trying to process all the information. "She did what? She said she was sorry?"

It was a bombshell.

"Yes," she answered. "Heather said she was sorry that the Nebraska outbreak had occurred. She said that she knew better and tried to stop it. But that she had been given too much responsibility for her education so it was not her fault. She said that she tried to make changes but that she couldn't change everything."

There was an exception to the Nebraska rules of evidence that allowed a jury to hear defendants' confessions. It was all I could think about. Unlike several other states, Nebraska had not enacted "I'm sorry" legislation as yet, which could have given Heather immunity to apologize. As a result, Heather's statements were enormously significant to prosecuting the hepatitis C cases. Suddenly, after all this time, we had a confession. It was an earth-shaking revelation.

"Why?" Jill finally broke my train of thought.

In thinking about Schumacher, I had tuned her out completely.

"What?" I asked.

"Why do Schumacher, Prochaska and Javed still have licenses to practice medicine? It has been nine months since the outbreak became known."

I had been so caught up in fighting the hepatitis C lawsuits that I had never even thought about medical licenses. What was even more concerning to Jill was that Linda Prochaska was currently employed as a nurse at an Omaha Hospital. By this time, we had already taken Nurse Prochaska's deposition, and I was far from impressed with her. It was obvious to me that she had played a large part in the outbreak at Javed's clinic. The "I was just following orders" defense fell short of what I expect from healthcare providers. In Jill's opinion, she was a danger to society who shouldn't have been working with patients. I strongly agreed.

In practicing law as a medical malpractice attorney, I have found that there are certain things that I simply have to live with. One of those things is that sometimes I am virtually powerless to accomplish some of the things that victims of malpractice want. Almost uniformly, people who are injured by the negligence of a medical provider want an apology. Many times, if the medical provider had simply apologized, the injured person would never have filed suit. At some time during every plaintiff's case, they ask me to force the defendant to apologize. I had never seen this happen. The law does not force apologies from defendants no matter how serious the negligence, and it is almost unheard of for a healthcare provider to apologize as Heather had.

One of the second most powerless moments in a malpractice attorney's life is when a client asks that a doctor's license to practice medicine be revoked. Even in cases as extreme as the one against Dr. Javed, I had never seen it happen through a lawsuit. The only option Jill had was to file a licensure complaint with the Nebraska Health and Human Services' Division of Investigations.

She left my office and went home. Within an hour, I got a phone call from her. She had already written her letter to the state, requesting the license revocations of Javed, Prochaska and Schumacher. The following day, it was mailed.

We didn't know it at the time, but a number of other victims had already written to the state in October 2002, asking that the state take away the medical licenses of Javed, Prochaska and Schumacher. After months of letters and phone calls, the Division of Investigations finally gave a report to the Board of Physicians and Surgeons regarding the license of Tahir Javed. The board recommended that Javed lose his medical license, and this recommendation was forwarded to state attorney general, John Bruning.

Usually, the attorney general would quickly prosecute such a recommendation. This was not the case with Javed, however. Months passed without action. Finally, several victims initiated a letter-writing campaign to the attorney general, requesting action on Javed's license. Hundreds of letters were sent to the attorney general and members of the Nebraska legislature. Despite public pressure, the wheels of bureaucracy continued to move very slowly.

I soon learned, however, that when Jill Watson was involved, things happened. I couldn't imagine how she would get it done, but I should have known from that very moment that it was only a matter of time before licenses were revoked.

A few days after Jill sent off her letter to the state, I heard from her again.

"What are you doing this afternoon at two o'clock?" she asked.

"Why?"

"A TV news station from Omaha found out about my letter to the state and they want to run a piece on it. Come get me at my house and we will meet them at the park at two o'clock."

I have never been one of those attorneys that enjoys being on the nightly news, but when Jill asked, I couldn't deny her request.

That evening, the Omaha TV station ran a story telling the eastern half of the state that Dr. Javed and his nurses still had their licenses to practice medicine. They tried to contact Nurse Prochaska to comment, but she refused their call. The television broadcast must have gotten the attorney general's attention.

On July 22, 2003, the state of Nebraska filed a petition to revoke Dr. Javed's license to practice medicine. To a person, my clients were overjoyed. As discussed in Chapter 33, the Nebraska Hospital Liability Act often pitted the state against injured plaintiffs. Because the plaintiffs felt betrayed by the state, it was refreshing to the victims when the state finally took steps to take away Javed's license. Even though Javed was in Pakistan, likely never to return, it was nice that the state made the gesture. It seemed as though the state was going to do something solely for the benefit of the victims. It was going to make the results of its investigation public and tell the whole world that Javed was no longer welcome as a Nebraska physician. I didn't know it at the time, but our faith in the state's intentions was misguided.

When I, as an attorney working in the civil courts, want to get information in a lawsuit, my options are fairly limited. My power to question witnesses and collect documents is only as broad as the court allows. I can have subpoenas issued that command hospitals or doctors to turn over records, and I can take depositions of witnesses to ask them what they know. The only real threat that I can make to someone who refuses to respond is along these lines: "Well... If you don't give me the records, then I'll go tattletale to the judge and he might get mad at you." It is usually not very intimidating.

The state of Nebraska, however, plays a different game, with different rules altogether. When the state conducts an investigation—like the one Nebraska Health and Human Services Division of Investigations conducted to revoke Javed's license—state officials can be much more intimidating. Government officials can flash their badges and get things done that all the civil trial lawyers in the world cannot.

The state conducted an in-depth investigation before they filed their charges. By law, their case file was protected from my subpoena. As they used their vast powers to collect information about the Nebraska outbreak, my co-counsels and I were anxious to find out what they had learned. At that point, we still did not know many facts about the Nebraska outbreak. We didn't know how we were going to prove our cases at trial. The state, on the other hand, had all the facts because of their licensure investigations.

We sat for hours, debating how we could get our hands on the evidence they had, but legally, there was no way. The Nebraska statutes protected every bit of evidence in their files. The public could not get access to it because it was part of an "ongoing investigation." The good news was, however, that the upcoming revocation hearing was open to the public. This meant that we could go to the hearing and watch as the state investigators testified about the details of the Nebraska outbreak. We could get copies of the documents they offered into evidence. After the hearing, it would all be public record, no longer protected by statute. Finally, after an endless wait, the license revocation trial was set. All we had to do was wait until the day of the hearing to learn all the details that we were struggling to find out on our own.

What happened next further convinced me that Nebraska law, as it was currently written, was unfair to victims of malpractice. In the days before the hearing to revoke Javed's license, the state entered into a settlement agreement with Javed wherein he voluntarily relinquished his license to practice medicine. As a result, the hearing never took place, and the state never had to share its information on the outbreak with the outbreak victims or their attorneys. I was not privy to the settlement negotiations between Javed and the state, and I do not know what Javed got, if anything, in return for volunteering his license. I know that Javed had previously bragged to a Pakistani newspaper that Nebraska would not revoke his license, and I also know that the state of Nebraska never called for the extradition of Dr. Javed. The FBI called me to tell me they were calling off the criminal investigation against Javed within a month of Javed's agreement to give up his license. No criminal charges were ever filed against Dr. Javed by the state of Nebraska either.

On September 29, 2003, Dr. Javed reached a settlement agreement with the state of Nebraska wherein his license to practice medicine was voluntarily surrendered. In that document, he admitted to the following:

1. Gross negligence regarding patient care
2. Unprofessional conduct
3. A pattern of negligent conduct
4. A violation of confidentiality between a patient and a physician

Nurse Prochaska continued to work nine more months as a nurse at an Omaha Hospital after Dr. Javed lost his license. On March 22, 2004, nearly seventeen months after the outbreak became public knowledge, she voluntarily surrendered her license for an indefinite period of time. Once again, the state's investigation was sealed. When Prochaska voluntarily surrendered her nursing license, she temporarily gave up her career. The state did not file criminal charges against Nurse Prochaska for her involvement in the Nebraska outbreak.

It is possible that Nurse Prochaska—the head nurse who caused the largest outbreak of hepatitis C in American history—will once again be providing medical care to Nebraskans. Since the license was surrendered for an "indefinite period of time," she has the option to petition the state for reinstatement two years after revocation. If and when she reapplies, there will be no public hearing and no notice to her victims or the public.

All totaled, the state of Nebraska spent more than 550 hours investigating the outbreak and documented over 1,000 pages of interviews with doctors, nurses, administrators and other healthcare providers. The entire investigation was paid for by the Nebraska taxpayers, although they were never entitled to see the results of that investigation.

Heather Schumacher, RN

In 2006, another formal complaint was filed against Heather Schumacher's license. The complaint included parts of her deposition wherein she testified under oath about her own improper port flush procedure and her observation of Linda Prochaska's improper port flush procedure. She admitted seeing it happen, and even doing it herself. As a licensed healthcare provider, Heather was mandated by Nebraska law to report her first-hand observations of Linda's pattern of negligent conduct under Nebraska Health and Human Services System Title 172 NAC 5.

The Nebraska Board of Nursing made a recommendation regarding Heather's license. The language of the recommendation was never disclosed to the public. The recommendation was passed on to the attorney general's office. The attorney general's office declined to take any type of licensure action. The attorney general has not responded to inquiries as to why no action was taken against Heather's license. To her credit, Heather cooperated with the investigators during their investigation. She was the only person involved in the Nebraska outbreak who has ever apologized for her part in the outbreak.

Leslie Mayberry, RN, and Marissa Winke, RN

Complaints were also filed against the licenses of Leslie Mayberry and Marissa Winke, the two nurses who conducted the audit of the Fremont Cancer Center on behalf of the Missouri Valley Cancer Consortium. The MVCC audit resulted in a five-page report in which they outlined improper nursing procedures. The complaint was based on their failure to report what they had observed to authorities, as mandated by Nebraska law, Nebraska Health and Human Services System Title 172 NAC 5.

Nebraska Health and Human Services (NHHS) Division of Investigations interviewed the two nurses as well as other healthcare providers. They turned over their investigative report regarding Marissa to the Board of Nursing. The board made a recommendation to the attorney general's office, although the terms of the recommendation were not disclosed to the public. The recommendation was forwarded to the attorney general's office. The attorney general's office dismissed the complaint without any action against her license. The attorney general has not responded to inquiries as to why no action was taken against Marissa's license.

The NHHS Division of Investigations determined that Leslie Mayberry "had no first-hand information" about the substandard nursing practices at Javed's clinic. NHHS declined to open a full investigation into the matter and no action was taken against her license.

Rodney Koerber, MD, Gerri Means, RN, and Fremont Area Medical Center

The state's investigation into the Nebraska outbreak did not trigger an investigation into the actions of Dr. Rodney Koerber, MD, or Gerri Means, RN.

In November 2006, a licensure complaint was initiated against Rodney Koerber and Gerri Means. The basis of the complaint was that Koerber and Means did not report the hepatitis C cases from Javed's clinic as a related cluster, as required by NHHS Chapter 1 Title 173. NHHS Division of Investigations investigated the complaints and forwarded its report to the Board of Physicians and Surgeons for Koerber and the Board of Nursing for Means. The respective boards made their recommendations to the attorney general's office. The recommendations were passed on to the attorney general, who declined to take action.

JoAnn Erickson, who investigates hospital complaints on behalf of the Nebraska Health and Human Services Division of Investigations told us that the hospital was not investigated for its role in the Nebraska outbreak. Mike Leibert informed us through his legal counsel that the Fremont Area Medical Center was investigated by NHHS. Mr. Leibert stated that there was not enough evidence or information to indicate that the hospital violated a law or regulation that would result in a sanction. Therefore, a full investigation was not opened.

The records from the respective investigations are sealed, and will never become available for public inspection. Out of the seven licensure complaints filed in connection with the Nebraska outbreak, only two were actually disciplined.

Non-mandated Reporting

As discussed before, licensed healthcare professionals in Nebraska are mandated by law to report first-hand observances of substandard medical practices. However, *any* citizen may (although they are not required to) make a complaint against a licensed healthcare provider. First-hand knowledge is not required. In other words, doctors, nurses, hospital administrators, housekeeping employees, patients and family members could have filed licensure complaints reporting their concerns at any time, even if they did not have first-hand knowledge. If this had happened, the extent of the Nebraska outbreak may have been minimized or perhaps even prevented.

The complaint procedure against licensed healthcare providers is found on the Nebraska Health and Human Services Website at www.hhs.state.ne.us.

CHAPTER 24

■

Javed's Life in Pakistan

"Here is a Pakistani doctor's novel way of Jihad: To kill the kuffar (infidels), he uses no guns or bombs. His weapons are plain, planned negligence and his targets, hapless American sick people, among whom he spread hepatitis C virus. An UNPRECEDENTED case of gross, criminal negligence that can put the whole medical profession to shame has been committed."

—*The Patriotic Chronicle*

Dr. Javed proved that he was a master of deceit. Despite all that, he still had supporters in Fremont who remained loyal to him. He was so charming and likeable that even after he left, some people refused to believe that he betrayed them. The sad reality was, however, that when he fled Fremont in July of 2002, his twisted story continued.

The Continued Deception

When Javed took his diplomas from his office wall and left the Fremont Cancer Center, no one suspected a thing. He simply closed the door to his office, and the clinic continued to see patients. Many of them were still in the middle of ongoing chemotherapy. In the days before he left he took great steps to make sure the Fremont Cancer Center would continue to run even though he was gone. At first glance, his actions seemed to be caring and compassionate for his patients. As usual, however, Dr. Javed's actions were deceiving.

Several months before he left, Javed called an acquaintance from medical school, Dr. M. Salman Haroon, to offer him an associate position in his office. Dr. Haroon practiced oncology in a town just across the Iowa border, an hour away from Fremont. Haroon agreed to leave his own practice and come to Fremont to join the Fremont Cancer Center at the end of the summer.

On Friday, July 12, 2002, Javed called Haroon again, this time in tears. It was only one day after Dr. Tom McKnight had demanded an explanation from Javed about four new hepatitis C cases. Javed explained to Haroon that his mother had suddenly fallen ill and was concerned that she may not survive. He said that he had to leave immediately to return to Pakistan and asked that Haroon join the Fremont Cancer Center as soon as possible.

While Dr. Haroon and he were only acquaintances, Haroon felt sympathy for Javed. Haroon was also an immigrant from Pakistan who had left his family behind to practice medicine in the United States. Javed's tears struck a chord with him. Haroon's mother had passed away in Pakistan some time earlier. Because of the distance, he had not been able to return there before her burial. Haroon immediately agreed to take on the enormous task of running the clinic until Javed could return. In exchange for Haroon's immediate assistance, Javed promised that upon his return he would make Haroon a partner in the practice. Haroon's patients in Iowa would be cared for by his former partners there, so he agreed to come to the Fremont Cancer Center earlier than originally planned.

The day Javed left, he mailed a letter to all his patients, informing them that Dr. Haroon would run his clinic until he came back. His letter was an assurance that even though he would temporarily be absent, his patients would be well cared for. Seemingly, these last-minute arrangements benefited no one other than his patients. The truth of the matter would soon be learned.

Dr. Haroon began working as the oncologist at the Fremont Cancer Center in early August 2002. Dr. Haroon cared for Javed's patients as though they were his own. As the weeks progressed, Haroon began to wonder when Javed would return. With an issue as sensitive as a mother's illness, Haroon did not want to be a burden. He didn't want to call Javed in Javed's time of crisis to bother him with issues of work. When the sixth week passed, Haroon finally felt he needed to contact Javed to find out when he would be returning. Haroon also was becoming concerned about his compensation. Haroon was able to reach Javed by phone, but Javed was evasive.

Before he had left, Javed had told Dr. Haroon that he would be paid a percentage of the profits from the Fremont Cancer Center until Javed returned. What Haroon did not know was that before fleeing to Pakistan, Dr. Javed had set up a system wherein all the profits were routed directly to himself in Pakistan. During the entire time Haroon cared for the Fremont Cancer Center patients, Javed reaped the profits. Even after Javed left the country to flee the disaster he had left behind, he had found a way benefit.

Though innocent, Dr. Haroon will forever be linked to the site of the largest hepatitis C outbreak in United States history. He is embarrassed to be introduced as the Fremont Cancer Center oncologist at seminars and social gatherings, even though he was a savior to the maltreated patients Javed abandoned. To date, Dr.

Haroon has received no compensation for his two months of work at the Fremont Cancer Center.

Javed in Pakistan

The story of Dr. Tahir Ali Javed and the hepatitis C outbreak is so strange, it appears surreal. Upon his returned to Pakistan, his story became even more unbelievable. No one could have imagined the rigged elections, drive-by shootings, gunfights, political nepotism and anti-American propaganda to come. To understand the depth of what took place next, it is important to understand the political system in Pakistan in the summer of 2002.

In many respects, Pakistan (officially known as the Islamic Republic of Pakistan) has not seen much change in the past thousand years. Much of the nation is still rural and divided along tribal lines. Less than one-half of the population is literate, and over ten different national languages and dialects are spoken within its borders.

In 1999, the country fell under the military rule of self-appointed president Pervez Musharraf. Musharraf took control of the country in a military coup. The country, which is approximately twice the size of California, is divided into four geographical regions know as provinces—Punjab, Sindh, Balochistan and the North-West Frontier. Musharraf ruled the republic through his federal government. The four provinces of the country were each governed by chief ministers. The regional governments were elected in separate elections. The federation controlled national affairs such as military, currency and international policies. The provincial governments each controlled their own local affairs.

Sometime shortly before or after Dr. Javed fled Fremont, he placed his name on the ballot to become a member of the provincial assembly of Punjab. He was elected to the assembly after his return to his homeland, essentially as a state legislator. Less than one month later, on January 2, 2003, chief minister Chaudhry Pervaiz Elahi gave him an even higher political position when he appointed Javed as the minister of health for the Punjab region of the Islamic Republic of Pakistan. Less than six months after causing the largest outbreak of hepatitis C in United States history, Dr. Javed was one of the highest-ranking officials in the Punjab Pakistani government.

Javed's Challenge to Nebraska

By September of 2003, Javed had been the highest-ranking medical official in Punjab province for nine months. On September 3, 2003, Pakistan's *Daily Times* questioned Dr. Javed about the Nebraska outbreak. He told the newspaper that "there is currently an anti-Muslim campaign in America that is also targeting educated Muslims."

He told the paper that it was ridiculous to blame him for the Nebraska outbreak since hepatitis C takes more than three years to develop, and challenged Nebraska to try to revoke his medical licenses in New York and Nebraska. He also denied the allegations that he had sexually abused one of his former patients (Individual #7).

Twenty-seven days after his comments in Pakistan's *Daily Times*, the FBI caught up with him and questioned him about the Nebraska outbreak. In this interview, he was apparently not so flippant. Again he denied his part in the Nebraska outbreak. This time, he did not blame a United States anti-Muslim conspiracy. He defended himself by arguing that complaints had not been filed against him until after he had left the United States.

Dr. Javed's licenses to practice medicine in Nebraska and New York were subsequently revoked despite his boastful challenge. Following the revocations, he was questioned once again by Pakistan's *Daily Times*. In that interview, he denied knowing anything of his license revocations, and claimed that his lawyers in the United States must have entered into the license revocations without his consent. The *Daily Times* subsequently ran another article pointing out that even though Javed claimed not to know anything of his license revocations, he had signed the revocation documents himself as part of a settlement with the state of Nebraska. Another Pakistani newspaper questioned Dr. Javed's integrity. On November 14, 2003 *The Patriotic Chronicle* stated: "Here is a Pakistani Doctor's novel way of Jihad: To kill the Kuffar (infidels), he uses no guns or bombs. His weapons are plain, planned negligence and his targets, hapless American sick people, among whom he spread Hepatitis C virus. An UNPRECEDENTED case of gross, criminal negligence that can put the whole medical profession to shame has been committed."

Javed's New Power

Upon taking his new position as health minister, Javed immediately began to wield his power in a very public way. The Punjab Health Department traditionally conducted inspections of drug stores to assure they were not selling expired or stolen drugs. Usually, low-level inspectors conducted the inspections. It was unheard of for the minister of health to conduct them himself.

Once Javed took power, however, he began conducting armed raids of these drug stores. The raids were conducted after the local media had been alerted so that the new health minister would look good in the news accounts.

The storeowners claimed that these armed raids were in violation of Pakistani law. In one of these raids, the Lahore High Court agreed, and ordered the reopening of several drug stores that Javed had ordered sealed at gunpoint.

A Bloody Reelection Campaign

In the summer of 2005, Javed was up for reelection in Punjab. He eventually won the election. To win the election, he allegedly had his followers torture supporters of a political opponent in an effort to keep them away from voting stations, according to local news reports. Javed also allegedly had several of his supporters break into a voting station at gunpoint and open six ballot boxes. His opponent's votes were removed and replaced with votes for Javed, according to those same reports. The election officials at the polling stations filed reports at the local police station, confirming the incident.

The election turned bloody when the discord escalated to gunfire. In August 2005, members of Javed's entourage were gunned down on the way to a polling station. Six armed men sprayed Javed's entourage with gunfire. A young man who was apparently an innocent bystander was killed in the shooting. Later, Javed's house was sprayed with gunfire as well, although no one was injured in that exchange.

Charges were filed against Javed by one of his political opponents. The charges were eventually dropped without ever being reviewed on the merits of the case. They were dropped because the signatures on the charging documents were not property notarized.

Nepotism at Work

Following the reelection shootings of 2005, Javed reportedly wanted to have his father appointed as the nazim of Narowal. Essentially, it was the head official of a district within Punjab. A political opponent, at the same time, decided that his own father should be appointed to the same position. Both men wrangled back and forth, allegedly exploiting their political influence, but eventually, Javed's father won. Government officials allegedly abducted Javed's father following the appointment. His final fate was never reported.

Pakistani Physicians Demand Javed's Resignation

Eventually, a group of Pakistani physicians from Punjab called for Javed's resignation as minister of health. According to news reports, they complained that he was simply not doing his job. They claimed he was not "streamlining" Punjab hospitals as promised, and that he had only given "lip service and press statements" to the issue. They also complained that he had been placing inefficient and corrupt people into administrative posts and hospital management boards. Javed declined the demand to resign.

Getting Rid of the Quacks

Sometime after Dr. Javed became the health minister for Punjab, he participated in a public seminar to address health issues related to his region. Ironically, one of the topics was hepatitis. Untrained, unlicensed healthcare workers were giving immunizations to citizens in rural villages and reusing syringes and needles.

One speaker at the seminar said, "It is their [the victims'] ignorance that they become the victims at the hands of quacks who utilize and reuse syringes. We can control hepatitis and other infectious diseases by getting rid of the quacks…"

Dr. Javed then added to the speaker's thoughts by proclaiming that all the "quacks" had been eliminated from *his* province.

CHAPTER 25

The Plaintiffs' Committee, As Explained by Travis

I once had a disgruntled client who was tired of having her case linger on endlessly in the court system. In a moment of understandable frustration, she told me that the fastest way to bring something to a standstill was to get two lawyers involved. Although I have always tried to prosecute my cases as quickly as humanly possible, I understood her frustration with the legal system, and I initially agreed with her. Today, I know that she was wrong. There is a far more effective way to bring progress to a dead crawl: appoint a committee of lawyers.

Shortly after the Nebraska outbreak became public, eighty-nine victims found and hired attorneys to file their lawsuits. At this point, the victims became "plaintiffs" and Dr. Javed, Nurse Prochaska, Nurse Schumacher and Fremont Area Medical Center became "defendants." Initially, some newspapers reported that the Nebraska outbreak had caused as many as 120 lawsuits to be filed, but those reports were incorrect. The fact was that in their mad rush to the court-house, some lawyers had filed their plaintiffs' cases twice.

Some District Courts in metropolitan areas handle dozens of civil trials each day. The Dodge County District Court was far from being a metropolitan area court, however. In Dodge County, there was only one District Court judge. Along with the regular caseload of divorces, felonies and other civil matters, he could have probably handled only three or four medical malpractice trials in an entire year. With the Nebraska outbreak there were suddenly eighty-nine plain-tiffs claiming damages, and the Court was swamped with more cases than it could have tried in twenty years.

To add to the confusion, at the time these cases were filed, the District Court was in the midst of major changes. The previous judge, F.A. Gossett III, was on his way off the bench, as he had been appointed to the Federal Court in Omaha. He was a good, no-nonsense judge who had been on the bench for a decade, and he wasn't intimidated by anyone. He had a wonderful way of cutting to the root of a matter and would have done a solid job of tackling the bulging civil docket. Unfortunately for Dodge County, those same qualities had made him a good candidate for the federal bench, and he was moving up.

The incoming judge, John Samson, was a younger man who had been the part-time county attorney in a neighboring county. He had just been appointed by the governor to replace Gossett but he had not yet reached the bench.

With the filing of the hepatitis C cases, our little town was suddenly swamped with out-of-town lawyers. Some of them were the finest plaintiff and defense attorneys in the state. There was huge trepidation by the lawyers. There were many tenured judges in the state who would not be able to handle the onslaught that was about to hit the unproven judge on the Dodge County District Court bench. While most people picture judges as they are portrayed on television, attorneys understand that judges are just people. Most experienced trial attorneys have seen young, inexperienced judges pushed around by much older, seasoned trial lawyers who practice before them. These older, locally famous, aggressive attorneys often start sentences with, "In all my thirty-five years of trying cases, I have never…" Irrespective of what they are proposing or whether or not they are correct, the judge will often defer to their experience.

Plaintiff lawyers from all over the area called me to find out what I knew about John Samson. Would the new judge be able to handle cases of this magnitude? Could the "big city" lawyers bully him? Was he pro-plaintiff? Pro-defense? No one knew if he could handle the largest series of lawsuits in Nebraska history the first day on the job. I had handled a case or two against him when he was still a practicing attorney. It was impossible for me to guess how he would handle the daunting job. I had always known him to be even-tempered and honest. Unfortunately, that was more than I could say for some of the lawyers swarming into our little city.

After Gossett left the bench, a retired District Court judge, Judge Buckley, came out of retirement to handle the courtroom until Samson arrived. Judge Buckley had spent a career on the bench and saw the unbelievably cumbersome workload Samson would face the first day he arrived. Buckley did not want to make rulings in the hepatitis C cases, since he would not be there to see the cases to completion. He was scheduled to be off the bench and back into retirement within weeks.

The first pressing task for the plaintiff attorneys was to take depositions. At a deposition, the parties and their lawyers gather with a court reporter to take the sworn statement of a witness. The lawyers take turns asking questions, which the deponent answers under oath. Depositions can sometimes last for days but in most cases, only a few hours. They are usually recorded only in writing but sometimes videotaped as well.

From the outset, the number of cases was causing the plaintiffs' lawyers fits. Eighty-nine plaintiff cases all shared many of the same witnesses. Depositions had to be taken of the Fremont Cancer Center employees as well as hospital doctors, nurses and other staff. There were so many people who had valuable information to our cases that it was essential that we immediately begin taking their statements. If an important witness passed away before he or she was deposed, valuable information would be lost forever—information that could prove our cases. It was imperative that we begin depositions.

The obvious problem was the logistics of deposing witnesses for the eighty-nine cases. Did each nurse have to take a day off work eighty-nine times to give her deposition in eighty-nine different plaintiffs' cases? Furthermore, if she were to give her deposition only once, was it fair for all plaintiffs to benefit from it, while only one plaintiff paid the costs of the deposition? Each deposition would cost between $1,000 and $2,000 just for the transcriptionist. Some witnesses were able to charge for their time. Some of those fees would be as much as $5,000 to $10,000. If all plaintiffs would get to use the depositions in their cases, but only the plaintiff taking the deposition paid for it, a disincentive would have been created wherein every plaintiff's attorney would hold back for someone else to pay the costs. It was the first of many logistical problems Nebraska had never seen before.

Judge Buckley saw the problem, and although he did not want to get involved in Samson's cases, he solved it with the stroke of a pen and announced it as a "Christmas gift to the incoming Judge Samson." He could not legally order the cases to become a class action lawsuit under Nebraska law. Instead, he issued an order consolidating all the cases for discovery purposes only. Under this order, he protected all the witnesses from multiple depositions, and he eliminated plaintiffs' attorneys' fears of paying more than their share in costs. At the time, I thought it was a wonderful stroke of genius. The only downside was that a steering committee to oversee the consolidated "plaintiffs committee" needed to be created to coordinate depositions, discovery costs and the workload. It seemed to be a solution to all the complicated logistics. Time would prove otherwise.

In the Beginning

From the outset, the abominable plaintiffs' committee was a bungled mess. The first meeting was to be held at a conference room in a local hotel. All the plaintiffs' attorneys were supposed to attend. I hoped that we could all get together and discuss a coordinated effort and fairly divided workload to prepare our cases for trial.

While Judge Buckley had ordered the sharing of depositions, I held out hope that we could openly share *all* evidence and information about the cases. I turned out to be naïve. In reality, several attorneys felt they had a disincentive to cooperate with the rest of us. The Merritt decision had not been released (see Chapter 26). Hence, some plaintiffs' attorneys didn't share information in the hope that their cases would be stronger than the rest, and that they could win a larger share of the limited defense funds. After the Merritt decision was rendered, this reluctance was alleviated and information was shared more liberally. However, a year went by without shared information.

A notice about the meeting was sent out to all lawyers, and immediately, my office began receiving faxes back. Attorneys asked me to reschedule the meeting because they had a conflict with the appointed time. So, my partner and I rescheduled it and sent out a new notice. The result was the same. Once again, we got letters, faxes and phone calls from other attorneys, asking to reschedule. Of the thirty-some plaintiffs' attorneys who needed to attend, there would inevitably be four or five who could not attend on any given day. In desperation, I started calling each of the plaintiffs' attorneys, asking if we could schedule the meeting on a Saturday to avoid business conflicts. I made only two calls before I was told that would not work either.

"Saturday is the day for Nebraska football," I was told.

In the end, the meeting was scheduled so far in advance that it ended up delaying depositions for months. The ultimate disappointment was that when the meeting did take place, only a dozen or so attorneys appeared. I began to wonder if some of the plaintiffs' attorneys simply did not care about their plaintiffs' cases. My suspicions were verified when one of the twelve or so attorneys who did appear commented that they did not intend to actively prosecute their plaintiffs' case. They would pay their clients' shares of the costs, but were simply going to "lay back and ride the coattails" of those of us who were intent on doing right by our clients.

"You guys have twenty cases," I was told. "I only have a couple. You can do all the work because you have a much greater stake in the proceedings. Besides, these cases aren't worth much anyway."

It was a sad commentary.

Since it was impossible to get thirty lawyers together at one time, a smaller steering committee was created. Its responsibilities were to schedule depositions and speak for the plaintiffs as a whole in any minor procedural matters. The five law firms that had the most plaintiffs' cases each had a seat on the committee. An additional sixth seat was added for a plaintiffs' attorney who did not have very many cases, but whose age and experience was well-respected. My law partner and I represented nineteen of the eighty-nine Nebraska outbreak victims—the second-largest number of victims represented by any firm—and so my partner, as my elder, received the second seat on the committee.

Categories and Mock Juries

I would venture to say that at least ninety percent of all the work in the first two years was done by less than ten percent of the plaintiffs' lawyers. While a handful of us were spending every weekend plowing through reams of medical records, preparing for depositions and trying to figure out what had happened, the rest of my colleagues were nowhere to be seen. Along the way, the plaintiffs' committee held regular meetings, but few plaintiffs' attorneys ever attended. Dozens of depositions were taken, but most plaintiffs' lawyers only showed up sporadically at best. Some never showed up at all.

Once every couple of months, I would receive a phone call: "…my client asked me yesterday what was going on in his case… So, what's going on?" The few of us who were working were not just working for our clients, but were working for all the plaintiffs. However, we were not paid for our efforts by the uninvolved plaintiffs' attorneys.

One afternoon in the fall of 2004, I received a correspondence. The defense lawyers wanted to meet as a group with all the plaintiffs' lawyers and discuss a "global" settlement. The idea was that we would all meet and negotiate a single dollar figure that the defense would pay in one lump sum to the larger plaintiffs' committee. The cases would all be dismissed, and the plaintiffs' attorneys would have to distribute the money among the plaintiffs.

The only catch was that none of the plaintiffs could opt out of the settlement. If any plaintiff disagreed, the entire settlement would be cancelled. It was a genuinely stupid idea. The first time I heard it, I knew it would be an enormous waste of time. There was no way in the world the eighty-nine plaintiffs would all agree. Furthermore, even if they did, how in the world could the plaintiffs' attorneys agree to a settlement award for each plaintiff? It was not as simple as dividing that number eighty-nine ways. Each plaintiff had different damages. The disease had killed some. Others were yet to die from it. Some would fight the disease on their own, without need for treatment. Others had died from cancer soon after they were diagnosed with hepatitis C. Still others would endure months of costly, difficult treatment. No two cases were the same. Under the proposal, the plaintiffs' committee would agree to a single number as a global award and then fight with each other over whose plaintiff had more damage than the others. It was an unethical recipe for disaster.

Almost to a man, the other plaintiffs' attorneys who had been working these cases and I wanted to reject the proposal and continue working on the cases. Suddenly, however, the dozens of other plaintiffs' attorneys who had been "riding coattails" became very interested in the cases. The next plaintiffs' committee meeting had an unprecedented turnout. I saw faces that I didn't even know had cases. It was obvious that the coattail riders thought that the end was near.

Evelyn's lawyer, Matt Miller, and I argued against the proposed settlement talks. We were overwhelmingly outvoted. We were going to move on to the group settlement, even if a few of us considered it grossly unethical, immoral and unjust for our clients.

The group had spoken, but now there were new problems. Since we were going into a group settlement, we had to have some way to categorize the victims so we could figure out how we were going to distribute any settlement we would receive. I found the concept of categorizing victims repulsive, but there was no point in further objection.

If the categorization was to be done, someone had to do it. Since my colleague, Jim Brown, and I had done more work on these cases than anyone else, and since we knew the cases better than anyone else, we were burdened with the unholy task. It was not enough that I knew the facts of my cases. Suddenly, I was expected to know the facts of all the victims' cases. So at the conclusion of the meeting, Jim and I spoke up.

We asked for a summary of each plaintiff's information from each plaintiff's attorney. The summary didn't need to be very long, but it needed to include their client's basic information. We simply needed to know who the victim was, their age, their health, whether or not they still had cancer, whether or not they were married, number of minor children, etc. As unbelievable as it sounds, I eventually had to create an information cheat-sheet so that attorneys would know what information they needed to ask their clients.

I was shocked to find that after two years of ongoing litigation, many of the "coattail riders" had not even bothered to collect their own clients' medical records. Some of the attorneys did not know if their clients still had cancer, or if they were married, or if they had children. By then, I had spent time in my client's homes. I knew the names of their children. I had some of them over to my house for dinner. Yet as shocking to me as it was, some attorneys could not even tell me their clients' names. They had literally done nothing to prosecute their plaintiffs' cases, and had instead only waited with hope that the defense would someday throw money at them. With the settlement talks looming, they thought that day had arrived.

After two weekends of reviewing everyone else's cases, Jim and I came up with a rudimentary way to categorize the victims and their damages. There is no real way to value what suffering is worth, but we simply tried to do our best as the great plaintiffs' committee had asked. We spent hour upon hour weighing one case's damages against another. We took into account everything from the patient's current health, to whether or not they had a family. We tried to honestly value each case, considering the factors a jury would have been allowed to consider.

With the loathsome task of categorizing victims behind us, we now had only one more obstacle before us prior to group settlement talks—we needed to know how potential juries from Dodge County would value these cases so that we had a benchmark to compare the offer from the defendants. As the defense was prone to remind us, Dodge County jurors had a low per capita income, and their jury verdicts were often low. As with most low-population, blue-collar, farming communities, Dodge County jurors tended to have a "get over it" attitude toward plaintiffs. Nebraska does not value injured plaintiffs like most states. They don't believe a person's life is worth much unless he is the breadwinner of a family supporting young children. Furthermore, they tend to doubt that a physician would injure a patient.

So, the plaintiffs' committee decided to schedule two groups of regular Dodge County folk to sit on two secret mock juries. The steering committee hired a jury evaluation expert, who charged somewhere around $35,000. He then coordinated the selection of approximately thirty random mock jurors. Jurors were paid $30 for their day.

The steering committee rented a hotel meeting room under the name of a fictitious organization for two weekends and put on mock trials. Since we did not know if the mock juries would favorably value the cases, we did not want anyone to know what we were doing. Only plaintiffs' lawyers were to be allowed to know of the mock juries, or to sit in and watch. Yet, before long, it seemed like everyone knew what was happening.

The major concern was that the plaintiffs' committee did not want to skew the award by putting on a half-baked defense. Since all the plaintiffs' attorneys wanted to see high mock verdicts, there was a concern that the plaintiffs' lawyers who were playing defense lawyers in the mock trials would not be as thoroughly prepared as the real defense lawyers would be at trial. So, special care was taken by the steering committee to select and prepare the mock defense cases. Although I was never actually a member of the steering committee, one of the other active plaintiffs' lawyers and I were asked to fabricate facts of the two cases. We created fake plaintiffs, since we were ethically precluded from using facts about real clients.

Finally, the day of the first mock jury came. Once again, I was amazed to see the large number of plaintiffs' attorneys present. The mock jury was taken into a room by themselves, while video cameras broadcast the events into a second room where the plaintiffs' attorneys sat, eagerly hoping for enormous mock verdicts.

"Alright," it was announced to the room of plaintiffs' lawyers. "The mock jury is in the other room, waiting."

I had just arrived. Since it was a Saturday morning, and we were all to be locked in our room far away from the mock jury, I simply wore a pair of blue jeans and my old, grey cowboy boots.

"Mock defense team, are you ready?" someone asked.

"We are ready."

On my way in, I heard one of them mention that the mock defense team had spent the better part of two weeks preparing for the mock trial. They were not going to skew the mock verdict by being unprepared.

"Mock plaintiffs' team…"

No one answered, and we all just looked around.

"Mock plaintiffs' team?" There was another pause. "Oh Jesus," I heard someone say, "Don't tell me we don't have a mock plaintiffs' team."

The steering committee had coordinated the event, hired the twenty-four mock jurors, rented the hotel meeting room under a fictitious name, prepped the mock defense team, and spent $30,000 hiring a mock jury evaluation expert. Apparently, they had forgotten, however, to appoint someone to put on the plaintiffs' case to the mock juries.

I put my head in my hands in disgust.

"We cannot cancel now," I heard a voice say. "We've spent too much money to cancel. The jury is waiting!"

For a moment, there was an awkward silence.

"Travis can do it," another voice said.

"Yeah, he knows these cases better than anyone," another agreed.

I was honored that they had chosen me, and of the thirty or so lawyers in the room, I had certainly spent more hours than anyone else working and learning about the cases. Even so, the entire situation was extremely frustrating. I felt that the plaintiffs' committee had let me down. More importantly, they had let the plaintiffs down. They had just paid a jury analyst more money than most plaintiffs made in a year, for an event that they had obviously been under-planned. It was the plaintiffs' money, spent for the purpose of determining the value of the plaintiffs' cases. The mock valuation was to be used as a bench-mark for settlement talks. They had taken the time to book the rooms, and bring donuts and coffee, yet they forgot to pick a plaintiff's counsel. It was a mistake that undoubtedly cost the plaintiffs.

I borrowed a legal pad of paper and began writing my opening statement to the jury as I walked the twenty feet from our room to the mock courtroom. As I sat there in my blue jeans and weathered cowboy boots, feverishly scratching notes on my legal pad, the fake defense counsel put on a wonderful presentation. They had a slide show with charts and graphs. They stood there with their silver pointer, quoting statistics found in *this* medical journal by *that* doctor. They had a statistical breakdown of how hepatitis C has historically been treated and "cured." They did a great job, well-prepared and well-presented.

Then it was my turn. I did the absolute best I could, but it was hard to compete with the high-tech, computer-aided slide show the mock jury had just seen. I spoke off the top of my head for about half an hour. When I left the room and returned to my fellow plaintiffs' attorneys, they commented on how well I had done.

"You couldn't have done better even if we would have given you two weeks to prepare," one comforted me.

The fact was that I felt horrible. I had done my best, but my presentation on behalf of the plaintiffs would have been much better if it had been prepared.

Juries are nearly impossible to understand. One jury could issue one verdict, and a different group of people would find completely differently. Mock juries are even harder to figure out. As I was speaking to the mock jury that day, I decided that I didn't like the mock jury system. The whole system seemed to be flawed. Everyone around me was putting stock into the belief that these people would tell us exactly how much money the hepatitis C cases would bring at trial. Plaintiffs were going to rely on their fake verdicts to determine how much money they should take in settlement.

Yet, the mock jury wasn't getting all the information a real jury would get. I tried to convince the mock jury to give a fake amount of money to a fictional plaintiff whom they never got to see. They knew they were not real jurors. They knew that there was no real plaintiff. In a real courtroom trial, the jury would have gotten to spend at least an entire week watching the plaintiff. They would see for themselves how the plaintiff suffered with his or her injury. It was impossible to persuade the mock jury that they should feel sorry for a plaintiff that didn't exist—particularly since I had no time to prepare my presentation. It was absurd.

The first mock trial came back with a verdict just less than $100,000 and the second mock jury came back with a verdict just under $200,000. The benchmark had been set disappointingly low. The plaintiffs' attorneys' once-excited mood was now solemn. Their skewed expectation of becoming millionaires from the Nebraska outbreak was shattered.

The Day of Group Settlement

There was a flurry of activity in the days before the group settlement talks. A tree's worth of faxes shot back and forth. The cases had now been valued. In many attorneys' minds the only issue remaining was getting the defense to write a check.

I thought we'd had a good turnout for the mock juries, but the turnout for the group settlement was even better. Suddenly, plaintiffs' attorneys that I hadn't seen in years appeared.

Two days before the group settlement, Jill Watson and I spoke. She was always very interested in how her case was progressing, and wanted to be abreast of new developments. She, like all the eighty-eight other plaintiffs from the Nebraska outbreak, had been notified that the settlement talks would take place.

"My husband and I want to go with you," she said.

The steering committee had voted on the issue and had decided that none of the plaintiffs' lawyers would bring their clients to the settlement talks. My impression was that some attorneys simply didn't want the plaintiffs getting in the way, but I'm not sure why the decision was made. Once again, however, I disagreed with the plaintiffs' committee.

"You know what, Jill," I said, "if anyone in the world deserves to be there, it is *you* and Brian. None of the plaintiffs' committee members have hepatitis C. If you want to be there, you come and sit beside me. Let them try and throw us out," I added indignantly.

When the day cam, I walked into to a crowded room of attorneys with Jill and Brian by my side. Instantly, I got curious and even upset looks from many of the faces around the room.

I was quickly pulled off to the side.

"What are they doing here?" I was asked.

I gave the same response I had given to Jill.

"They have more right to be here than anyone else. None of us got hepatitis."

Soon, Jill, Brian and I were seated around the long conference table with each and every plaintiff's attorney. There were at least forty-five other attorneys in the room.

"I haven't seen most of these people at any of the depositions," Jill commented at one point.

I was too embarrassed by my colleagues to comment at the time.

The settlement talks were scheduled to take place through the mediator. Within a few minutes, he entered the room. He was essentially a very high-priced messenger, carrying offers back and forth between the plaintiffs' attorneys and the defense.

"The defense will pay $14.5 million," he finally got to the point.

Immediately, attorneys at the far end of the table started doing the math. It felt like we were at an auction.

"That means $160,000 apiece!" one said.

The plaintiffs' attorneys debated the offer endlessly. Some wanted to take the money irrespective of whether or not it was just or ethical. The same attorneys who didn't know anything about their own clients a month earlier now wanted to accept the offer. It was the very reason people disparage attorneys.

Matt Miller and I objected. How could we even consider accepting a settlement on behalf of all the victims when we didn't know how we would split it among them? How could the attorneys accept the group settlement without consulting with their clients? A few of the attorneys in the room agreed. Still, a segment of the group wanted to accept the offer.

"If you don't believe we have the authority to accept this offer," one of them finally asked me from across the room, "how do you believe we have the authority to reject it?"

It was one of the moments in my life when I felt completely justified in my actions. I looked at Jill.

"Well," I said aloud, for the room to hear, as I stood looking down to where she sat quietly by my side. "It only takes one client to reject the deal and the whole thing is off. Jill is the only client here. Jill, will you take $160,000?"

"Not in a million years," she answered as she stood beside me.

Instantly, I saw the far end of the room deflate as the three of us headed for the door.

I went back to my office, demoralized by the fact that the two prior months' worth of work had been for nothing. What bothered me even more was that all the work had been foisted upon me by a group I did not respect or support, in a strategy in which I did not believe. The only good thing that came from the plaintiffs' committee was that it had enabled us to share the costs of depositions. Even then, last I heard, not all the plaintiffs' attorneys paid their share.

Later, I received a phone call from my colleague, Jim Brown. If anyone had done more work than I had in the preparation of the hepatitis C cases, it would have been Jim Brown. He felt like I did. The group settlement talks had been a ridiculous waste of time, and the plaintiffs' committee was as well. The plaintiffs' committee would never again lead this plaintiffs' attorney. With the majority of discovery having taken place, the plaintiff's committee quietly fizzled out and died.

CHAPTER 26

The Merritt Decision

The most important lawsuit concerning the Nebraska outbreak did not involve hepatitis C. In fact, the most important lawsuit that was filed was not even filed by a victim of the Nebraska outbreak at all. It was filed by the state of Nebraska.

A cultural shift regarding medical malpractice had worked its way into the American way of life beginning in the 1960s. Gradually, more and more medical malpractice lawsuits were filed against healthcare providers. In response, medical malpractice insurance companies raised their rates. Physicians found themselves paying more and more for malpractice coverage.

When malpractice rates are perceived as too high by physicians, three things can happen:

1. Physicians practice defensive medicine by ordering unnecessary tests and prescribing unnecessary medications. Defensive medicine drives up healthcare costs.
2. Physicians restrict their practices. They stop delivering babies and performing other high-risk procedures. Restriction of physician practices results in making healthcare inaccessible.
3. Physicians simply retire from active practice, rather than pay the increased malpractice liability premiums.

As a result, in 1976, Nebraska passed the Nebraska Hospital Medical Liability Act (NHMLA). The NHMLA attempted to keep physicians' malpractice premiums low by setting up a new system that capped malpractice insurance companies' liability. To do so, it shifted the rest of the burden away from insurance and created a pot of money called the Excess Liability Fund.

Under the NHMLA, a physician was still required to have malpractice insurance, but only enough to pay $200,000 to an injured patient. Once the malpractice insurance carrier paid out the first $200,000, the remainder of the patient's awarded damages were paid by the Nebraska Excess Liability Fund (NELF). The injured patient's total recovery was capped at $1.25 million at the time of the Nebraska outbreak lawsuits.

By requiring physicians to only carry malpractice insurance to cover damages of $200,000 per claim, malpractice insurance companies had limited exposure. Physicians' premiums for their insurance were kept low, and physicians bought the rest of their coverage by making payments to the NELF. In 2004, physician exposure was increased statutorily to $500,000 per claim for a maximum of three claims per year, and the cap was raised to $1.75 million.

The NELF collected money through a surcharge assessed on every physician in the state of Nebraska. Although it was funded by physicians, it was solely administered by the state of Nebraska. The state hired legal counsel whose responsibility was "to aid in protecting the fund against claims." This meant that the state of Nebraska was an adversary of the outbreak victims.

Shortly after the hepatitis C cases were filed in the spring of 2003, the state of Nebraska did something that was absolutely shocking. Since it administered the Nebraska Excess Liability Fund (NELF), it was obligated to pay the victims with NELF funds. The state of Nebraska filed a lawsuit of its own, asking the Court to rule that it didn't have to pay all the plaintiffs' claims. The state's argument was that under the plain language of the Nebraska Hospital Medical Liability Act (NHMLA) of 1976, the state only had to pay those plaintiffs who had already received their first $200,000 from Dr. Javed's insurance. Since Javed only had insurance totaling $600,000, the state asked for a ruling that it only had to pay three plaintiffs. It would save the state millions of dollars, even though it would leave the remaining eighty-six Nebraska outbreak victims without any recovery. They would be on their own to collect damages from Dr. Javed, who was in Pakistan.

The lawsuit filed by the state had four parties: the state of Nebraska (Plaintiff); Dr. Javed (Defendant #1); The Medical Protective Company (Defendant

#2); and lastly, the victims of the Nebraska outbreak as a group (Interveners). The parties' relationships to one anther can be diagramed as thus:

Parties to the NELF Lawsuit

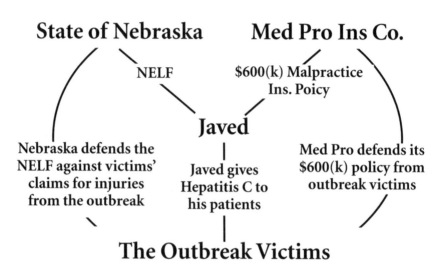

State of Nebraska

NELF

Nebraska defends the NELF against victims' claims for injuries from the outbreak

Med Pro Ins Co.

$600(k) Malpractice Ins. Poicy

Javed

Javed gives Hepatitis C to his patients

Med Pro defends its $600(k) policy from outbreak victims

The Outbreak Victims

In order to practice medicine in Nebraska, Javed had purchased malpractice insurance totaling $600,000 in coverage. The unlucky malpractice insurer was the Medical Protective Group (commonly referred to as "Med Pro"). When the Nebraska legislature passed the Nebraska Hospital Medical Liability Act, the state of Nebraska became the administrator for the Nebraska Excess Liability Fund. In other words, the state became liable to pay injured plaintiffs from the Excess Liability Fund for any amount of damages they suffered at the hands of their doctor above $200,000, and up to $1.25 million.

Since Med Pro's liability was capped by the insurance policy with Javed at $600,000, the state of Nebraska suddenly realized that it may have to pay all the damages suffered by the remaining eighty-six victims. To avoid this responsibility, the state filed a lawsuit against Dr. Javed and Med Pro. The victims of the Nebraska outbreak (through their attorneys) intervened in the lawsuit, since their futures hung on the Court's decision. Here is a summary of the arguments by each party:

The state of Nebraska: The state argued essentially three things. 1) The NELF should not have to pay eighty-six of the Nebraska outbreak victims, unless Dr. Javed paid their first $200,000 in damages. Since Javed was in Pakistan, the state hoped to avoid paying the remaining victims altogether. 2) Med Pro should have to pay for the legal defense of Dr. Javed, even after it paid its policy limits. The state did not want Med Pro paying policy limits and leaving the state, through the NELF, with the obligation of paying for Javed's legal fees. 3) The Nebraska Excess Liability Fund was going to be insolvent if they had to pay Nebraska outbreak victims and therefore should not have to pay.

Med Pro: Med Pro argued that once it paid out its policy limits, it had no duty to defend Javed. Ironically, Med Pro's argument was based upon a prior case, which had been decided by the Nebraska Supreme Court several years earlier, called *Carman Cartage v. Ohio Casualty Insurance Company*. In that case, Travis had represented Carman Cartage Company and argued the case to the Supreme Court. He'd lost that case when the Supreme Court ruled that Ohio Casualty did not have a duty to defend once it paid policy limits.

Now, it turned out that the case was resurfacing again. If Med Pro was correct in its reading of the Carman Cartage case, it could pay policy limits and leave Javed to "defend himself." Since he was in Pakistan and likely never to return, it would have left the plaintiffs with no one responsible for the outbreak. Luckily, the Court did not read *Carman Cartage* the same way Med Pro did, and Med Pro had to remain as Javed's legal counsel.

Dr. Javed: Javed (represented by his malpractice insurance attorney) argued that he didn't care who paid the Nebraska outbreak victims as long as he didn't have to do it. The unstated fact, however, was that even if a judgment was issued against him personally, there was no way a plaintiff could collect from him in Pakistan.

The Nebraska outbreak victims: The interveners argued that the legislature did not intend the NHMLA to keep eighty-six of the Nebraska outbreak victims from recovering their damages while the Excess Liability Fund had millions of dollars in reserve. The Nebraska outbreak victims were just victims of malpractice and should be compensated.

The case was filed in Lancaster County District Court. It took a year before the case was decided. Judge Merritt ruled that Dr. Javed's position was correct, and that while he had created the entire Nebraska outbreak, under the NHMLA, he had no personal responsibility to pay for it. He then went on to rule on the bigger issue. Judge Merritt wrote, "As a result of the court's determination herein that Dr. Javed has no personal obligation to pay final judgments…the Excess Liability Fund is obligated to pay all final judgments…after the proceeds payable under the Med Pro Policy have been paid."

While the NHMLA may have been short-sighted, it was certainly not designed to leave eighty-six of the eighty-nine injured hepatitis C victims without compensation. As a result, the Nebraska Excess Liability Fund ultimately had to pay for Javed's misdeeds. Contrary to the state's fear, the NELF did not go bankrupt from the Nebraska hepatitis C outbreak. In reality, the Nebraska outbreak had little effect on the overall health of the fund at all. Pakistan's *Daily Times* reported on February 28, 2005 that an unnamed Nebraska lawyer estimated that the total payout of the hepatitis C cases would be $9.2 million—less than one-fourth of the amount regularly kept in the fund.

In an article in the *Omaha World Herald* that was released after the decision, the state of Nebraska explained their attempt to leave the Nebraska outbreak victims without recovery.

"I had to pose these questions simply to have some resolution of what were, I think, ambiguities in the language of the act [NHMLA]," Nebraska insurance commissioner Tim Wagner said.

Despite the "ambiguities" of the NHMLA, the argument never should have been made.

CHAPTER 27

■

Travis Reveals
the Plaintiffs' Trick

While the plaintiffs' committee was failing miserably at every turn, several plaintiffs' attorneys were able to work together effectively. Our greatest moment of achievement came on the day when the Court was to set the first three cases for trial.

For a long time, I debated with my co-counsels how the Court *should* decide which of the eighty-nine cases would go to trial first. I emphasize the "should" because in reality, we had little or no control over the issue. The ultimate decision was up to the Dodge County District Court. It was an issue of great importance, however, since the Court only had the capacity to hold two or three cases of this size per year. With eighty-nine total cases, I did not want my clients to be waiting for years before they got their day in court.

Several options were put forth, and each had its own problems:

1. The Court could set the cases for trial in the order they were filed. The upside of this option was that it was completely unbiased. No plaintiff could complain that they were being treated unfairly if they had to wait several years for their trial. The problem with this system was that it could have made the Court try more cases than it would have had to otherwise. Ideally, Judge Samson would have had to try only a few cases before the parties were able to settle the rest of the cases by using the initial court cases as benchmarks. Under this system of setting cases for trial by

order filed, the Court would have to try a number of cases in which the plaintiffs had survived the disease before it would try a case wherein the plaintiff had died from the disease. The parties would have no way to value what a jury would give to the family of the deceased until a jury had come back with that answer, possibly years down the road. In addition, it was no secret that some of the plaintiffs' lawyers who had filed cases early on had no experience trying medical malpractice cases. They had no desire to go to trial against the monster defense team that had been assembled. The fear was that if the inexperienced attorneys were forced to try their cases, they would lose miserably and set a bad precedent.

2. The second option was to break the cases into groups based upon damages. All the members of group A elected not to undergo treatment (presumably because their cancer was very advanced) and therefore had the smallest damages from infection with hepatitis C. Group B was composed of victims who cleared the virus, but only after the interferon treatment. The treatment was six months of suffering and $30,000 to $40,000 in treatment costs. Group C was the most unfortunate victims. They had either died from the disease or had failed treatment and would likely die. The hope was that by grouping the plaintiffs by approximate damages, we would try only three cases. By trying one from each group, we would then know approximately what the cases were worth to Dodge County jurors. With this information in hand, we could hopefully settle the remaining cases rather than try all eighty-nine of them. One problem with this system was that it grouped plaintiffs in broad and imprecise categories. However, the even bigger problem with this system was that we had no plan for who would decide which particular case would be tried from each group. If the plaintiffs' attorneys picked the individual cases, they would pick the strongest case in each category in hopes of getting the biggest judgments. If the defendants picked the plaintiff cases, they would choose the weakest cases—ones with the least amount of damages.

In the end, the Court decided upon an equitable but complicated solution. The plaintiffs would be categorized into the three categories—A, B and C. The three plaintiffs' firms with the most cases would pick a total of twelve cases (four cases from each firm). Each plaintiff's firm was to include in their choices at least one plaintiff from each of the A, B and C categories. The defense team would then pick one case from each category to be tried.

The only requirement of the defense was that they pick the plaintiffs' cases so that each of the three main plaintiffs' firms got to try one of the three cases. The idea was that both sides would have some control over which cases would be selected so that neither the plaintiffs nor the defendants had the ultimate ability to skew the cases in either direction.

The plaintiffs' ultimate goal was to make sure that my C case was tried— for everyone agreed that it had the largest damages. If my co-counsel and I could land a large verdict with that case, it was thought that the other cases would benefit from higher settlement offers. It took us a while to figure it out. Then, with some math, we figured out a perfect solution so that *we* got to pick the cases *we* wanted tried.

Davis, Bennington & Brown (my group)	Law Firm 2	Law Firm 3
A	A	B
B	A	B
B	A	B
C	B	B

My firm chose two B cases, one A case and the C case we really wanted to try. Another firm chose several As and a B, stating it did not have a C case. The last firm only chose Bs by stating that everyone they represented was in the category B.

As the defense was forced to pick one case from each category, and each plaintiff's firm could only try one case, we had taken the choices away from them. In the end, they were forced to pick my C case, an A case from Law Firm 2 and a B case from Law Firm 3. It was the first, last and only time the plaintiffs' attorneys worked together as a team successfully.

CHAPTER 28

■

The Glenn Doescher Story, As Told by Travis

I am ashamed to admit that the first time I met Glenn Doescher, I was not impressed with him. He was a truck driver, working longer hours than the state of Nebraska knew. I didn't understand his pit-bull attitude or why he was all business. By the time I'd met Glenn, I had spent the better part of three months meeting continually with the victims of the Nebraska outbreak and their families. They walked in my office one after another and were scared and uncertain of what to do.

Glenn Doescher was not scared. He spoke of his situation very coldly. It was as if it were no surprise, and he had known about it all along. The first question he asked me was not about his future. It was much more to the point.

"I know this thing is going to kill me. What kind of attorney's fee do you charge?" he asked. "And you had *better* be willing to negotiate that fee."

What I didn't understand at the time was how his entire life had simply been one horror story after another. I had never met him before that day when he walked in off the street unannounced. I did not know that he had been kicked around by life way too often to be scared of a disease that could kill him. He had faced that all of his life.

Glenn was one of the few victims of the Nebraska outbreak who never had cancer. He was born with hemophilia—sometimes called the "the royal disease" because it is associated with Queen Victoria of England, who was a carrier. Hemophilia is a blood disorder that prevents a person's blood from clotting.

Glenn was a forty-five-year-old man who had spent his entire life missing out on daily activities that most of us take for granted. To Glenn, a small cut or bruise could potentially be fatal. Over the years, his hemophilia had kept him in and out of hospitals, receiving countless blood products. His staggering medical costs had forced his family into perpetual poverty.

Finally, in February of 2001, Glenn's hemophilia had led him to the Fremont Area Medical Center. In a moment of weakness, wanting to spend quality time with his youngest son, he had done the unthinkable—he'd gone on a short bike ride with Jared, down the street and back again. The next morning, he had woken up to find that he had blood in his urine. It was a horrible sign. The simple bike ride had caused blood vessels in his bladder to burst. In a normal person, the vessels would have clotted within minutes. His hemophilia didn't let that happen, though. Instead, he continued to bleed inside his own body, where no Band-aid could reach.

Glenn immediately went to the emergency department at the Fremont Area Medical Center and was checked into the hospital. Within a few hours of being bedridden, he was introduced to his new physician—the hospital's rare blood disorder specialist, Dr. Tahir Ali Javed.

Under Javed's care, Glenn received blood product infusions called "factor 8." Hospital nurses administered it through an IV line, along with saline. Factor 8 promotes blood clotting. Within a few days, Glenn's internal bleeding stopped and he was released from the hospital. He had to return for follow-up factor 8 infusions, though, and since Dr. Javed had his clinic in the hospital, Javed suggested that Glenn's final treatments all be given at the Fremont Cancer Center.

When Glenn had left Dr. Javed's care, he'd had no idea that he was infected with hepatitis C. When he'd received a notice from the state of Nebraska saying that he needed to be tested for hepatitis C, Glenn wasn't really surprised. Prior to the letter from the state, he'd had no inkling that his own physician might have given him a disease, but it really wasn't shocking. It was just another example of life kicking him when he was down. What was fairly surprising to him was that after his hepatitis C test results came back, he was found to be negative. He went home that night and showed his wife, Lynn, and the kids the letter from the state of Nebraska.

"I am happy to inform you that your blood has tested **NEGATIVE**," it said. "...Based on this information we are confident that you **ARE NOT** infected... No further testing or medical care is necessary..."

It had been the first time in his life that anyone had ever told him that no further medical treatment was necessary. It had been an unexpected blessing, so he and his family had rejoiced. It had not lasted for long. A few months later, he had read in the local newspaper that the state, which had been so certain in their prior testing, had announced that those who had previously tested negative would have to be retested because the first test results may have been wrong. Suddenly, life had been more predictable again, and with his retest, his skepticism had been vindicated. The prior state testing had been inaccurate, and he did indeed have hepatitis C3a, just like all the other Nebraska outbreak victims.

Glenn's Legal Dilemma

When I received Glenn's medical records from the Fremont Cancer Center, I was not surprised to find that they were poorly kept and incomplete. I was learning that poorly kept medical records were a common trend at Javed's clinic.

Glenn's entire medical record contained only one page of nurse's notes from his factor 8 treatments. In very poorly scribbled handwriting, the records reflected that Glenn had only received one factor 8 treatment, and that it was not even given at the Fremont Cancer Center. Glenn was adamant that the records were wrong. He told me at great length every detail of his four visits to the clinic to receive factor 8. He remembered where he had sat within the clinic and how the nurse had given him a saline IV before starting the factor 8 drip. He remembered his oldest son, Jake, sitting beside him while he took his treatments. He even remembered Raegene, one of the nurses who had worked on him. How could it possibly be that his medical records from the clinic did not show him ever receiving treatment at the Fremont Cancer Center during the timeframe of the Nebraska outbreak?

I met with him again and again to go over his memories in tedious detail. His remembrance of the events was unyielding. Raegene had given him saline IV, and it didn't make any difference to him if his medical records showed it or not. It made a huge difference to me.

Medical malpractice lawsuits in the state of Nebraska were hard to win. Until a dozen or so years prior, it had been almost unheard of for a plaintiff to win a malpractice case, no matter how blatant the negligence. The truth of the matter was, juries didn't believe that a doctor would hurt someone, and they did believe that plaintiffs would say anything to get rich quick. While times may have changed a little, one rule that had remained was that if something did not appear in your medical records, it did not happen...period. Absent some miracle to explain why his records were incomplete, there was no way for him to prove that his hepatitis C3a came from the cancer center.

Dr. Mark Mailliard, the chairman of gastroenterology at University of Nebraska Medical Center, studied the Nebraska outbreak after it became public. He studied the statistics on hepatitis C in North America and in particular, hepatitis C3a in Nebraska. He told me that there was only a 1.68 percent chance that Glenn's hepatitis C3a had come from anywhere other than the Nebraska outbreak.

Statistically, hepatitis C3a is extremely rare in our part of the world, and it would be even rarer that Glenn would have coincidentally contracted the exact same rare strand of hepatitis C that all the other Nebraska victims had in the same timeframe. To win a medical malpractice case, Glenn only had to prove that it was "more than likely" that it had come from the Fremont Cancer Center.

To Nebraska jurors, however, that 1.68 percent chance could have given them all the doubt they needed to find against him. After all, Glenn was a hemophiliac. He had received blood transfusions repeatedly over the years. Some of those transfusions had come during the 1980s, when doctors were not screening the blood supply for hepatitis C. If even one juror doubted that Glenn got his hepatitis C from Dr. Javed, the results of his lawsuit could be disastrous.

In April of 2005, I finally gained insight into the quandary when Raegene Lawson gave her deposition. It turned out that Raegene was not a nurse. Raegene was a certified nurse's assistant. Put bluntly, the only education she had was a two-week course on emptying bedpans, giving baths, taking vitals and getting patients in and out of bed. She had no formal training in giving shots or infusions like factor 8, or in writing in medical records.

"Did you have any formal education after high school?" my co-counsel, Jim Brown, asked at deposition.

"No," she answered flatly.

"You did work at Javed's office?"

"Yes."

"What training and education did you have to be able to work there?"

She thought for a moment.

"I had previously had a seventy-two-hour certified nursing assistant course at the Platte Valley Community College."

"Is that CNA? Is that what that stands for?"

"Yes."

"Is that a licensed position?"

"It's just—you just get a certificate. It's not a license."

"Are you trained in vascular access skills at all?" he continued to question her later in the afternoon.

"No."

"Drawing blood, anything like that?"

"No."

"Are you trained or do you have the capability of giving oral medications?"

"No."

"What did you do at the Fremont Cancer Center?"

"I put patients in the rooms, you know, taking vital signs."

"Did your job ever change?" he pressed her further.

"Well, I started running labs on the Celldyne machine… I started to give the growth factor shots," she went on. "…And they also taught me how to flush a port."

I think everyone in the room was shocked. Suddenly, Glenn's story did not sound so crazy.

"Who decided you should be doing that?"

"Dr. Javed and Linda… Dr. Javed had taken me to his office and said they wanted me to start giving the growth factor injections."

"You weren't trained at the Platte Valley Community College," Jim stuttered a little with surprise, "to give injections, were you?"

"No."

I could tell that Jim was flabbergasted.

"How did you calculate the dose?"

With her lack of formal medical training, it was hard to imagine that she had been put in charge of giving medication to patients who were entrusting their lives to Dr. Javed.

"At first, we kind of just went with a general 'everybody got the same dose."

"Did Dr. Javed ever instruct you to reuse a single dose vial?"

"Yes."

"And did you do that?"

"Yes."

As the deposition continued, I was aghast. Finally, Jim passed the questioning on to me.

"When you flushed patients' ports, was it noted in the record that you had done the port flush?" I asked.

I had never seen Raegene's name noted on any of the victim's records.

"If it was for their chemotherapy, no. Linda wrote the note, 'Port flush, needle discarded.'"

A Sacrifice for the Greater Good

When I was in college and deciding what to do with my life, I narrowed my choices down to medical school or law school. In the end I choose law school because I never wanted to be in the position of telling someone that they were going to die and that I was powerless to do anything about it. As fate would have it, I did that very thing on January 13, 2006. It was the day I told Glenn that he was likely going to die from his hepatitis C before I could get his case into the courtroom and get him the money he needed for a liver transplant.

When I'd first met Glenn, he'd been a remarkably healthy-looking individual, considering his circumstances. He'd told off-color jokes and looked alive. Over the years I'd spent working on his case and plodding through the judicial backlog caused by the Nebraska outbreak, I'd seen his health fade to the point that his spark was all but gone. There were no more jokes or smiles. His eyes were sunken and his skin became a lifeless grey-yellow.

I got a phone call from his liver specialist, Dr. Mailliard.

"The short of it is," he said, "Glenn is dying. His body is shutting down. I cannot tell you when, it may be this weekend, or next year, but within a year or so, he will be dead if he doesn't get a new liver."

Hepatitis C had destroyed his liver to the point that it was barely functioning. Now toxins, which are normally filtered out by the liver, were building up in his bloodstream. His blood was becoming poisoned, his complexion was becoming jaundiced, and he walked around in a perpetual mental haze. The same toxins that were turning his skin yellow had also begun to cloud his memory.

Glenn had been bedridden during treatment for hepatitis C with six months of symptoms resembling a severe flu. Interferon was the $40,000 treatment for the virus—but unfortunately, it had no effect other than to make his mental haze worse. The financial strain was compounded by the fact that he had no health insurance, and he had become too sick to drive his semi truck. It left him with only one option. He had to sell the only thing he owned of any significant value—his big rig. With a family to consider, he had no option but to swallow his pride and turn to food stamps to feed his family. But there was a glimmer of hope. He had been placed on the liver transplant list.

Normally, a patient has to post a bond of $250,000 to be put on the liver transplant list. Glenn didn't have $25 to his name, much less a quarter of a million. Nevertheless, he was put on the list because the other victims of the Nebraska outbreak were going to hold a fundraiser for him. His family was optimistic.

As his fundraiser was in its planning stage, I continued to admonish him that he could not talk to the media about his case. Judge Samson's gag order prohibiting us from talking to the press was still in effect. The Court told us that if anyone violated the gag order it would likely order a change of venue in all the cases. The understanding was that if there were any more news coverage about the outbreak, it might have been impossible to find a jury of unbiased people in our county or the surrounding counties. Two-thirds of the cases had settled, but the rest were still awaiting trial. A change of venue would have potentially been devastating to the remaining plaintiffs. If venue was changed, it would likely be sent further west, into rural Nebraska. None of us wanted that.

About one week before we officially announced the fundraiser, a local television station from Omaha caught wind of it. In typical media fashion, they contacted Glenn directly, without first speaking to me. If they had, I would have told them we couldn't talk to them. Instead, they asked Glenn to talk about his ailment, and how he needed money for his transplant. By that point in the interview Glenn had probably not violated the strict letter of the Court's order. What came next clearly did.

"I need $350,000 for a liver transplant and the defendants are only offering me $25,000," Glenn complained.

The following day, I spoke to Evelyn, a member of the fundraiser committee. I told her that I had admonished Glenn not to do any interviews but that he did not follow my directive. The fact of the matter was that Glenn was dying and needed a liver transplant. He was very ill from his failing liver, and it was causing him to have serious memory problems. He simply could not remember anything from one moment to the next. Even though he and I discussed it repeatedly, he forgot about the gag order.

Evelyn and I discussed the potential likelihood of him speaking to the media again, and how that would hurt all the remaining victims who still had cases on file by causing a change of venue. We knew that in Glenn's medical condition, there was no way he could remember my admonitions and that if we announced the fundraiser publicly, he would be swamped with media.

With all this as a background, I called Glenn and told him that the fundraiser committee had decided to cancel the fundraiser. It was a sacrifice for the greater good of all the remaining plaintiffs who needed verdicts to ensure that they could pay for their own medical costs, but it was heartbreaking for me. In typical fashion, Glenn shrugged it off and accepted it as though he had somehow known that life was going to let him down once again.

The following day, I received a phone call from his liver specialist, Dr. Mailliard.

"Did you know the fundraiser has been cancelled?" he was clearly perplexed. "Glenn has been taken off the transplant list because he can't put up the money."

I knew the seriousness of the situation.

"Yes, I know. But what else can I do?" I mumbled.

"All I can think of is that you can contact the director of the business office at the med center. If you call him and explain the situation, maybe he can put a hold on collecting the fees until Glenn gets done with his lawsuit. Because I'm telling you, otherwise, he won't live to see his trial date."

"Can I use your name?"

"Absolutely." He didn't even hesitate. "You can tell them that both the transplant surgeon and I want to see Glenn get his liver, even if he cannot pay for it. The medical community as a whole feels terrible about this outbreak. We are still in shock that it was caused by a fellow physician. We also feel terrible that we didn't fully understand the outbreak until it was too late for Dan McGill and Cheryl Gentry. Now that we do know what is going on, we want to make sure that none of the other outbreak victims die while waiting for a liver."

I got off the phone and immediately called my co-counsel, Jim Brown. As a retired physician himself, Jim knew the gravity of Glenn's situation. He was shocked when I told him Glenn was taken off the transplant list. I told him I was going to contact the business office at UNMC. Jim had been around the block before. He had been in practice as a medical malpractice attorney much longer than I had, and I instantly noted his skepticism. It was unbelievable to me that Glenn's life was coming down to asking a state-funded hospital for a quarter-of-a-million-dollar handout. Jim agreed it was our only option, but I could tell he was thoroughly convinced it was a waste of my time.

For three days, I called the business office at UNMC without connecting to the director. As precious time was slipping away from Glenn, I asked the director's secretary in frustration if there were any other way I could get in contact with him. She gave me his email address, and I wrote out the situation in detail to him and begged him to call me.

By this time, Glenn was falling into depression. I spoke with him every day, and he continually asked me what he was going to do. I could tell he was starting to give up, but I insisted that he hold out hope, even as slim as it may be.

On the fourth day, I finally got a return phone call from the man in charge at the UNMC business office.

"Don't get me wrong," he said, "we expect to get paid, but we'll go ahead and transplant Glenn as soon as a liver comes available. We'll wait on payment until he can get the money together."

I called Glenn back. It was his first good day in a long time.

Glenn Suffers Memory Loss

Despite the deplorable condition of Glenn's medical records from the Fremont Cancer Center, I was confident that we could still prove his case against Dr. Javed. Over the years I had met with him on numerous occasions to hear him recount his story of taking treatments, even though his medical records did not show him doing so. The only piece of our case that was missing was his sworn testimony that he indeed did receive treatment there.

His treatments had flowed through the IV tubing with a mixture of saline. The saline had obviously been contaminated, like it had been with all the other Nebraska outbreak victims, and he, like the other victims, had contracted hepatitis C. All he had to do was retell the story in court like he had done to me so many times. As time went on, I saw his memory begin to fail him. It became paramount that his testimony be taken under oath before trial. Four years after he had contracted the virus, he finally got the chance to tell his story in a deposition.

One of the first questions in depositions is always about the plaintiff's family.

"Are you married?"

"Yes," Glenn answered.

"How many children do you have?"

My jaw nearly hit the floor when Glenn could not, for the life of him, remember how many children he had. The answer was five, but he didn't know it. I sat there quietly as his deposition continued for another seven hours. He couldn't remember his children's names, or his ex-wife's name. He couldn't remember much at all. When the time came for the critical issue of his treatment inside the Fremont Cancer Center, he couldn't remember that either. His mind was a blank.

The failed interferon treatments and his failing liver had caused his mind to fade. The razor-sharp Glenn I had known a couple years previously was gone. He described the Fremont Cancer Center vaguely, but in reality, he was describing an amalgamation of each and every treatment center he had ever been to in his life. He tried to describe the nursing staff, and the clinic's location within the hospital, but it was all wrong.

With his flawed testimony, we could not prove that he was in the clinic for treatments. We needed something else. We looked for the Fremont Cancer Center billing records to prove when Glenn had been in the clinic and for what he had been charged. Unfortunately, all the billing records had been destroyed. Our options were limited.

Glenn's Liver Fails

In March, I saw Glenn at my office. He had terrible news. His hepatitis C and his failing liver had taken the last step toward death—liver cancer. If he didn't get a liver transplant soon, he would die. Even then, it may be too late. If the cancer spread, it would likely be just a matter of time even if he did get the transplant.

On May 9, 2006, I received a phone call that was a mixed blessing. Glenn was going to have a chance to live, at the expense of someone who had died in an accident. I could hear the nervousness in his voice as he told me that the transplant team had just paged him. He was going to get a liver. The concerns now were that he survive the surgery, and that all the cancer be removed during surgery.

The following day, I went to see him at the University Hospital Intensive Care Unit. The instant I saw him, I was delighted. The grey skin color I had come to expect was gone. He was unconscious from medications, but his skin was a lively pink. He had survived the transplant and his new liver was working. From someone else's tragedy, Glenn was given another chance. He had been cut open from hip to hip, and he had a wire hanging out the side of his neck, connected to a monitor in his heart, but he was alive. His ever-faithful wife, Lynn, was at his side.

"The cancer?" I asked.

"They think they got it all before it spread." She smiled through her glassy, joyful eyes.

We stood over his bedside and spoke a few moments before I left them alone once again. She told me two stories—both made me fight back my own tears.

She told me how their six-year-old son had grabbed hold of Glenn's leg when she'd loaded him up to take him to the hospital. Jared had refused to let him go, crying that he might never see his daddy again.

She then told me how she knew she had to be strong for Glenn. She said she had never cried once during the past four years, since his diagnosis of hepatitis C. Then, as she sat there in the waiting room, and she was finally given the news that his operation had been a success, she broke down and sobbed like a baby. Seeing the loving look on her face as she told her story led me to believe that even after all Glenn had been through, in many ways, he was a very lucky man.

CHAPTER 29

■

The Bob Ridder Story, As Told by Travis

I met with Bob Ridder and his wife, Verena, in July of 2004 to discuss the prospects of including his story in this book. Bob and Verena were both very soft-spoken, private people, and were initially reluctant. He eventually agreed to allow me to tell his story as long as I complied with three requests.

First, he wanted to make sure that this book conveyed the suffering that he and the other Nebraska outbreak victims had gone through, and continue to go through. I told him that my co-author was, in my opinion, doing just that. Second, he made me promise that Evelyn and I would not withhold any of the truth as to what had happened to cause the Nebraska outbreak. I promised him we would not. Lastly, he asked that when I tell his story, I simply stick to the facts. He didn't want any literary hype or big-word jargon. With those three requests in mind, here is Bob and Verena's story.

Bob Ridder had been diagnosed with cancer in July of 2000. He was a farmer by birthright, and he was a tough, stoic man. Without much hesitation or complaint, he had entered chemotherapy treatment and by Christmas, he had been told his cancer was in remission. As the new year, 2001, had begun, Bob and Verena had thought the worst was behind them. The cancer treatments had been tough, and although he'd decided that he was no longer going to actively farm the ground himself, he would continue to raise cattle.

On October 13, 2002, the Ridders had gotten a letter from the state of Nebraska, telling them that Bob needed to be tested for hepatitis C. A few days later, on October 18, 2002, he'd complied with the state's request. He'd been told that he would have the results back in two weeks. Two weeks later, he still hadn't heard back from the state or his physician. Another week had passed without a test result, so he'd finally called his physician. His physician had confirmed the worst. Bob was a victim of the Nebraska outbreak.

Immediately, Bob's doctors had begun to monitor the hepatitis C. It was aggressively attacking his liver. If he did not take action soon, his liver would be irreparably harmed, or worse, the hepatitis C would cause liver failure or even liver cancer. On January 31, 2003, he'd begun interferon and Ribavirin treatment to combat the disease. The first day he'd taken the drugs, he'd developed a terrible headache. He'd been sick for the next two days. The co-pay had been $750 for the first round of drugs from the pharmacy. With the first day of treatment behind him, he had only had 182 more days of treatment to go.

Over the next couple of months, Bob's reaction to the drugs had become severe. He had continued to make trips to the doctor's office for blood draws, and he'd fought to keep working every day, but his condition had continued to worsen. The side effects of the drugs had been progressively making him sicker and sicker. Each time he'd taken another dose of the drugs, his reaction to them had been worse. Before long, he'd become too sick to work some days and had begun quitting work early on others. His headaches had worsened, fatigue had set in, and he'd begun to fall into depression.

Bob had grown up on his family farm, just south of Dodge, Nebraska. It had been his father's farm before he passed it onto Bob. Bob had spent fifty-four years on that farm. Verena had lived there as his wife for thirty-one years. Before Bob had been diagnosed with hepatitis C, he'd had no plan of ever letting the homestead get out of his family. Under normal circumstances the idea would have been unthinkable.

However, with the debilitating side effects of the hepatitis C medication, he and Verena knew they couldn't care for the cattle. They'd known that the surrounding farmers would undoubtedly help him if his condition didn't improve, but Bob and Verena hadn't wanted to rely on the kindness of others to survive. They'd held out hope as long as they could, but the reality of the situation had been apparent. They'd felt they'd had no option, and in the spring of 2003, they'd decided to sell the homestead and the cattle. It had been a crushing blow that had been hard to take in his weakened condition, but Bob had kept his chin up the best he could. If it had to be, then it had to be. That was all there was to it. Despite his weakened condition, he still had to support his family, so he'd worked as a laborer for a business in town.

In March, the interferon treatments had taken such a toll on him that his blood counts fell dangerously low. In addition to his normal treatments, he'd begun taking two other drugs, Epogen and Neupogen, to boost his blood counts. The new drugs had increased his blood counts, but he had not felt any better.

By April and May, Bob had hit an all-time low. He had been more ill than he had ever been. Even his chemotherapy treatments for cancer had not made him feel as bad as the treatment for hepatitis C. He had been missing more and more work—something that he had never done in his entire life. Later, in his journal, he wrote about those months of his life. He wrote:

> I went to work most days, except for the days I was too sick to leave the house. Most mornings after trying to eat breakfast I would sit in the recliner and wonder if I should go to work or not. It was hard to get the strength to go to work, but I figured I couldn't miss too many days because I had too many bills to pay from the drugs and it didn't do any good to stay home because I wasn't going to feel better. It kind of got your mind off how bad you felt when you went to work. There was evenings when I came home from work when I would just stay in my pickup and put my head on the steering wheel because I didn't have the ambition to go in the house.

In June, Bob's niece had her wedding. Bob had been too sick from the treatments to enjoy it with the rest of the extended family. His birthday had come, then Father's Day, and then his anniversary. They had all passed without celebration. He had simply been too sick.

July 11, 2003 had been moving day. Bob had been sick from the interferon and Ribavirin, and he'd had a splitting headache. Still, without complaint, he'd loaded up the last of his life at the farm and moved with Verena into the village of Dodge, to a house around the corner from their church.

He'd woken up the following Sunday morning and was miserable. Another horrible side effect of the hepatitis C medications had overtaken him, and he had been suffering from a yeast infection on his tongue. It had been swollen and coated with a white film. As he and Verena had been walking to church that morning, Bob had been at one the lowest points in his life. He had been suffering physically, emotionally and financially. He had lost his family farm, his physical relations with his wife were gone, and he was so miserable all the time that he felt his interaction with his grandchildren was changing.

As they had walked the few blocks to church that Sunday morning, he'd felt comfort in knowing that the church was still there for him. It was one thing that had remained constant for him in a time when everything else had been falling apart. With the church in sight, he and Verena had walked up the hill before Mass. Halfway up the hill, Bob had run out of energy. He had given everything he'd had to simply walk the three blocks from his house. The hill had been too much for him. Physically, he couldn't walk up the hill.

"Should I walk back and get the car?" Verena had asked.

It had been the final straw. He couldn't even walk up the hill to church, and his wife's concerned offer just highlighted how sick was. It had seemed like life was over.

As the weeks went by, Bob had tried to keep his chin up, but it was difficult. He was not the kind of man who had ever given up on life, but it had not been easy. Verena had been suffering too. One afternoon, he'd come home to find her sobbing. Weeks earlier, she had taken a hepatitis C test, to make sure that Bob hadn't given the disease to her before they'd known he had it. She had sat in the kitchen, sobbing, holding the notice that her test result was negative. She didn't have the disease. It hadn't mattered, though. She had not been crying tears of joy. She had been crying tears of frustration.

"I'm never taking another one of those tests and waiting for the results," she'd told him through her tears.

Finally, in July 2003, Bob had taken his last interferon shot. The preceding year had been the worst of his life. Even after the treatments had ended, he'd still been sick for another month and half. His physical ordeal had finally been coming to an end, but his hard times were not over yet.

The Only Hepatitis C Trial

When Bob had first been diagnosed as one of the victims of the Nebraska outbreak, his doctor had told him to hire a lawyer and file suit against Dr. Javed. As he was finally starting to feel better physically, after the interferon treatment, his trial date approached. Every other plaintiff before him had settled his case. When the defendants' lawyers approached Bob and Verena about settlement, they spent a long time debating what they should do. If they settled their case, they would get out of the legal system and could finally move on with life.

The problem that the Ridders struggled with was that if all the plaintiffs behind them also settled their cases, the world would never know of the Nebraska outbreak or what happened to cause it. Bob and Verena spoke with their children. The kids agreed. There was more than money on the line. This was an issue of principle. The acts that led to the Nebraska outbreak needed to be known. If a trial was the only way to get the facts out, then they would go to trial even if it cost them everything they had left. The world needed to know.

For weeks before the trial, the Ridders couldn't sleep. Bob's stomach was upset. He was not the "suing type." This was different, though. He felt he was standing up for all the victims of the Nebraska outbreak. He was going to trial to tell the world that what had happened to them was not fair. If his family hadn't supported him, he wouldn't have done it. But this wasn't about the money anymore. It was about standing up for justice.

"We [the Nebraska outbreak victims] can live with the fact that we had cancer," he later told me. "We can deal with the fact that maybe we caused it ourselves. Some of us smoked and caused it, others of us got it and don't know why, but we can live with the fact that we may have done something to cause it. But we didn't cause our hepatitis C."

From the first day of trial, Bob and Verena knew something was wrong. They didn't understand it at the time, but it was not at all what they had expected. According to the Ridders, their attorney had, without their knowledge, allowed the Fremont Area Medical Center out of the lawsuit. Bob was told it was done to make it easier to pick a jury.

"Since half the town seems to either work there or know someone who works there, it will be nearly impossible to pick an unbiased jury," he was told.

It was hard to swallow and he didn't believe it. Nonetheless, the hospital was not on trial. The other defendants admitted they were liable for Bob's injuries, even though at no time did they apologize. The entire trial turned into a debate over whether or not he had damages from his hepatitis C. Days went by and no one ever told the jury about bags of saline, or who was responsible for the Nebraska outbreak. Instead, the defense wanted to talk about how Bob and Verena had stopped having sexual relations since the discovery of his hepatitis C. It was an unexpected embarrassment for them both.

"Our marriage is still good," Verena said from the witness stand. "But not in every way it should be."

They had been married for forty years, but now she was afraid of contracting her husband's disease.

"There's always still a chance," she said. "I work in a daycare. I work with babies. It's a contagious disease."

The defense attacked her fear as irrational. When asked if there was a chance of Verena contracting Bob's disease through sexual transmission, the defense's expert witness replied, "The answer is a resounding 'no.'"

"We went to trial thinking the outbreak would all come to light, and that everyone would know what Javed and the hospital had done," he said later. "Instead, all they wanted to talk about was my sex life."

Although the newspapers painted Verena as neurotic for her fear of sexual transmission of the disease, it was later found that her fear was very rational. Approximately one year later, it was discovered that one of the outbreak victims had indeed transmitted the disease to a committed sexual partner through sexual relations.

In the end, the Nebraska outbreak story never truly came to light. The entire reason Bob went to trial evaporated before his eyes. The only vindication he got from his trial was the time he got to mention to the jury that he thought that Dr. Javed was "chicken shit" for running out of the country to avoid prosecution. Even that bit of redemption was short-lived, as the judge quickly struck the comment from the record and told the jury to disregard it. One afternoon, he caught up with Nurse Prochaska in the elevator outside the courtroom. She denied him any closure to the tragedy.

"I was just following orders," she told him coldly.

The jury awarded Bob and Verena $685,000. When the media looked for Bob and Verena after the verdict came in, they were nowhere to be found because they had returned to work for the day. Before the month ended, the defendants filed an appeal to the judgment that threatened to hold the case in appeals for years. During the entire appeals process, the money awarded by the jury would be held by the defendants. Bob and Verena had no vindication, no money from their verdict, and, most importantly, the story of the Nebraska outbreak had not come to light and would not come to light through their case. It seemed as if it had all been for nothing.

With everything seemingly lost, the Ridders gave up the fight and settled their case with the defendants, just to bring the litigation to an end. It was all very anticlimactic. All he was left with was a reduced settlement check and the lingering side effects of the interferon—as of the time of the writing of this chapter, he still suffers from continual fatigue and short-term memory loss.

The Ridders' experiences left them untrusting of all professionals, including attorneys. When I met with them to discuss this book, it was not surprising that they were leery. We spoke for hours, and I saw that once they understood that Evelyn and I were trying to tell the truth about what happened, Bob became re-energized. At the end of our meeting, Bob shook my hand and I could see that he was deeply touched to learn that after all the fighting he had done, there was still hope that the story of what had happened to him would come to light. As we parted, he gave me his personal journal and told me that I should read it before writing his story.

Bob wanted more than anything to have the victims' story of the Nebraska outbreak told. It is only fitting that he tell it himself. The last page of Bob Ridder's private journal reads:

> I feel so sorry for anyone who went through what I and my family went through because of the hepatitis. I used to put all my trust, and my life, in the medical profession. Not anymore. I hope the people who caused these problems truly realize what they have done. People have already died and more will die because of them. The pain and suffering of these families will never stop. You would have to be a part of one of the families to understand the pain, worry and anxiety this whole thing has caused. I could never take those treatments again. It was too hard. I thank God for my loving family and friends who were my support.
>
> —Bob Ridder

CHAPTER 30

Evelyn Talks About
Her Health Challenges

*"[They're] not feeling like a rose during that twenty-four weeks [of treatment]...
They cannot focus well. [They] may get depressed. They get very irritable and have
a short fuse."*

—Dr. Eugene R. Schiff, MD
(Expert witness testimony, October 13, 2004)

At the risk of sounding like I have been keeping company with attorneys too long, I want to start this chapter with a disclaimer. This chapter is the story of *my* health issues. In this chapter, I am not suggesting that my story is the same story as *all* hepatitis C patients. Many people with hepatitis C have an easier time coping with their disease and its treatment. Some have an even more difficult time than I had. I am sharing my story as an illustration of the treatment and course of one case of hepatitis C.

As with the other victims of the Nebraska outbreak, my health journey was impacted by the original diagnosis of cancer and its subsequent treatment. Because chemotherapy took away our bodies' ability to fight infection, we were at a disadvantage compared to those who have not had chemotherapy. In addition, the stem cell rescue permanently altered my immune system and undoubtedly affected my ability to tolerate the interferon/Ribavirin treatment for hepatitis C.

It has been six years since my last occurrence of breast cancer and I consider myself cured. I realized my dream of seeing Alex graduate from high school and cried as he cited me as a source of strength and inspiration in his valedictory address. With any luck, I will see Alex graduate from college as Dr. Javed predicted.

Deciding on Treatment

I needed to recuperate from the stem cell rescue for quite some time before hepatitis C treatment was advised. Since liver biopsies showed only mild inflammation and no cirrhosis, we felt safe in waiting until I was stronger.

The stem cell rescue was done in February 2002. In December 2002, a strange thing happened. Within the period of a few days, my joint pain became much, much worse. I walked and felt like an old woman. A blood test showed that my liver enzymes had gone down to near-normal levels.

Dr. Gilroy, my liver specialist, was cautiously optimistic.

"Here's what I think is happening," he explained. "The stem cell rescue wiped out your immune system in February. That caused your viral load—roughly, the amount of virus in the body—to go up. Your immune system is now reconstituting itself. It has recognized the virus and is fighting it. If we are really, really lucky, your immune system will win the fight and you will clear the virus. You'll just have to ride out this period of extreme joint and muscle pain and we'll check your viral load in a month or so."

To support my body in its fight against the virus, I imagined it as the site of a football game, with the home team (my immune system) competing against the visiting team (hepatitis C). I visualized the scoreboard showing the home team beating the visitors 100–0. I was very hopeful that the virus would be defeated.

Gradually, the extreme joint aches lessened to a more tolerable level. With great anticipation, we awaited the results of the blood test. It showed that the viral load was less than 7,000 IU/ml. At the time of the hepatitis C diagnosis, the viral load was 2,000,000 IU/ml.

"This is good news, don't you think, Richard?" I asked Dr. Gilroy hopefully.

"Well...somewhat. Your joint pain may be less for awhile," he cautiously responded. "But I'm afraid you did not clear the virus. If you had cleared the virus, you would have an undetectable viral load. We can check it again in a month, but please don't get your hopes up."

My hopes were already up. We were disappointed with his prediction but hoped that he would be wrong and that in a month, the viral load would be undetectable. He wasn't wrong. A month later, the viral load was still detectable. After working through the disappointment, we shifted our hope to clearing the virus through treatment.

Tom and I talked about the pros and cons of treatment with Dr. Gilroy on several occasions. The argument in favor of treatment was that it was the only way to completely eliminate the virus from my system so I could be a "healthy" person again. The argument against it was that it could be a very grueling treatment. If I were to go through the six months of physically taxing treatment only to have an occurrence of terminal cancer, I would have suffered needlessly and lost six months of life. In addition, I could conceivably live a very long time with the virus with minimal symptoms. Despite the fact that all the other Nebraska outbreak victims who had finished the six-month treatment had cleared the virus, there were no guarantees. I might be the exception because the stem cell rescue had permanently compromised my immune system.

Dr. Gilroy reviewed pertinent research regarding hepatitis C treatment in immunocompromised patients with us. He opined that given my compromised immune system, I would have about a fifty percent chance of clearing the virus.

"Well, mates, what we have here is three intelligent people trying to make a well-reasoned decision," he concluded.

After some thought, I spoke up. "This whole hepatitis C outbreak was not born of well-reasoned decisions," I observed. "I'm going to put reason aside at this time and go with my heart. I want to go ahead with the treatment. I want to be healthy and well again."

Six Months in Hell

Treatment began in February 2004. The treatment consisted of four pills of Ribavirin every day and one shot of pegylated interferon weekly in my abdomen.

Within two weeks, I felt terrible. Every fiber of my being ached. My upper arms hurt so badly, I could not lift a comb to my head to comb my hair. My aching ankles and feet made every step painful. My arms and legs felt like lead pipes hanging from my torso. My neck and shoulders throbbed. Pain pills, although somewhat helpful, added to the fatigue.

Nausea and diarrhea were constant companions. I was constantly thirsty. Most days, I drank more than the recommended one gallon of water per day, but even then, my thirst was never abated. My dry skin and dry eyes were unbearable.

I was extremely weak, fatigued, and chronically cold and short of breath. A walk across the parking lot from my car to the door of my office left me gasping for breath. The shortness of breath was likely due to the plummeting red blood cell count. I had to start the dreaded growth factor shots to produce more white and red blood cells, which added to the joint pain.

My blood counts continued to drop despite the growth factor shots. The anemia began to make me lightheaded and faint. One Sunday in May, I passed out in church. Tom brought me home early and the boys came home in a separate car after Mass was over. I was lying on the couch resting when they came home. Alex poked his head over the back of the couch and whispered to me.

"Mom?"

"What?" I whispered back, keeping my eyes closed.

"How do you feel?"

"Terrible."

"Here's some good news that might cheer you up."

"What?"

"You know how you like the word 'swimmy'? You can start using it again. You can say 'My head feels swimmy.'"

I opened my eyes and looked at his earnest face, ringed in curls. I hoped intensely that I would see him graduate from high school the following year, but given how awful I felt, I wasn't confident that I would.

The days were long. All of our boys were away at school and Tom routinely worked twelve- to fourteen-hour days. It became unsafe for me to be alone in my own home. There was a strong chance that I might pass out as I made the frequent trips from the couch to the bathroom. I didn't want to add "head injury due to fall" to my list of ailments. When I passed out during a visit to Dr. Osborn, he declared that something had to be done. He consulted with Dr. Gilroy and it was decided that since the growth factor shots were not keeping my blood counts high enough, I should have a blood transfusion.

The thought of having a blood transfusion scared me to death. I knew that the chance of being exposed to hepatitis C through a blood transfusion in 2004 was one in a million, but nonetheless, I was paranoid about receiving another dose of the virus I was fighting so hard to eliminate. However, I also knew that unless I had twenty-four hour nursing care, I could not continue the treatment regimen. If I did not continue the treatment regimen, there was no chance I would clear the virus.

We consulted with the Red Cross blood bank and shared my worries. They agreed that given the emotional trauma of the Nebraska outbreak, directed donation had merit. The blood bank agreed to arrange for the drawing, testing and safe delivery of a blood transfusion donated by donors who had no risk factors.

First, we turned to family to find blood donors. Curtis and Tom weren't my blood type, so they couldn't donate.

Luke matched my blood type. However, he was not a potential donor because he was worried about hepatitis C himself. Four months previous, Luke had called at 3:00 a.m., from his apartment in Spain. "Do you think I am at risk for contracting hepatitis C?" he asked Tom. "I just cut myself on my roommate's razor while putting my toothbrush in the medicine cabinet." While I was engaged in the fight of my life against hepatitis C, we were also on pins and needles, wondering if Luke's test results would come back positive for the same virus.

That left my baby, seventeen-year-old Alex. He was my blood type and had no risk factors. I needed one more donor. My siblings, nieces and nephews began to scramble to determine their blood type. My sister, Marilyn, was a match. We could proceed.

It took several weeks to process the necessary paperwork through the Red Cross, obtain the donations and have them processed for me. Although I was weak, I still had enough life in me at the time to pick a fight with Tom. We were sitting on the couch, discussing the blood transfusion. Luke was home on break from medical school for a few days and was in the adjoining kitchen, making a sandwich.

"Tom, I am not having the transfusion at the hospital," I stated adamantly.

"Ev, you know I can't take a day off work to drive you to Omaha. If you have it at the Fremont hospital, I can check on you several times during the day. Dr. Osborn can check on you, too."

"I'm not going there. The outpatient department is now in Javed's former office. I am not going to sit in the same room, in the same recliner where I *contracted* hepatitis C to receive a blood donation which I am scared to death about to *combat* hepatitis C."

"You'll be fine there," Tom said reassuringly. "You can take a pain pill before you start and then you'll probably sleep through the whole thing. We'll request Marlene to be your nurse and she'll watch you and fuss over you and make sure you are comfortable."

"No," I refused. "Tom, you've got to let me start making my own health decisions." I made my weak voice as forceful as possible. "This is my life and I'm making this decision. I am going to Omaha for the transfusion. And furthermore, if it comes to the point that I need a liver transplant, I'm making that decision on my own, too. And I'm telling you right now, I am not going to have a liver transplant. You're just going to have to let me go at that point."

"Hold it! Wait a minute," Luke interrupted. He had heard enough. He pointed his table knife with mayonnaise on it at Tom. "Dad, Mom does not have to go to the Fremont hospital for the transfusion. Do you want her to have flashbacks and post-traumatic stress disorder? I'll take her to Omaha for the transfusion and sit with her."

There, I thought to myself smugly. *I was right.*

"And Mom," Luke continued, waving the mayo knife in my direction. "You are not to talk about a liver transplant at this time. That's just not fair. We are expecting that you will clear the virus and never need a liver transplant. We are just looking at one day at a time for right now."

Luke put down the knife forcefully and looked at us expectantly. Tom and I swallowed hard, looked down at our laps and said meekly, "Okay."

There was a palpable paradigm shift taking place in the room. Our child was parenting us, his parents. Suddenly, we felt very incompetent.

"We were under a lot of stress," Tom consoled me later in private.

"Oh, yes, it was a difficult time," I agreed.

But from that time on, we discussed every healthcare decision with Luke.

The blood transfusion gave me some much-needed strength and improved my blood counts for a time. Even though I continued to receive growth factor shots, my blood counts continued to gradually drop. It was decided that the dosage of Ribavirin and interferon should be reduced. For most of the six months of treatment, I could not tolerate the full dosage.

There are growth factor injections that stimulate red blood cell and white blood cell production. However, at the time of the treatment, there was no injection that would stimulate platelet production. My platelet count dropped to the dangerously low level of 29,000 (greater than 135,000 is considered normal). We worried that I would cut myself and the bleeding would be hard to stop, or that I would fall and hit my head, causing a bleed in my brain. In addition, the diarrhea, pain and fatigue continued relentlessly.

"You've got to take better care of yourself," Dr. Gilroy admonished me at an office visit in the fourth month of treatment. "I want you to stop losing weight, stop exercising and lay on the couch as much as possible."

How often does anyone hear *that* from a doctor?

Despite following Dr. Gilroy's advice, I continued to lose weight. The diarrhea caused me to lose about twenty-five pounds. The silver lining of the dark cloud of diarrhea was that I returned to the weight I had been on our wedding day and I was able to wear my wedding dress at an anniversary party.

We had a family party to commemorate our twenty-fifth wedding anniversary in July. We renewed our vows at a special Mass. Our joy was intensified by the loving support surrounding us. We knew we were very blessed to have such loving family and friends.

However, hepatitis C pricked even this happy event. When the priest offered me the communion cup during Mass, I took a sip. Through the rest of the evening and into the next month, I worried. Would the alcohol in the sip of wine damage my liver? With that one sip, had I undone all the effort and suffering I had gone through to regain liver health?

Finally, the six months ended on August 10, 2004. We were happy and optimistic. We anticipated that I would feel much better in a few months and that all the health issues of the previous four years would be laid to rest.

Several weeks later, Tom came home from work to find me at my usual place, lying on the couch.

"I have something to tell you," he said softly.

I knew this was an ominous signal, but for the life of me I couldn't guess what he would say.

"Did something happen to the boys?" I finally asked with trepidation.

"No, they're fine. You did not clear the virus."

"What do you mean?" I sat bolt upright, puzzled.

"You did not clear the virus. You still have hepatitis C."

"How do you know that?"

"Don't you remember?" Tom asked. "Dr. Osborn drew a blood sample when you were in to see him last week and sent it in for a viral load."

"Did you talk to Gilroy about this? Are you sure?" I searched his face for answers. "Maybe we should draw another specimen. The test at the halfway point showed no detectable virus."

"Yes, we're sure. Yes, I talked to Gilroy," Tom answered sadly. "He sends his sympathies. I'm so sorry, Ev."

"He sends his *sympathies*? Well, that's fine, but what is he going to *do* about it?" I demanded.

"Honey, there's nothing any of us can do. There are no more treatment options. I'm so sorry," Tom repeated.

I just couldn't believe it. After the "no detectable virus" result three months into treatment, I never gave it a thought that I wouldn't clear the virus. I was completely disheartened. I wondered if I would have cleared the virus if I had undergone treatment before the stem cell rescue. Would I still have the virus if authorities had warned us of the risk of hepatitis C in the Fremont Cancer Clinic in the summer of 2001 and I had undergone treatment at that time?

Tom and I sat together in shock on the couch a long time. We couldn't talk, we couldn't cry. Our lives had taken a sudden turn. Through the three years of cancer and hepatitis C treatments, we had always been confident that we would regain our full, healthy lives someday. Today, we had to acknowledge that our lives would never be the same. Hepatitis C would always be in the background, darkening our plans and compromising the quality of our lives.

Six More Months in Hell

We found it difficult to share the bad news with others. We softened the news as much as we could. We explained that although the treatment had not been successful, my viral load had decreased and so hopefully, the symptoms of joint aches and fatigue would decrease.

Curtis came home during a break from St. Louis University in October. He seemed fine when he arrived and resumed his usual rounds of visiting friends as soon as he returned to Nebraska. One day, he was on his way out the door when he turned to me.

"Uh, Mom, I was wondering. Could I go to counseling?"

I looked up in alarm from the newspaper I was reading. He had never made such a request before. I hadn't noticed that he was troubled. I didn't know what to make of his request.

I have learned over time that difficult conversations with my sons are more productive if I let them take the lead. So I proceeded with caution and tried to structure my responses in a way that would encourage him to open up to me.

"Sure, honey."

There was a long pause. I looked at Curtis quizzically. He looked down at the floor.

"Anything you want to tell me?"

"No, no. I just feel sad. I'm just so sad."

There was even a longer pause.

"Classes going okay?"

"Yeah, fine. Actually, they're pretty easy this semester. So far, I have a 4.0."

Curtis shifted his weight from one foot to the other, fidgeted with the car keys in his pocket and avoided my eyes.

"And…how are things with the girlfriend?"

"Oh fine, she's fine. That's all fine."

I paused again to contemplate while Curtis continued to avoid my eyes. I just couldn't read the situation. Curtis was an effervescent, fun-loving but sensitive twenty-two-year-old. I knew there was some good reason why he was feeling blue. It was troubling and worrisome that he didn't feel comfortable sharing the source of his sorrow with me.

Cautiously, I asked, "Curtis, are you worried about me?"

He started to cry. I walked over to him and put my arms around him.

It was heart-wrenching for me as a mother to have my man-son, who towered over me, weep in my arms like a baby. I was the cause of his sorrow and I didn't know what to do to comfort him. All I could do was rock him back and forth as he wept and recite the blessing I have frequently given my sons throughout the years: "May God bless you and keep you, may God's face shine upon you, may God look upon you kindly and give you peace."

My words just made him sob harder. After a soul-searing eternity, a new thought came to me.

"Curtis, do you remember everything I said when I told you I didn't clear the virus?" I asked. "I also told you that Dr. Gilroy said that chemotherapy tends to make liver cirrhosis worse. I've had a lot of chemotherapy and I still don't show any liver cirrhosis. So we can be very optimistic that the disease will progress very slowly and maybe I won't show any liver damage at all for a long time. And hopefully, by the time I do, researchers will have found a new, more effective treatment."

Curtis jerked his head back and looked at me.

"No, I don't remember you saying that. He really said that? I guess I stopped listening after you said you didn't clear the virus."

His brown eyes locked with my blue eyes and the gaze spoke volumes. Our eyes said that we loved each other very much and that we would work through our grief together. Finally, Curtis spoke.

"You shouldn't have to go through this, Mom," he said sadly.

"I know it, honey," I answered softly.

He wiped the tears from his eyes and took several deep breaths.

"Well, I'm really happy to hear your prognosis, Mom...really glad."

He took another deep breath and fished in his pocket for the car keys.

"Well, I'll be going then. Don't wait up for me. Love ya," he said as he pecked me on the forehead. The sorrow clouding his face had lessened.

I didn't recover as quickly as Curtis. I sat down on the couch and pondered our bittersweet exchange. On the one hand, I was strengthened by Curtis' deep concern for me. On the other hand, I was miserable to see him so distressed. In spite of everything, I was profoundly grateful for the opportunity to be a parent, and I intensely hoped that I could continue that role for many years.

In January 2005, I started the new year by having the yearly scans to detect cancer. The prep kit for the CT of the abdomen and bowel worked *very* effectively. I came home after the scan exhausted from the previous night in the bathroom.

I fell into bed and into a sound slumber. The next thing I knew, Tom was shaking me awake. I squinted at the clock and wondered why he was home in the middle of the day.

He sat on the bed. I could tell he had been crying.

"I have some thing to tell you," he sobbed. "There is a spot on your liver."

"It's cancer?" I asked, although I knew the answer.

"Well, we don't know for sure. But we do know that hepatitis C is a major cause of liver cancer. I'm not going to sugarcoat it. I'm afraid it is cancer."

He began to sob. I sat up and pulled him close to me. We have an unspoken arrangement in our marriage. Only one of us can decompensate at a time, and at that time, it was his turn. He cried for some time, then sat up and rubbed his eyes.

"I'm so sorry, Ev."

That was the signal that it was my turn to cry. He pulled me against his chest and all the betrayal, anger, powerlessness, sorrow and fear of the past four years came out in great gasping sobs.

When we visited the Mayo Clinic for a second opinion in January 2001, we were told that a cancer metastasis after an initial breast cancer diagnosis was disastrous. If that should happen to me, doctors would not offer hope for a cure but would set a goal of keeping me comfortable for as long as possible. Our worst fear of a cancer metastasis was realized with this apparent diagnosis of liver cancer and had likely been fueled by hepatitis C.

Unfortunately, Tom had to go back to work. We said our goodbyes to each other. Not, "Goodbye, I'll see you later," but, "Goodbye. It has been a blessing to be your spouse. I will do my best to be as patient and brave as I can be in the next months. I want you to be happy after we part. I'll look forward to our reunion on the other side."

I walked Tom to the door and waved as he drove down the driveway. I then walked to the couch and sat there, staring at the blue-grey carpet. I was not angry or sad or fearful. I was in shock. It felt like a low-level electric charge was running through my body, short-circuiting every emotion and rational thought.

I don't know how long I sat there. The next thing I knew, I had the telephone receiver to my ear.

"Ev, I just talked to *Mark Stevens*," Tom rejoiced. "He looked up your previous scans in the basement. You had that spot on your liver three years ago. He thinks it is a hemangioma. So it's nothing. You're fine. No cancer!"

"What… Who… Who is this?" I stuttered, not understanding what he'd said.

"It's Tom. Mark Stevens says you're fine!"

"Who's Mark Stevens?"

"Ev, you know Mark," Tom said patiently. "We ate supper with him and his wife last week… The radiologist."

"Why does he think I am fine?"

"Ev, listen to me," Tom spoke slowly and carefully as he drew from his years of experience of sharing life-altering news with patients. "The hospital got a new CT scanner. It has better resolution than the previous one. Today it picked up a little spot on your liver. Mark searched through the archives and found that that spot was on your liver three years ago. They did an ultrasound at that time and found it was a hemangioma. So, it's not cancer."

I tried to say something but no words would come out of my mouth.

"Ev, do you understand me?" Tom finally asked.

Again, I was speechless as I tried to wrap my mind around this information.

"Ev, say something. Answer me," Tom commanded.

A third time my mouth tried to form words, but nothing would come out.

"Ev, do you need me to come home?" Tom asked forcefully.

His question startled me into a reaction. In the twenty-three years that we had been in Fremont, there was only one time that Tom had left an office full of patients and come home in the middle of the day. That one time had been one hour earlier.

"No. I'm okay," I finally answered. "You think I'm okay?"

"Yes, you're fine."

"I don't need any additional tests or anything?"

"No."

"There's no liver cancer?"

"No."

"So, now what?" I asked, still befuddled. "What should I do now?"

"Just go back to your 'perfectly normal life,'" Tom answered, echoing the common misperception about the Nebraska outbreak victims.

We hung up. I went back to the couch and sat there a long time, again staring a hole in the blue carpet. I didn't know what a "perfectly normal life" was but I was pretty sure I didn't have one.

I had had two big shocks within an hour. After the first shock, I could feel no grief or any negative emotion. After this second shock, I could feel no happiness or any positive emotion. I was numb. I walked around in a daze for a week. It was impossible to concentrate on work or a coherent conversation.

The night terrors started shortly thereafter. I had long, terrifyingly real dreams that caused me to wake up screaming. Strangely, Tom was the one who was threatened in these dreams. It was Tom who was being trampled by horses or falling through the ice on a lake or sitting in the chemo recliner with IV tubing and needles attached. I would wake up screaming in fright. I would rush to the phone to call him to see if he was alright, sobbing so hard he couldn't make out what I was saying. He had to reassure me over and over that he was fine.

I couldn't shake off the anxiety that these dreams stirred in me. Despite my best efforts to think of something else, I found myself running over the details of the dreams again and again. I began to obsess. What if something did happen to Tom? How could I take care of the boys? How could I take care of myself? I didn't have a good answer to these questions and my trepidation increased out of control.

One morning in March 2005, I stumbled to the kitchen to fix myself some oatmeal. While it was heating, I swallowed my morning pills. Among the pill bottles was the pain medication (Propoxyphene HCL) that I took for joint pain. I opened the bottle and counted the pills.

At that point, one of the pills skittered out of my palm. I turned to pick it up from the counter and caught sight of my reflection in the microwave. I was stunned by my appearance. Even in the distorted reflection of the microwave, I saw that I looked very disheveled and extremely depressed and I was clutching a handful of pain pills! The vision pushed me into much-needed action. I put the pills back in the bottle and picked up the telephone. When Dr. Osborn's receptionist answered the phone, I asked for the earliest possible appointment.

Dr. Osborn prescribed antidepressants for me. I found them to be a miracle of modern medicine. Within a couple of weeks, the night terrors stopped. I also sought counseling to help with the depression with my good friend, Jean Riggins, a licensed mental health counselor. She helped me see that I had been very sad for a very long time. She helped me adjust to and accept my situation.

I stopped obsessing about the future and the possibility that I may not see my sons walk down the aisle on their wedding days or hold their children in my arms. I was able to see my sons as they were in the present and enjoy their caring, fun-loving, ways. I developed a new appreciation for the wonderful relationship that Tom and I shared. I realized that I was, indeed, a very lucky woman.

Living With Hepatitis C

For me, living with hepatitis C is like having the flu twenty-four hours a day, seven days a week, three hundred sixty-five days a year. Like a flu virus, the hepatitis C virus causes fatigue and muscle and joint aches.

Do you recall the last time you had the flu? You tossed and turned all night and woke up in the morning thinking, *Oh, I'm so tired and achy—I must be coming down with the flu.* But you decided to go to work and try to get through the morning. At noontime, you stretched as you thought to yourself, *I must be coming down with the flu. I'm so tired, weak and achy.* So you put your head down on your desk and napped a bit but decided to try to get through the afternoon.

As soon as you could, you headed home after work and then took up residence on the couch. At nine o'clock in the evening, you dragged yourself to bed, where you had another fitful night's sleep. In the morning, you thought, *I must be coming down with the flu.*

And so it goes that day and the next day and the next day and the next day for those with hepatitis C. During our days of fatigue and joint pain, we wonder when the serious problem of liver cirrhosis will begin.

There are ways of coping with the symptoms of hepatitis C, and fortunately, these methods are getting better all the time. A diet rich in protein and low in iron and fat is helpful. Alcohol must be eliminated completely. A balance of rest, exercise and activity is important.

Finding a proper balance of rest and activity is most difficult for me. Sometimes I overestimate my stamina and do too much. Then, I have to pay the price of increased fatigue and joint/muscle pain. Sometimes I don't push myself enough and then pay the price of needlessly missing out on activities that enrich my life. Finding this balance is important for my physical comfort and my mental health and for strengthening relationships with my loved ones.

My physicians and I search for medications that will improve my quality of life. I am on medications for sleep, pain and depression and find these medications helpful. However, taking all these medications plus a daily chemotherapy pill causes me to worry that I am taxing my already stressed liver.

People infected with hepatitis C must have hope for the future. We hope that researchers will find a new, more effective, less challenging treatment that will cure hepatitis C. We hope that there will be no more instances of healthcare transmission of hepatitis C. We hope that everyone will be screened and take preventative measures to stop the spread of hepatitis C. We hope that a vaccine will be discovered that prevents hepatitis C. And finally, we hope that you will join us in advocating for hepatitis C research and education so that these hopes turn into reality.

CHAPTER 31

■

Evelyn Tells
Her Litigation Story

I was completely naïve to the litigation process when the Nebraska outbreak was uncovered in 2002. Tom and I knew nothing about litigation or who to go to for help.

The most pressing issue, however, was not how to file a lawsuit, but whether to file a lawsuit at all. Javed had, after all, saved my life twice. He had been a trusted friend. Surely he'd had a good (or at least forgivable) explanation for the whole sorry mess. And as for the nurses? If they'd been acting on the doctor's orders, could one fault them for that? What about the hospital? Tom had cared for patients there day and night for twenty-one years. At first, I couldn't fathom filing suit against the hospital.

We were plagued with other questions. How had all this happened? Could it possibly happen again? What needed to be done so it didn't happen again, anywhere, anytime? We wrestled with these questions day and night.

We needed a fresh perspective. Tom remembered a casual acquaintance who made his living defending physicians in malpractice suits. Tom called him and briefly explained our situation. He listened sympathetically to our story and then said emphatically, "You need to hire an attorney to represent you."

"Are you suggesting that we file suit against Javed?" Tom asked, surprised.

"From what you have told me and what I have read in the newspapers, yes. You have a very strong case and this man needs to be brought to justice."

When Tom got off the phone, we looked at each other in amazement. A lawyer who defended physicians against malpractice was telling us that we should sue a fellow doctor!

In the past several decades, a growing animosity had mushroomed between doctors and plaintiffs' lawyers, directly related to the increase in malpractice suits against physicians. Huge distrust existed in both camps. Some doctors believed that plaintiffs' lawyers enticed patients to sue their doctors if the patients had even a very minor and unavoidable complication. Some plaintiffs' lawyers believed that doctors had a God complex and would admit no imperfection, even when negligence was obvious. Doctors thought that plaintiffs' lawyers convinced juries, with courtroom dramatics, to award outlandish awards to malingering plaintiffs. Plaintiffs' lawyers believed that all juries sided with "the good doctor" no matter how blatant the malpractice.

Defense lawyers were hired by malpractice insurance companies to represent doctors. Some malpractice insurance companies distributed sensational propaganda about runaway jury verdicts and innocent physicians being stripped of all their personal assets, even though these dire outcomes very seldom happened. Through these half-truths, the insurance companies rationalized outlandish malpractice insurance premiums.

Adding to our discomfort was the combative nature of litigation. Litigation placed the opposing parties in adversarial positions. It was a system that stressed deception rather than accountability.

Tom spoke after we digested all these thoughts a bit.

"Well, *if* we decide to sue, how in the world do we find a personal injury lawyer?" he asked. "We want one who is upright and honest. We need a person who will represent us with integrity, conviction but equanimity. And, given how gossip flourishes in this small town, we want one who is not from Fremont. We don't want to fuel any rumors by being seen walking into a lawyer's office in Fremont."

We considered the task ahead of us. There were pages and pages of personal injury lawyers in the Omaha phone book and probably just as many in the Lincoln phone book. Short of interviewing each and every one, it seemed unlikely that we would find a lawyer who would fit our qualifications.

Instead, we asked for recommendations from our professional associates in Omaha. Matt Miller's name was mentioned most often. After we interviewed him, we knew he was the right man for the job.

A Very Short Statute of Limitations

We bent Matt Miller's ear for three hours straight at the first meeting. We found him appropriately sympathetic, knowledgeable and rational. He helped us sort out our thoughts about filing suit against the defendants.

"Matt, what is the reason to file a suit? What will we gain? Is it just money?" I asked. "Money won't give me my health back. Will a lengthy litigation be worthwhile to us, given that we are financially secure? Regarding the defendants," I continued, "Javed is gone and not coming back. Nurse Prochaska is no longer working in Fremont. And as for the hospital, well, we think the hospital will work with us directly regarding important patient safety policies so that this doesn't happen again."

"That's a good question," he answered thoughtfully. "I'm glad that you are financially secure—most people are not. For you, this is an issue of justice. Litigation is the method that we have to ensure that the guilty parties take responsibility for their actions and that they do learn from this fiasco. To date, no one has challenged the guilty parties in a lawsuit. Someone needs to make the guilty parties accountable," he said vehemently. "Litigation isn't a perfect system, but it is what we have. I know this is a difficult decision for you. Why don't you think about it and get back to me? But I do want to caution you about one thing. The statute of limitations is two years. The defense will be sticky about this point and insist that the statute of limitations expires two years from the date that you were first treated by Dr. Javed. Odds are, the judge won't interpret the statute of limitations that way, but there's always a chance. So, when was your first chemotherapy infusion, Evelyn?"

"November 17, 2000," I answered.

"Okay, this is October 31, 2002. November 17 is on a Sunday, so we would need to file by Friday, November 15. I'm sorry you have to make a decision so quickly but I think it is best that you do. You can always file suit and then drop it later if that's what you decide. Why don't you come back and see me in a week? You may have thought of more questions," Matt offered.

In the Beginning

When our children were still at home, I worried that Tom and I would not have anything to talk about when our nest was empty. Our supper table conversations had always been with the kids. We talked about soccer matches, spelling lists and tree house projects.

Silly me. I didn't need to worry—we had plenty to talk about. I never could have imagined, though, that our conversations would revolve around THE LAWSUIT. The lawsuit conversations started November 1, 2002 and went on for more than five years.

After much emotional discussion, we decided that I would file suit against

Javed and Prochaska. It was very difficult to work through the issues regarding filing suit against Tahir Javed. We'd had great admiration for and loyalty to him for the years that he'd treated me. Within a few months, we'd had to face the fact that he had betrayed us and the whole community of Dodge County. Then, we'd had to take the next step and authorize the filing of the suit. It caused us endless discussions, tears and sleepless nights.

Because we are rather private people, we decided that Tom would not be a party in the suit. We hoped that by leaving him out of the suit, our life would be shielded from public display. We also decided at that time that I would not file suit against the hospital. Even though the hospital president admitted to Tom that "the hospital has some liability," we felt loyalty to the hospital and we were sure that we could work together with the administration to examine the situation and correct any deficiencies on the hospital's part.

Matt was sympathetic with our reticence to sue the hospital but again, he was concerned about the statute of limitations. He suggested that we file a Nebraska Political Subdivision Tort Claims Act (NPSTCA) notice—a formal letter to the hospital that informed them of an intention to file suit. If we filed the NPSTCA notice now, before the statute of limitations expired, it would enable us to sue the hospital down the road if we changed our minds.

"If you don't do this," Matt pointed out, "what will you do if the hospital refuses to listen to your concerns?"

"Oh, the hospital will listen to us," I answered confidently. "But okay, if it isn't binding, then go ahead and file the notice. Tom will call the hospital and set up a meeting with administration to talk about policy and procedure changes so this kind of thing won't happen again."

"Actually, why don't you let me call the malpractice insurance lawyer who is representing the hospital to set up the meeting?" Matt replied. "It's the proper protocol in this sort of thing. I'll get back to you next week with the meeting time."

Tom had been on the medical staff at Fremont Area Medical Center for twenty-one years. We'd thought he had a good relationship with the administration and board of trustees. We were eager to meet with them to share our ideas about patient safety policy changes that would benefit the community and prevent this type of disaster in the future.

Fremont Area Medical Center, through their legal counsel, refused to meet with us. We were incredulous.

"Are you sure you understood the hospital's lawyer correctly?" I asked Matt.

"Yes, I'm sure. I'm sorry," he answered. "They probably were scared off by the NPSTCA notice."

"What do you mean, 'scared off'?"

"They interpreted it as a definite decision to file suit. They didn't want to say anything in a meeting that could be held against them in a court of law."

"We weren't asking them to say anything. We were asking them to listen. Plus, we were quite willing to have their legal counsel present."

"Yes. Regardless, their decision is not to meet with you."

"Well, what do we do now? How do we get them to listen to us?"

"I think you have two options. You can write them a letter or you can authorize a formal suit against them. I'm here to help you sort out those options if you need a sounding board," Matt offered.

After much more emotional discussion with Tom and Matt, I did both.

The Evil Mr. Pie

During the litigation process, Tom and I attended several depositions. As I sat through some depositions and read the written transcripts of other depositions, I admired how articulate, knowledgeable and clever the attorneys were. Begrudgingly, I grew to respect some lawyers on the opposite side of the litigation. There was one I did not respect, however. He was the stereotypical aggressive, argumentative lawyer.

During one very quarrelsome deposition, my frustration with him grew. I began to daydream about a drive-by pie-throwing. As I watched him verbally abuse a plaintiff's lawyer, I imagined sneaking up to the conference table with a cream pie behind my back. When I reached his chair, I launched the pie in his face before I quickly ducked out of the room.

The thought tickled me so much that I giggled out loud. Several very serious, very dignified attorneys in the room shot questioning looks at me. I slunk down in my chair and struggled to stifle my giggling. The harder I tried, the more I giggled. I could feel the stern looks from the business suits in the room so I kept my head down and started to cough. I quickly exited the conference room and went into the restroom, where I laughed so hard that tears rolled down my cheeks.

After some time, I stopped laughing, blew my nose and wiped my eyes. I looked at myself in the mirror and thought about how bizarre the situation was. I was in the women's restroom, dreaming about embarrassing a man who was arguing with another man over technicalities. The financial and emotional well-being of eighty-nine suffering human beings would be impacted by the outcome of these arguments. I couldn't speak for myself, and I could not sit down with the defendants to work through the issues of our disagreement. The feelings of powerlessness and injustice were chipping away at my composure.

From my perspective, Mr. Pie was ruthless and cold-hearted toward the plaintiffs. He did not see us as fellow human beings with feelings, families and futures. We were problems that he had to attack and dispose of as quickly and cheaply as possible. When the Nebraska outbreak was over, he would go back to his ritzy Omaha law firm and never think about us again. The long-term welfare of our community was of no concern to him.

"Why is Mrs. McKnight so angry?" Mr. Pie asked my attorney one day, late in the litigation process.

This question came after three years of recorded testimony by plaintiffs and their treating physicians describing the betrayal, stigma, anxiety and physical discomfort that hepatitis C had brought us. Even if he believed only half of what our physicians described and discounted everything that the plaintiffs said, it was incomprehensible to me that he didn't have an inkling of the distress that we endured.

Shortly after we began collaborating on this book, Travis asked me if I was disgusted with all lawyers based on the actions of Mr. Pie. The answer was and continues to be, "Of course not." Granted, Pie's behavior was despicable. There are members of every profession that behave badly. However, I have seen, through Travis Bennington, Matt Miller, Jim Brown and other lawyers, how decent some attorneys are. Skillful and upright attorneys abound on both sides of every legal issue. It is the duty of litigants to engage principled legal counsel and to direct them ethically.

Fighting for Reform

My case was not chosen as one of the three category cases to go to trial, but one by one, those cases settled out of court. New cases were scheduled. One by one, those cases settled, too. My case became the next one scheduled to go to trial and was assigned a court date in June 2006.

Matt asked us if he could bring Jim Brown into the case as co-counsel. I readily agreed. I had seen Jim in action in depositions and was impressed with his wealth of knowledge. He had been a family physician for years before he'd gone to law school, and now had many years of experience as a plaintiffs' lawyer. As a physician, he had been compassionate and skilled in medicine; as a lawyer, he was passionate for plaintiffs' rights and versed in nuances of the law.

Matt and Jim called us into Matt's office in Omaha several times to keep us abreast of developments. They brought up the option of mediation.

In mediation, the two sides sit down with a professional mediator, who helps the parties reach an agreement for a monetary settlement to be paid to the plaintiff. The defendants are not required to declare guilt or innocence.

"What are the advantages of mediation?" I asked.

"If the mediation is successful, you will be finished with the lawsuit within a month or so, rather than a year or more. You will avoid the public scrutiny and emotional drain of a trial," Matt answered. "You will have one day of discomfort—the day of mediation—rather than the three weeks of distress of a trial."

"Through mediation, is there any way that the causes or lessons of the Nebraska outbreak are examined by the affected parties—or by anyone, for that matter?"

"No. As the system is designed now, it is simply a coming together to discuss a monetary settlement. You'll have a chance to tell your side of the story to the mediator in order to help him understand, but no one else will hear your story. The only way to shine a light on this sordid affair is to take it to trial."

"Then we will take it to trial," I said while Tom nodded his head in agreement.

Defense attorneys asked for mediation time and time again. Jim often crossed paths with them at depositions.

"Why won't Mrs. McKnight come to mediation? What does she want?" one attorney asked. "Money is no object," he emphasized with shrugged shoulders and upright palms.

"It will take more than money to get her to settle," Jim retorted.

"Like what? What else is there?"

"The McKnights asked the hospital board of trustees to meet with them regarding necessary patient safety policy changes at the start of this litigation. That would have been a beginning of a dialogue. They want to see some changes made at the hospital so this sort of thing never happens again," Jim replied courteously.

"Tell you what. Have her write up her list of demands," the defense attorney offered. "I'm going to go out on a limb and speak for all the defendants and say we'll take a look at them."

Tom and I were moving Alex to the University of Notre Dame when Matt called us and relayed the defense's offer to entertain non-monetary terms. On the sixteen-hour drive to and from South Bend, Indiana, we brainstormed our ideas until we came up with a list of twenty. We put it into a letter dated August 22, 2005 and sent it off.

We discussed the defense's response with Matt and Jim a month later.

"Evelyn and Tom, you have received the defense's reply. What do you think of it?" Matt asked.

"Matt," I told him, "of the twenty requests, one was agreed to, eleven were answered with, 'Well, maybe, with qualifications,' and eight were flatly refused. That isn't good enough. I don't understand why defense is fighting us on improvements that would safeguard against an outbreak in the future. I'm ready to proceed to trial."

"Are you sure? Defense has indicated that they put a lot of time and effort into this reply. A trial will be hard on everyone."

"Yes, I understand. Regardless, our decision is to go to trial," I affirmed, as Tom nodded his head in agreement.

A Visit From Board Members

"Two hospital board members are coming to visit with me after clinic hours tomorrow," Tom said to me at the dinner table one evening in November 2005.

"Oh, really? Do you think they are coming to talk about the lawsuit?" I asked.

"No, definitely not. No one from the hospital has ever mentioned a word to me about the lawsuit. I'm sure it is a courtesy call. Board members visit with physicians sometimes to see how everything is going. If they were going to talk about the lawsuit, they would ask for you to come."

The two board members were rather new appointees. We had known both since we'd first moved to Fremont twenty-four years earlier. We respected them both very much.

They were waiting in Tom's private office for him when he finished seeing patients the next day. There was no small talk about families or the weather. They cut right to the chase.

"Tom, what will it take to settle the lawsuit? We want to see this matter put to rest."

"What will it take?" Tom asked. "Didn't you see a copy of Evelyn's letter regarding patient safety policies?"

"Yes, we did. But you know, she asks for things we cannot do. The administration has spent a lot of sleepless nights thinking about it. We just can't do all the things she asks for."

"Oh." Tom paused. "I see." He paused again. "I guess I don't understand. I don't think there was anything in our list of demands that was extraordinary. We think the demands will make the hospital better."

There was an awkward silence. Clearly, the two men disagreed with Tom about the demands. After a brief discussion of other hospital matters, they stood up, thanked him for his time and left.

Tom sat back in his chair and reflected. How bizarre. He had spent much of the last twenty-four years making rounds, delivering babies and sewing up lacerations at Fremont Area Medical Center. He had spent so many hours there that I had virtually been a single parent to our three sons. He had always promised me that we would make up for lost time during his retirement.

Now, our retirement together was in jeopardy because of the hepatitis C I had contracted within a private physician's clinic within the physical confines of the hospital. Even more incredibly, I was suing the hospital where he had spent so much of his life.

My Deposition

My deposition was scheduled for January 12, 2006. The plan was that my deposition would be first and when it was finished, Tom's deposition would begin. If we were lucky, both would be completed in one day. I prepared by reviewing my symptom diary and my personal notes and by making a list of how hepatitis C affected me. I didn't need to bother. The defense wasn't very interested in these issues. They had other topics on their minds.

I was very nervous before the deposition. I knew that I had done nothing wrong and that I would speak the truth. I also knew that the defense attorneys were very skillful at confounding witnesses and twisting their words.

Present at the deposition were the risk management supervisor from the hospital, the court reporter, seven attorneys and me. Two attorneys represented me, two represented the Nebraska Excess Liability Fund, and one represented each of the other defendants—Prochaska, Javed and the hospital. After the court reporter had me swear to tell the truth, Javed's attorney stated that he would not allow Tom in the room. He had that right because Tom had not filed the lawsuit with me. As Tom left the room, I had a sinking feeling in my stomach. How could I do this without him? He was always a source of courage for me. Just seeing the determination in his face gave me strength.

I got through the deposition, all nine hours of it, but it was very draining. During the first four hours, the defense attorneys asked a few questions about the effects of hepatitis C, and then quickly moved on to questioning me about my property holdings, my audiology practice and my understanding of my prognosis, regarding both cancer and hepatitis C. These were easy questions that I could answer. They also asked many questions about Tom. How many patients did he see in a day? How many babies did he deliver in a year? What medical staff committees had he been on and when? What financial arrangement did he have with the hospital? I had enough on my plate managing my own life. It was way beyond me to keep tabs on Tom's superhuman existence.

Consequently, for more than an hour, my response to these types of questions was "I don't know."

About halfway through the morning, we moved on to other topics, such if I was angry that I had been given a disease that could kill me. The morning concluded with questions about how many people from Dodge County had sent me get well cards during my chemotherapy. At lunch, Tom grilled Jim, Matt and me about the deposition. The deposition was held in the conference room at his clinic and he had spent the morning in his office, thumbing through notes to prepare himself for his deposition and being nervous, both for himself and for me.

Mr. Pie took over questioning in mid-afternoon. He referred to my request to meet with the board of trustees regarding patient safety policies at the start of the lawsuit in January 2003. He asked me what concerns I had at the present time.

I outlined five concerns that I could come up with extemporaneously. One by one, Mr. Pie dissected these concerns. And one by one, by complicated and convoluted questions, he confused and attempted to discredit me. It was a very draining and humbling three hours of questioning. As he continued to attack my position on needed improvements in hospital policies, I couldn't help but wonder why there was so much resistance to improvements that would prevent another such tragedy.

As the hours dragged on, my responses became progressively weary. Finally, Matt stopped the questioning at five o'clock, for a break. He took me aside for a private conference.

"Evelyn, you are doing great, but I can tell you are getting tired. Do you want to stop for the day?"

"Am I making too many mistakes?" I asked.

"No, you're doing fine. You are doing very well."

I looked at him suspiciously. I didn't know if I should believe him. After hours of hostile grilling, my defenses were up. At that moment, Mr. Pie had caused me to distrust everyone in a business suit—even Matt, who I trusted explicitly during every other moment of our association.

Finally, about five-thirty, the questioning was turned over to another defense attorney. He asked me in several ways how much money defense would have to pay me to settle the lawsuit and give up my fight for improvement.

I wondered why he was asking about money when my primary motive in the lawsuit was to improve patient safety in Dodge County. No matter how many times I asked for positive change, the real issue was still money.

"So, I'm going to repeat it. How much?" the lawyer asked again.

All eyes were on me, waiting for a response. I was well aware of what was expected of me. I had been a doctor's wife my entire adult life. Everyone in the room, except my own lawyers, expected me to be loyal to the local healthcare providers and let them off easy, with minimal damages.

From the first moment that I understood that I had a legitimate claim for damages, at the start of litigation three and a half years earlier, I had decided that any money I received would be used for doing good. As defense asked me again and again about how much money I wanted, I decided that I was going to get as much money as I could. I would use the money for patient advocacy.

"The cap," I answered evenly. "$1.2 million…the cap."

I had just asked for the maximum amount allowed by law in Nebraska. The defense attorneys were speechless at my seemingly outlandish request.

"No further questions," they stated one by one.

The deposition ended abruptly, nine hours after it had begun.

Tom's Deposition

Tom's deposition took place on February 9, 2006. Mr. Pie was very congenial and called him "sir" and "doctor." It made me livid that Pie had mistreated me so egregiously but was ingratiating to Tom.

As I listened to the proceedings, I tried to puzzle out why Pie was being so cordial to Tom but had ripped me to shreds. The only explanation I could come up with was that as a malpractice defense lawyer, Pie represented physicians. It would have been politically incorrect for him to be nasty to Tom, a physician. I was not a physician, I was a plaintiff. He saw it as his duty to berate me.

The deposition started at nine o'clock in the morning and continued into the afternoon without a lunch break. The three defense lawyers politely questioned Tom. Eight times, the hospital's attorney used the term "cover up" in questioning Tom about the hospital's behavior in response to the reports it had fielded of improper procedures in Fremont Cancer Center.

"You can call it a cover up, or you can call it not bringing the information forward, but I call it a cover up, if that is the name you want to put on it," Tom agreed.

"We've talked in detail," the lawyer said, "and I used the word before you did, Doctor, so don't think I'm putting this word in your mouth, of a possible cover up by the hospital in relation to Dr. Javed in the hepatitis C outbreak. Have we discussed every way that you believe that there may have been a less than full and frank discussion of those issues with the appropriate medical staff committees?"

Tom tried to remember all the things that the hospital knew regarding problems in Fremont Cancer Center. He listed them one after another.

"Do you have any information that—and again, it's my word, not yours—that this cover up or lack of providing information to the medical staff committees was motivated by the development of Health Park Plaza?" the hospital attorney continued.

As I listened to this exchange, I wondered if the hospital's lawyer knew something we didn't know. We had never accused them of a "cover up." The only thing we ever alleged in litigation was that they had liability—that they'd had information from numerous sources, for an extended period of time, but had failed to act.

The Campaign for Mediation

Several weeks later, Matt and Jim asked us to come into their Omaha offices for a conference. We thought that they would simply update us on how litigation was progressing. Instead, we got a powerful argument in favor of mediation.

"I spent time with the defense lawyers at several recent expert witness depositions," Jim began. "With the strength of your depositions and the strength of the expert witness depositions, I think we should consider mediation. I'll tell you why. They have asked several times if your list of demands from August 22, 2005 still stands. They appear more willing to negotiate regarding the patient safety points. I think you are the only plaintiff who can get them to make changes and I know you want to see things changed. These are issues that neither a judge nor a jury can award. If we go to mediation, however, I think we can get them to agree to your patient safety demands.'

"And," Matt continued, "I don't think the defense wants to take your case to trial. They may wait until we are walking up the courthouse steps, but I believe that they will admit guilt rather than have you two tell your story on the stand. They don't want this on the front page of the newspaper. Instead, they would admit guilt by wrapping it up in a nice big bow. By this, I mean they would issue a finely crafted press release. It would say something like, 'The hospital recognizes the great suffering in the community because of the actions of one doctor and one nurse as related to the Nebraska hepatitis C outbreak. Rather than add to the emotional and financial suffering of this community by reliving the horrors of the Nebraska outbreak for several weeks in a court trial, we have opted to admit liability. We believe that this action will facilitate the healing that this community deserves. The hospital will continue to provide compassionate care that the community can trust.'

"So," Matt concluded, "we think we should resubmit your list of demands to the defense. We'll see how they respond. If they are willing to negotiate, we will set up mediation. Remember, if we get to mediation, we can always walk out at any time if we feel the defense is being unreasonable."

Tom and I looked at each other.

"Okay," I said rather reluctantly. "But I've heard that in mediation, the monetary award is kept confidential. Will there be a confidentiality clause on the non-monetary points? We want the world to know that the plaintiffs are not just interested in money."

"Oh, no, just the monetary award will be confidential. There is no precedent to require the non-monetary points to be kept confidential," we were assured.

"Okay, we'll consider mediation, but you tell the defense they'd better come into this with a spirit of cooperation. Otherwise, we are all wasting our time," I stressed.

"Agreed." Matt and Jim nodded.

Tom and I went home and reviewed the initial demands of August 22, 2005. We modified a few of them and sent them to our attorneys. Again, there were twenty steps we wanted the hospital to implement.

A few days later, we got a response from our attorneys.

"They said they are willing to negotiate your changes," Matt said. "They said they agree to all twenty *in theory*."

We were overcome with optimism. We felt like we were finally making progress. We were ready to go to mediation.

The Telephone Survey

A few days later, Tom called me at my office.

"You won't believe what Dr. Beacom just told me," he said angrily. "Someone is conducting a telephone survey. They ask questions like, 'Do you know Dr. McKnight? Do you know anything about a lawsuit involving Evelyn McKnight? Is Dr. McKnight your physician?' This just makes my blood boil. I'm ready to call off the mediation!"

"Wait! What does this have to do with the mediation?" I asked in surprise.

"I don't know for sure, but I bet defense is gathering information to see if they can get the case moved out of the county. If they have a lot of evidence to show that we are too well-known in the county to have a fair trial, they will use it against us in mediation to get us to settle. But why don't you call Jim and Matt and ask them what they think?"

Jim and Matt were just as furious as we were. They asked if I could get specific questions from someone who had taken the survey. I asked around and found someone who agreed to talk to me. Her husband was the superintendent of a neighboring school district. I took careful notes and then submitted them to Matt and Jim.

Jim called the hospital's attorney and asked that the telephone survey be dropped. The hospital's lawyer sent an email around to all the other defense lawyers, asking that the survey be stopped immediately.

We soon found out that the Nebraska Excess Liability Fund (NELF) was conducting the survey "to collect data to know if the Ridder case and subsequent cases should be moved out of Dodge County." It didn't make sense. The Ridder case had been tried five months earlier. It was over and done with. My case was the next one on the docket.

The telephone survey was repulsive. I've never felt so betrayed and so robbed of my right to privacy. What was just as offensive was *who* was conducting the survey. The NELF's lawyers were conducting it so they could get my case moved out of Dodge County. Since my husband was a Nebraska physician, he was required to pay into the NELF. The state of Nebraska, as administrator of the NELF, was using my own money to fight against me.

March 22, 2006

The day of the mediation finally arrived. Both Tom and I were nervous. We continued to hope that the hospital would finally accept our proposed twenty non-monetary points.

When we arrived, we were ushered into a large conference room. The mediator was the retired dean of Drake Law School in Des Moines, Iowa. Matt had recommended him because of his reputation for fairness.

The mediator, Linda Prochaska's attorney, the hospital's attorney, the hospital's in-house legal counsel, and the attorney representing the state of Nebraska and the NELF were all there—even though we were not suing, nor had any quarrel with, the state of Nebraska. Some members of the hospital board of trustees and administration were present. As always, Dr. Tahir Javed and Linda Prochaska were conspicuously absent.

The mediator gave a few opening comments stressing cooperation and patience. Then, he asked if anyone had any comments.

"Folks, I want to say that I feel terrible. We all feel terrible about what happened," Nurse Prochaska's attorney said.

"I want to say also on behalf of Fremont Area Medical Center that we feel terrible about what happened in a private physician's clinic," the hospital's lawyer said.

Tom and I nodded in acceptance. It was the closest thing to an apology that we had heard in three and a half years. I wished with all my heart that the other victims would have heard the "apology." They needed to hear it as much as I did.

We were split into camps. The defense was in one room and we were in another.

The mediator met with us first. He asked us to tell our story. He made notes and seemed sympathetic. Again, he asked us to be cooperative, patient and flexible.

He then met in private with the defense. He was with them for close to an hour before he returned.

"Well, folks, I believe I have an understanding of both sides of the situation. The defense is offering you this amount," he slid his note pad to us.

"You tell them we are not going to let them waste our time. I'm insulted with that number!" Tom shot back.

"Just a minute, Tom," Matt said. "This is a bit of chest beating on their part. This isn't their final number. Let's give them another chance. "

The day progressed slowly. The mediator would go to the defense, spend half an hour with them and then come back to our room to give us the offer. We would discuss it and counter-offer. Their offer would go up a nickel, and the mediator would then talk us into reducing our demand by a dime. The bartering went back and forth. When we broke for lunch, we weren't ready to leave the bargaining table but we were certainly tired of the procedure. Matt and Jim urged us to have patience, reminding us over and over again that if we couldn't reach an agreement today, we would have no hope of getting our twenty non-monetary points implemented.

About mid-afternoon, the process came to a crawl. The mediator was spending longer and longer in the defense's room but was unable to get them to make a fair proposal.

The mediator came into our room at about three o'clock in the afternoon. I could tell by his body language that he didn't have good news for us.

"The defense is saying they won't go any higher," he said. "Will you accept their last offer?"

"No," Tom and I said in unison. "I guess it is time to go home."

"Now, just a minute," Matt said to the mediator. "Are they aware of the damage to the hospital's reputation if Tom and Evelyn are brought to the witness stand? Have they discussed that in their room?"

"Yes, and they say they have a strong defense."

"Well, I'd like to know what it is," I stated.

"They haven't spelled out the particulars so I don't know what it is. Mr. Ridder's award has been brought up several times. They just don't think your case is worth more than his."

"However," Jim explained, "Bob Ridder and Evelyn do not have the same damages. Evelyn is ten years younger than he is, and did not clear the virus after six months of horrific treatment. Bob is virus-free. She doesn't have any treatment options left."

As gently as he could, the mediator turned to me.

"They have discussed your medical condition. They quoted a Mayo Clinic report. It said that since you have already had one recurrence of your cancer, you have an eighty-five percent chance of having the cancer come back again within five to ten years. They feel that you will die of cancer before the hepatitis C can do you any real harm."

I was livid.

"It's already done me real harm," I nearly screamed. "Every joint, every muscle in my body hurts. I grieve over the past, I'm depressed about the present, I'm anxious about the future. Hepatitis C has decreased both the quality and the quantity of my life. If they think it is no big deal, I'll trade my health status for theirs and they can keep their money."

"It's been four years since her last occurrence," Tom added his two cents worth. "She is in the fifteen to twenty percent who won't develop cancer because it usually occurs within the first several years."

Tom had finally had enough. He drew in a breath.

"You tell the defense this," he said coldly. "It has been so difficult for me to go to that hospital every day for the past three and one-half years of this lawsuit. I want to enjoy taking care of my patients in the hospital like I used to. The new highway bypass will allow me to get to West Omaha hospitals in twenty minutes. I have been seriously considering taking all my patients to Omaha. My partner will take his patients there if I do. Do they understand what that would mean to the hospital if one-fourth of their patients suddenly disappeared?"

The mediator capped his pen and sat back in his chair. The threat was serious and he knew it. He scratched a number out on his notepad.

"I think I can get them up to this number. Will you accept it?" he asked us.

"I have to think about it," I replied slowly. "Tom, will you walk around the parking lot with me? We can talk while we stretch our legs."

We bundled up in our coats and exited the building. We trudged around the parking lot arm in arm, dodging the patches of dirty snow.

Neither of us wanted to be the first to speak.

"Well, you know, we've always said it wasn't about the money, it was about patient safety," Tom finally broke the silence.

"Yeah, I know. It's just the principle of the thing. They tell us, 'Money is no object' and then they fight tooth and nail over every penny. Plus, the money will be used for patient safety, so it would be nice to get as much as possible," I complained.

"Yes, that's true. You know, I've been thinking about what might be going on in the other room. The lawyer representing the NELF is sitting in that room. I bet he is the one who is putting on the brakes. Now that everyone else has reached their insurance limits, the fund is the only one with a financial stake in this."

"I didn't think of that," I said disgustedly. "Another example of the state of Nebraska fighting against the victims," I snorted.

"Yeah, this hasn't been easy. It's been an emotionally draining battle for years now," Tom said with a heavy sigh. "It would be nice to get the hospital to make our changes, so that this sort of tragedy doesn't happen again. If we get those changes made, we can let the other victims know and future patients will be safe."

"Uh-huh, yes," I answered as I thought about the situation. My pace slowed until I stopped walking altogether. "Would you mind if I took a lap around the parking lot by myself? I just need a little more time," I said to Tom.

This time around the parking lot, I talked to my dad. Not on a cell phone, but in my heart. My dad had passed away eight years earlier. He had been a farmer all his life. He'd farmed with horses in his young years and then gradually changed over to tractors when they'd become affordable and efficient. Dad had had a reputation as a "horse trader." He'd prided himself in getting the best deal possible whether he bartered for a horse or a tractor or a combine.

Unlike Dad, I wasn't bartering about the value of a horse, or a tractor or a combine. I was bartering about the value of *my life*.

What was my life worth in dollars? I did not know. I did know that if I had the choice between all the money in the world and good health, I would take good health in a heartbeat. However, there was no way the defendants, or anyone else for that matter, could give me back my health. I had to accept that fact and move on.

"Dad," I said, as I pictured him in his overalls and straw hat. "Is this a good deal? Should I accept it?" As I walked, I knew what his answer would be.

When I came back to our mediation room and took off my coat, I could feel the stares from everyone in the room.

"I'll take it," I said softly.

Immediately, the room erupted in handshakes and smiles as the mediator and my attorneys hurried out the door to the defense's room.

Tom and I were left alone. We looked at each other. I began to cry. He did, too. It had been a long, draining journey for us.

"Now it will all be over," Tom whispered as he held me.

"It doesn't feel good," I answered. "It doesn't feel anything." I sighed. "But maybe in time, as the twenty points are implemented, we will come to some healing."

As slow-moving as the previous seven hours of the day had been, the remaining two hours went by in a flurry of activity. Lawyers scurried back and forth between the two rooms, hammering out the details of our agreement.

At one point, I walked down the hallway between the two rooms to go to the restroom. I approached two lawyers who were deep in a discussion with their backs to me.

"We're paying this woman way too much money," I overheard one say heatedly. "The next hepatitis C case better go cheap."

I was disgusted. I cleared my throat loudly so that he would know I had heard them. They didn't react, and continued their conversation without missing a beat.

Finally, my lawyers brought the handwritten document into the room and placed it in front of me. I read it, but I could not pick up the pen to sign it.

Throughout the years of the Nebraska outbreak litigation, a number of the other victims had told me that they were not financially able to bring their cases to trial. They had hoped that I would bring my case to trial, since I had the financial resources to pay the upfront expert witness and court costs. I knew Bob Ridder hadn't been happy with his trial. I felt that I owed it to all the other victims to make sure the story was told in court. I wondered if I would dishonor Dan McGill and Cheryl Gentry and let down all the outbreak victims if I let the details of the outbreak go untold. By signing the settlement, my case would be over and there was a strong likelihood the remaining plaintiffs would not go to trial, and the truth would never come out.

Matt saw I was indecisive. He pulled his chair close to mine.

"It is the right thing to do," he said. "I know it is hard for you. But in signing this, you have accomplished more good than ever would come out of a trial. In a trial, the ugly facts would come out in the newspaper, and everyone would be appalled for a time but nothing would change. This settlement includes promises from the defendants to change their ways. You have changed the way the hospital conducts itself forever—for its own good and for the good of the community. In addition, I think you may change the way we think about litigation and mediation throughout the country. As you talk about these twenty points, it will be a model for a more rational, civilized way to right some wrongs. Evelyn, I strongly believe it is the right thing to do."

I looked at Tom. He nodded his head. I picked up the pen and signed the document as I fought back tears.

"What happens now?" I asked.

"Now the defense will draft the formal settlement documents. Then it will all be over."

Four More Months of Bickering

A month went by before we received the formal court papers from the defense. When they finally came, we were taken aback.

The formal document said we couldn't discuss the non-monetary terms of the agreement. No one would ever know that the hospital had made changes because of the outbreak. The other victims wouldn't know that their suffering hadn't been in vain. I called my attorneys right away.

"Well, you're right," Matt said. "It has to be a typo. I didn't see that when I first looked at the document. We never agreed to that. I'll call the defense and get that taken care of right away."

It was not that simple. Defense refused to sign the document. They contended that *all* terms of the settlement were to be confidential—both the monetary and non-monetary terms. The argument dragged on for four months.

We exchanged countless correspondence back and forth with the defense. The confidentiality issue was a deal-breaker. We wouldn't budge and neither would they.

I was angry, anxious and emotionally worn out from the battle. One moment, I would decide to take the case to trial. The next moment, I was ready to give up. To complicate matters, Tom vacillated on the issue too, at times, in the opposite direction I was leaning.

The Compromise

In desperation, we asked three board of trustee members to meet with us. They listened respectfully as we gave our reasons for wanting to share the twenty non-monetary points with others. They said they would see what they could do.

We received a letter from the hospital dated June 5, 2006. They proposed a middle ground. We could say that non-monetary terms were agreed upon by both parties, but we could not list the specific changes we had demanded. However, the hospital also added a new clause.

"The McKnights have not indicated, and will not indicate, that the hospital caused or contributed to the hepatitis C outbreak and have not indicated and will not indicate that there was any cover up by the hospital as to this tragedy," it read.

"Wait a minute," I said to Jim after I read the letter. "I can't sign that. It is too restrictive. I may reluctantly agree not to talk about the specific changes the hospital has to make, but I want to be able to speak openly and honestly about the outbreak."

"You're right," Jim said resignedly. "I'll send them another letter."

The hospital sent us back a letter on July 7, 2006. They had rewritten the clause.

"The McKnights are not interested in hurting the reputation of the hospital and its employees and it is not their intent to do so," the settlement document read.

"What does that mean?" Tom asked our attorneys. "The wording seems awfully nebulous. We are afraid it will be interpreted in a way that will allow the hospital to sue us if they disagree with the way we tell our story."

"No, I don't think that the language is strong enough to bring suit over," Jim said. "It sounds to me like the language was added to appease a board member. I can't imagine it was added as a non-disclosure clause. I can't imagine that anyone would think it has any strength at all."

"We're going on vacation next week to Yellowstone," we said. "Can we wait until we get back to sign it? We want a little more time to consider the situation."

"Oh, sure," Jim agreed. "The agreement has been held up four months already. Another week won't hurt."

A Change of Heart—and Back Again

It was a long drive to Yellowstone National Park and after a while, the sagebrush scenery lost its novelty. We started talking about the lawsuit outside of Grand Island, Nebraska, and continued the conversation all the way to Yellowstone and back.

Tom drove and I made lists. We filled up nearly a whole tablet of paper with lists of advantages and disadvantages of signing the compromise versus going to trial. We prioritized the lists, gave each advantage and disadvantage a weighting factor and then computed each list's score. We made a summary page of our computations. By the time we reached home, I felt as though I had completed a college course in statistical analysis.

The value of the list-making exercise was that it enabled us to verbalize our feelings about the compromise. Yes, it was sane and reasonable to sign the compromise, but our stomachs tied up in knots whenever we considered agreeing. We interpreted this as intuition warning us not to sign. Intuition was not the sole factor in making decisions, but it was a worthy consideration. We decided we would not sign the compromise and therefore, we would go to trial.

I knew that our attorneys felt that it was a good compromise and I would have to convince them of our way of thinking. I wrote my arguments for going to trial as clearly and persuasively as I could and sent it to them in an email. Matt called me immediately and asked very politely if Tom and I would come to Omaha anytime soon—nights, weekends, just soon—so we could discuss our decision.

"Wait a minute, Matt," I interrupted his goodbye. "I value your opinion and I'm too impatient to wait. Will you give me a preview of what I can expect to hear on Saturday?"

Matt was the most persuasive speaker I knew. I listened for thirty minutes while he gave his convincing arguments for signing the document.

"Evelyn," he ended. "Perhaps the most important reason for signing the compromise is that you are passionate about working for the betterment of patient safety, for improvement in the malpractice system, and for hepatitis C advocacy. If you sever the relationships you have with the local healthcare system through an adversarial trial, I'm concerned that you will be tagged with a reputation for being unyielding and unreasonable. That reputation will follow you throughout the state and possibly the nation. Your efforts will be much less effective."

My head was spinning when I hung up. I sat down on the couch and stared at the blue-grey carpet in my living room, as I had done so many times in the past four years. I tried to make sense of everything I had learned while the Nebraska outbreak lawsuits worked their way through the judicial system. Slowly, I was able to formulate my thoughts about the compromise.

First of all, it looked as if the hospital board of trustees had authorized their lawyers to take the case to court. They had been pushed to their limit and would give no further. When it went to trial, only the judge would hear the case against the hospital since it was a county entity (see Chapter 34.) Since the judge was a county employee, I feared he would have political incentives to rule in favor of the county-owned hospital.

In addition, although I thought the hospital had committed malpractice, my opinion did not matter. Only the opinion of the judge mattered. The hospital did have arguments in its favor. The question of its guilt or innocence was up for debate. If the hospital was found to be innocent, we would be disheartened, as would most of the outbreak victims.

Secondly, the jury would not be seated during the case against the hospital. The jury would not hear what the hospital had done. They would only hear about my damages and make a decision as to how much to award me. Neither they nor the judge could compel the hospital to implement any of the important non-monetary points.

Thirdly, and perhaps most importantly, pushing the board of trustees any further would result in permanent and irreparable damage to the relationship we had with them and the administration. Taking the case to trial might have resulted in a reputation of being unyielding and unreasonable. That type of reputation could follow me throughout the state and the nation. My efforts in promoting patient safety and hepatitis C advocacy and improving the malpractice system would be less effective.

The debate in my head exhausted me. I laid down on the couch. Soon, I was snoozing. I don't know if it was wisdom or weariness that whispered in my ear while I slept. But when I woke up, I knew what was tying my stomach up in knots whenever I thought about signing the document. It was the disappointment of imperfection.

During the course of litigation, Tom and I could maintain hope that if we worked hard enough to achieve our goals and remained steadfast in our efforts, the end result would be "perfect." Patient safety in our community would be improved, we would have demonstrated a method of negotiating an agreement that met the needs of a maltreated patient and we would be able to share with the other victims the specific improvements that were made because of their suffering.

Once I picked up the pen and signed the document, however, we would have to give up the hope for a perfect outcome. We would not be able to share with the other victims how their suffering had improved healthcare in the community. We would have to accept an imperfect outcome. We had been interpreting imperfection as our intuition telling us that the compromise was all wrong. It wasn't all wrong—it was just a bit imperfect to our way of thinking. Although the compromise was imperfect, it was pretty good and deserved our agreement.

When Tom came home, I told him of my decision.

"I think you hit the nail on the head," he said, looking more at ease than I had seen him in a long time. "We'll sign."

We both breathed a sigh of relief. Four years after they began, our conversations about *THE LAWSUIT* seemed to be coming to an end. Or so we thought.

More Disputes

On October 19, 2006, Tom and I met with the risk manager at the hospital and the hospital's in-house legal counsel to plan for the execution of the twenty non-monetary points. It was a cordial meeting and we left with assurances that the points would be implemented and that we would be updated on the progress.

Time passed without further word from the hospital. Tom, Travis and I busied ourselves by launching a patient advocacy group which we named *Hepatitis Outbreaks' National Organization for Reform* (HONOReform). We founded HONOReform in hopes that we could make sure that no one ever had to suffer through a tragedy like the Nebraska outbreak again.

We arranged for a follow-up meeting with the hospital's Risk Manager on February 1, 2007. On the day before the meeting, our lawyer received word that the hospital would not attend because "the McKnights have violated the settlement agreement." The hospital had seen our Website for HONOReform and believed that it violated the settlement agreement by listing: 1) the name of the book; 2) the stated content of the book; and 3) the summary of the outbreak.

We were flabbergasted. We hadn't revealed the amount of our settlement nor had we divulged the specific patient safety changes we had demanded from the hospital, the two terms we were to keep confidential under the settlement agreement.

We immediately had our attorney write a letter to the hospital. He asked them: 1) Do you mean that you are not going to carry out the twenty non-monetary points or do you mean that you will execute these points without the McKnights' involvement? And 2) How exactly did the McKnights violate the settlement agreement? The letter Matt received back from their lawyer stated, "Please let me know your clients' position as to all of their violations of the non-monetary settlement agreement. When we get from you that information we can better respond to your inquiries."

Tom and I could see we were getting nowhere with the correspondence through the attorneys. We arranged a meeting with board members and the CEO, Mike Leibert, on May 31, 2007. I began the meeting by acknowledging that Travis and I were writing a book about the Nebraska outbreak.

"I want to end the book by praising the hospital for implementing the twenty non-monetary points," I stated. "However, at this point, I cannot do that. The only things I can talk about are these nonproductive letters that have gone back and forth."

The hospital representatives did not seem to be aware of the impasse. They agreed that the twenty non-monetary points were worthwhile and deserved to be implemented. Mike asked questions and took notes. Although the board members challenged me to write a balanced, fair book, the meeting ended on a positive note.

Several days later, we received a handwritten note from Mike, explaining the progress on one of the points. We were happy to receive the news. It looked as if we were moving forward together.

Regrettably, communication ground to a halt once again when the hospital filed suit against us to try to prevent publication of this book. After the lawsuit was dismissed, we asked the hospital to tell us if they had implemented the twenty non-monetary points. They wrote a seven-page letter back, describing the status of the twenty points. Happily, most had been implemented. The hospital finished their letter to us by saying, "We are willing to move forward with the Non-Monetary Settlement Agreement. In doing so, we hope that full discussion of the… [settlement document]…and how it relates to any book you intend to publish will allow us to continue to move forward in accomplishing the goals of the Non-Monetary Settlement Agreement."

CHAPTER 32

Travis Explains the Hospital's Suit Against the Authors

As Evelyn and I were writing this manuscript, we took great pains, as we have said, to make sure that we told the truth. We sorted through mountains of medical documents, legal records and witness statements. We also interviewed dozens of people who had information. The project took us over two years to complete. Along the way we were very careful to keep the contents of our manuscript as confidential as possible. For two years it was for our eyes only (with the limited exception of when we sent the book for possible licensing or publication). The only other people who ever saw parts of it were those who contributed to it.

For example, I met with outbreak victim Bob Ridder and took his statement. I wrote the chapter about him and then met with him again so we could make sure that I had the facts right. Evelyn and I did this time and time again as we met with Jill Watson, Glenn Doescher and many others. Each time we did, we only let them see the chapters written about them—no more, no less. We kept the contents of the manuscript secret because we did not want anyone to read it until we had completed our research and the story we told was accurate.

In the first week of June 2007, I threw away a nearly complete copy of our manuscript. At the time I dropped it into the garbage can beside my desk, I remember thinking that I should run it through the shredder. I even started to bend down to retrieve it, but I then thought that it would be silly to think that someone would go through my garbage to read our manuscript. So that afternoon, it left my office with the other trash.

I was shocked to learn that several days later, on June 21, 2007, the Fremont Area Medical Center (our local hospital) had filed a lawsuit to prevent us from publishing this book. The hospital's attorneys allegedly "received a copy of [the] book in a brown paper envelope" on June 12, 2007. They claimed the envelope had outbreak victim Jill Watson's return address. I knew that it couldn't have come from Jill and Jill later even signed an affidavit swearing that she'd never had a complete copy of the manuscript and had not sent it to the hospital.

As with everyone else that we'd interviewed, Jill had only been allowed to see the portion of the text that told her story. As a result, she'd never had more than the two or three chapters about her. She'd never had a complete copy of the book. No one but Evelyn and I, our vetting attorney, and potential publishers or producers ever had the complete manuscript. I interviewed everyone who had access to my office. None of them knew how a copy of it got out. To my incredulity, it was obvious to me that someone had gone through my trash looking for it. I cannot imagine who would want a copy of the book badly enough to dig through a dumpster, other than the hospital.

It took a couple of days after the filing of the lawsuit before we found out that we were being sued. When the hospital filed the lawsuit, they didn't let us know immediately. Instead, they went to the Court, without our knowledge, and convinced the Court to enter a restraining order preventing us from publishing the book. I was stunned to learn that we had not only been sued, but that an order had *already* been signed that prevented us from publishing this book. I was not a First Amendment freedom of speech attorney, but I knew the US Constitution wouldn't stand for banning the truth.

The hospital's lawsuit essentially claimed that the book contained some statements that were "inaccurate, false, malicious, negligent, salacious, scandalous, untrue and defamatory," although none of these "false" statements were specified in the complaint. The allegations went on to say that the contents of this book would "irreparably harm" the hospital if they became public.

In addition to the restraining order, they sued us for defamation of their character and casting a "false light" on the hospital. I never once feared a judgment against us on either of these actions, because I knew that the truth is always a perfect defense to these types of allegations. Just as importantly, however, I knew that we had not allowed any draft of our book to disseminate to the public. In my opinion, their lawsuit had no merit.

We discussed the possibility of counter-suing the hospital for filing a frivolous, bad-faith lawsuit against us, but decided not to do so. We also had several other options. One was to file a "slap back" lawsuit, which is when a wrongly sued author counter-sues the party who falsely uses the court system to violate their freedom of press. Another option would have been to contact the American Civil Liberties Union to take action on our behalf. A third option would have been to give the story to the media in hopes that the public would pressure the hospital to drop its lawsuit. After lengthy discussions, we decided not to take any of these steps in hopes that after some reflection, the hospital board would drop their lawsuit.

The hospital went on to allege that Evelyn, a victim of the outbreak herself, had violated the terms of her settlement with the hospital that she'd signed one year earlier, when she'd settled her Hepatitis C lawsuit. The language of her settlement had never stated that she couldn't write a book about what had happened to her. She'd promised to not tell how much money she'd received in the settlement. She never has.

In their legal pleadings, which are still public record at the Dodge County Courthouse, the hospital pointed to the language of the agreement, in which Evelyn agreed that she "…was not interested in hurting the reputation (sic) FAMC and its employees…" I knew that the judge would be able to see that that language couldn't keep her from telling her story.

Neither of us ever wanted to harm the hospital. All we wanted to do was to tell the world about the events that led to the largest hepatitis C outbreak in American history. We wrote the book to honor the victims of the outbreak, and to make sure that the wrongs that led to the outbreak would be remedied so that no one else would suffer the same fate. Hiding the events that led to this tragedy would only ensure future tragedies. Enough people had already died, and we wanted to let the world learn from the outbreak so no one else would lose their life in the future. Here again, since we were telling the truth, and had never let anyone see the manuscript, I knew she had not violated her agreement. After the lawsuit was on file, word passed to me through a fairly reliable source that an attorney for the hospital had said that the book "was going to cost the hospital millions of dollars." I was told that the hospital's attorney wanted me to also know that "the hospital was willing to go to any lengths to keep this book from going to print."

As it was reported to me, the attorney stressed repeatedly the words "any lengths." I never heard the message from the attorney himself, but I believed the person who passed it on to me. I took it as a personal threat, and knowing the gravity of the situation, it scared me. I spent some time looking over my shoulder and losing sleep at night. I closed the curtains in my home, and thought twice before going outside. I would tell myself that I was being paranoid, and then wonder if I was.

The whole ordeal was equally taxing on Evelyn. As if her being a victim of the Nebraska outbreak were not enough, she was now paralyzed with anxiety over the hospital's lawsuit. She couldn't sleep or eat. She lost entire days to paralyzing anxiety.

Within a couple of days, Evelyn and I hired a First Amendment specialist to defend our lawsuit. As an attorney, I hated the idea of paying attorney's fees (in the end, Evelyn and I paid $36,000 in attorney's fees to defend ourselves), but I was also smart enough to know that I had virtually no background in constitutional law. Other than classes in law school and occasional debates with fellow colleagues, my legal career had never dealt with civil rights.

Our attorneys immediately had a hearing to contest the temporary restraining order. The court, realizing that it had no legal basis to grant the order, dismissed the temporary restraining order on July 6, 2007. The remaining lawsuit for defamation was still left on file, but we were free to publish this book.

On July 18, 2007, with the defamation suit against us still pending, the hospital sent Evelyn a letter. "FAMC remains willing to move forward in a spirit of cooperation and healing," it read. "[The hospital wants] to move forward together for the betterment of the greater Dodge County community."

The hospital's defamation suit was legally interesting. One of our strongest constitutional rights as Americans is the right to free speech. Furthermore, telling the truth is never grounds for a defamation suit. Both principles are even more firmly protected when they involve citizens speaking out against the government. When an American, right or wrong, loses his or her ability to speak out in opposition to something the government is doing or has done, our American way of life breaks down. The freedoms and liberties we enjoy as Americans are based upon the fact that our government cannot arbitrarily censor those who do not agree with it. If it did, our freedom would end.

The Fremont Area Medical Center is owned by Dodge County, Nebraska. It enjoys the privilege of being a political subdivision of the state of Nebraska. It is part of the government, and therefore did not have the right to silence its critics. Put concisely, I do not believe it had the right to sue us for defamation.

As our attorneys prepared a motion to have the remaining suit dismissed, I learned some very surprising news. While I (as a malpractice lawyer) had elected not to defend Evelyn and myself in the lawsuit but instead had hired a First Amendment lawyer, the hospital had elected to have its medical malpractice lawyers file the suit. The first action they'd taken had been a huge error. When they'd gotten the temporary restraining order at the outset of the case, they'd entered our manuscript into evidence. They'd also entered Evelyn's "secret" settlement document into evidence. While it may have gotten them their short-lived injunction, it had also been a colossal mistake on their part. Evidence in civil matters is public record. While Evelyn and I had been careful to protect the manuscript from the public, the hospital had inadvertently given it to the world. Soon, word of the lawsuit leaked out of the courthouse. Everyone was asking me if I would give them a copy of the "tell-all book" we had written. I would always decline, often to hear, "Fine, I will just get a copy from the courthouse."

The hospital had given the world free access to the book, and Evelyn's "secret" settlement documents, which they wanted undisclosed. The irony was that for months, Evelyn and Tom had negotiated the terms of their settlement with the hospital. The entire time, the hospital had insisted that the twenty non-monetary points be confidential. This clause was the center of the hospital's claim that Evelyn breached the contract. Yet, in reality, the hospital had placed those same non-monetary points into the public record and had in theory, breached the contract themselves.

In the days before our motion to dismiss the suit, the hospital called our attorneys. They decided to voluntarily dismiss the suit themselves. The lawsuits to silence this book were over. That same week, I learned that the hospital's president, Mike Leibert, who had been the president of the hospital during the Nebraska outbreak, had tendered his resignation. Effective at the end of the year, he would be stepping down as FAMC president.

"It would appear from both a commitment focus as well as a personal health perspective that consideration should be given to a personal lifestyle change," his letter to local physicians read.

In the weeks before he announced his planned resignation, Mr. Leibert had also sent us a letter through his attorney, threatening a suit against us. Our attorney responded that any such lawsuit would be unfounded. We never heard from Mike Leibert's attorney again. We reviewed Mr. Leibert's letter, which made several claims of factual inaccuracies. We carefully considered and in some cases made revisions in response to those claims in preparing the book for final publication.

In the days following the dismissal of the hospital's lawsuit against us, Evelyn and I wrote to the FAMC Board of Trustees. Each member of the board had been given a copy of the unauthorized manuscript by their attorneys. We offered to review any evidence they might provide of factual inaccuracies that they claimed to have uncovered in their reading of the manuscript. Our only mission in writing this book was to tell the truth of what happened, and if we had indeed made any factual errors, we wanted them to tell us so we could correct them.

Several weeks later, we got a response to our letter, and we did make some changes to the book based upon the hospital's suggestions. We also included the hospital's point of view on some of the issues they raised, based upon their letter to us. In addition, we asked the hospital to provide us with several documents that they claimed were "missing" from the book. I had never known that these alleged documents existed. Months passed. To date, the hospital has not provided the missing documents.

CHAPTER 33

Travis Explains
the Legal Problems
of the Outbreak

Some people like to speak in unfounded generalities. They like absolute state-ments of fact that are true in every situation. One such statement that I, as a trial attorney, have heard time and time again over the years is that "the problem with this country is, there are too many lawsuits." In my entire life, I have never heard anyone say that lawsuits are indeed a good thing. Oftentimes, when I hear someone complaining about lawsuits, they follow their statement with the next logical step. If lawsuits are bad, then the plaintiffs who file them must have bad motives for filing them. They must be greedy.

During the years of legal proceedings resulting from the Nebraska outbreak, I have had the privilege of meeting many of the Nebraska outbreak victims. I represented roughly a quarter of them, and I met many others through the ensuing years of depositions, motions, hearings and other chance encounters. Personally, I try to avoid absolute statements about people, but I can say one thing about the victims of the Nebraska outbreak with great surety. The victims of the Nebraska outbreak were not "greedy plaintiffs." They were small-town neighbors, grandparents, fathers and mothers raising their children. They were almost uniformly blue-collar, Christian Americans. I never met a single one of them who was anxious to file their lawsuit. In fact, I met several of them who refused to do so.

There were 100 known victims of the Nebraska outbreak and only eighty-nine elected to file lawsuits. In spite of the fact that they were infected with a potentially life-threatening disease that could leave their families impoverished, ten percent of the victims and their families refused to file lawsuits. None of these plaintiffs were "looking to get rich" or "greedy" in any way. What I did see was a group of people who only wanted to make sure that if they needed the money to survive their disease, they would have it. These people were not lusting after new houses or new cars or a more affluent lifestyle. They were concerned that if they died from their disease, their children would still have food on the table—that is all.

Of the eighty-nine victims who did file lawsuits, each and every one of them sent letters (known as Nebraska Political Subdivision Tort Claims Notices) to the Fremont Area Medical Center and the state of Nebraska, asking for help before they filed their lawsuits. Each letter asked the Dodge County Board to compensate them for their financial losses. Of the eighty-nine letters received by the state of Nebraska and the Fremont Area Medical Center, to my knowledge none of them were ever answered. No one from the state or county wrote them back to deny their requests for relief. It was only after months of waiting with no response that each of these plaintiffs filed their lawsuits.

There are few struggles in life that are more vigorous than the fight over money. When an injured plaintiff files a lawsuit against the doctor who hurt them, people often think that the plaintiff is trying to take money from the doctor. People think the plaintiff is trying to get a court to take money from the doctor's bank account, or force him to sell his house to pay the plaintiff. This is not the case. When the Nebraska outbreak victims filed their lawsuits, they were suing insurance companies. In fact, the primary defendant, Dr. Javed, never saw the inside of a courtroom. When a defendant did not have insurance, they were usually dismissed from the lawsuits. It costs plaintiffs money to prosecute their lawsuit. The more defendants that are involved, the more costs are involved. If a defendant has no insurance, it is not cost-effective to leave them in the lawsuit, no matter how much responsibility they have.

Nebraska's Cap on Damages

To a person, the plaintiffs who walked through my office door looking for help had no idea how badly they would be treated in the litigation process. In the decades before the Nebraska outbreak, insurance companies and injured plaintiffs had been at odds over the issue of medical malpractice tort reform. Insurance companies had won that struggle, and the victims of the Nebraska outbreak had paid for those losses.

In 1976, Nebraska had passed the Nebraska Hospital Medical Liability Act (NHMLA), which had been intended to improve the medical malpractice situation in Nebraska. The act had created three major systemic problems for injured plaintiffs, like the victims of the Nebraska outbreak: 1) It capped the total recovery a plaintiff could receive from a jury *irrespective of what the plaintiffs' medical bills were*; 2) it placed injured plaintiffs directly at odds with the state of Nebraska; and 3) it was not designed to handle mass medical negligence.

At a glance, this system of capping recoveries may have seemed fair—$1.25 million was, after all, a lot of money. The problem with the system became evident as soon as patients were so seriously injured that $1.25 million would not pay for their *actual* damages.

For years, plaintiffs' attorneys, including myself, debated whether or not the NHMLA was constitutional. A challenge to the constitutionality of the NHMLA would require a unique test case. It would require a case wherein the shortcomings of the NHMLA were exposed. That challenge finally came in the tragic case of *Gourley v. Nebraska Methodist Health Systems, et al.*, 265 Neb 918 (2003).

In 1993, Mr. and Mrs. Gourley of Valley, Nebraska, became pregnant with twins. During her pregnancy Mrs. Gourley was under the prenatal care of her gynecologist/obstetrician, Dr. Michelle Knolla. During the thirty-sixth week of her pregnancy Mrs. Gourley informed Dr. Knolla that she had noticed a decrease in movement of her twin fetuses. Dr. Knolla told her not to worry about the change, as it was common and everything appeared normal.

Two days later, Mrs. Gourley again called to report the lack of movement. This time, she was referred to a physician at Methodist Hospital, where it was determined that one of the unborn children was suffering from bradycardia—a decrease in the fetal heart rate—and a lack of amniotic fluid. When the twin children, Colin and Connor, were finally born, Colin suffered from serious brain damage, cerebral palsy and significant physical, cognitive and behavioral deficiencies. After a lengthy trial, the jury found, on September 24, 1999, that Dr. Knolla and the OB/GYN group were both legally negligent.

Upon finding that Dr. Knolla and her OB/GYN group were negligent, the jury had to determine what amount of money it would take to compensate the Gourley family for their damages. As is all too often the case, no amount of money could ever truly compensate the Gourley family. So, the jury turned to the actual medical costs Colin would need over his lifetime.

At trial, a long-term healthcare specialist testified that the medical costs for Colin's care over his life expectancy would be $12,461,500.22. This amount of money only represented the actual out-of-pocket expenses the Gourley family would have to pay for Colin's care. It did not represent any emotional damages the family had, nor did it compensate Colin for the "normal life" that he would never have the chance to lead. The present-day value of $12,461,500.22, when adjusted to present-day costs irrespective of inflation, calculated out to be

$5,943,111. In the end, the jury awarded the Gourley family $5,625,000—slightly less than the expected actual costs to care for Colin over his lifetime.

Upon the jury's verdict, the District Court judge followed the Nebraska Hospital Liability Act and reduced the jury's award to the state medical cap of $1.25 million. The Gourley family pleaded with the court to allow them to keep the full amount of the jury's award, and to hold that the NHMLA cap was unfair and unconstitutional. After further deliberation, the court took a bold step in June 2000 and did just that. The court held that the cap was unconstitutional and that the Gourleys should not be limited by it. The defendants appealed and the case went to the Nebraska Supreme Court in February 2002.

The Nebraska Supreme Court deliberated on the issue for fifteen months before issuing their ruling on May 16, 2003. Nebraska has traditionally been a conservative state, and its Supreme Court has followed in that trend. Nonetheless, many observers were still shocked when the Court overturned the ruling of the District Court and upheld the cap as constitutional. Thus, the Gourley family only received a small percentage of their actual medical costs.

Justice Gerrard, in an almost apologetic concurring opinion, wrote:

> As I remain deeply troubled by the public policy choices reflected in the act, particularly the denial of economic recovery to negligently injured persons. *It is pointedly unfair, and may well prove unconstitutional, for the law of this state to safeguard a surplus of tens of millions of dollars in the Excess Liability Fund by denying negligently injured persons money for needed medical care and potentially condemning them to undue poverty.* (Emphasis added.)

Justice McCormack, in a partial dissent, devoted four pages of the opinion to a statistical analysis of whether or not the liability cap worked. He wrote, in part:

> It appears that at least one of the intended goals of the caps, to ensure reasonable malpractice rates, remains unmet—unfortunate news to the catastrophically injured such as Colin and his family, who can recover only approximately 20 percent of their medical costs *so that some medical providers can enjoy what they consider to be reasonable rates.* (Emphasis added.)

The second great inequity that was created by the NHMLA was the Nebraska Excess Liability Fund. The problem with the fund was that it was managed by the state of Nebraska. This meant that when a plaintiff sat down to negotiate a settlement in an injury case, he or she was no longer negotiating with the defendant or even the defendant's insurance company. The plaintiff was at odds directly with the state of Nebraska.

A system was created wherein taxpaying plaintiffs were fighting against their own state to be compensated for medical malpractice. A state has an obligation to protect the health and welfare of all its citizens. Yet under the NHMLA, an apparent conflict of interest was created wherein the state was concerned with the financial welfare of its physicians over and above the welfare of patients claiming malpractice.

A third drawback of the Nebraska Hospital Liability Act, which only came to light when the Nebraska outbreak occurred, was that under the NHMLA, a physician was required to keep enough insurance to pay for up to only three injured patients per year. It was inconceivable at the time the NHMLA was passed that a physician would injure more than three people in one year. Certainly, a physician wouldn't infect 100 people with a potentially deadly virus in only one year's time. It was short-sighted legislation that led to one of the biggest legal problems of the hepatitis C Nebraska outbreak—whether or not the state of Nebraska even had to pay the plaintiffs at all. This issue was so important, it is detailed in its own chapter. (See Chapter 26: The Merritt Decision.)

Punitive Damages

Many states allow an injured plaintiff to sue the person or company that harmed them for punitive damages. Punitive damages are essentially punishment damages. It is money awarded to the plaintiff to punish the defendant for the grievous act that caused the injury. The most well-known type of punitive damage award comes in cases wherein large corporations disregard the safety of their consumers in the name of profit.

When a mega-corporation has done a cost/benefit analysis showing that it will be cheaper to pay off a handful of families with burned children than to remake their baby clothing line out of safe, nonflammable material, punitive damages are often awarded. The idea is that if the corporation saved $50 million in product costs, but only had to pay the family a few hundred thousand dollars, the corporation would have profited millions of dollars. Oftentimes, when a jury awards punitive damages, they will simply award the injured family the profit that the corporation would have otherwise made based on their cost/benefit analysis. The hope is that by taking away a defendant's incentive (profit) to do wrong, people will not be hurt in the future.

None of the victims of the Nebraska outbreak could receive punitive damages because Nebraska does not allow punitive damages. Plaintiffs in Nebraska could only receive their actual losses. If these cases had occurred in many other states, they could have been worth millions of dollars each. As a result of Nebraska's ban on punitive damages, none of the outbreak victims could argue that the defendants should be punished (with punitive damages) for disregarding the safety of their patients. At the time of the Nebraska outbreak, the state cap on damages was $1.25 million. As a result of Nebraska laws regarding civil suits, however, the Nebraska outbreak cases were only worth a fraction of that amount.

Uninformed Juries

Oftentimes, on television or in the movies, fictional lawyers will make impassioned speeches to juries about justice and fairness. Those fictional juries are allowed to know the full truth about who the parties to the lawsuit are. They know that an insurance company backs the defendant. They know that the lawyer working for the defendant is paid by the insurance company, and they know that if they award damages against the defendant, the money will be there to pay the plaintiff.

Juries in those courtroom dramas do not have to feel the need to restrict a plaintiff's damages by what they feel the defendant can afford to pay. If they decide the plaintiff's damages are $50,000, they can award the full $50,000. They are not under the false assumption that the defendant will have to be financially burdened by the jury verdict. They do not reduce their verdict because of the "well, I know the plaintiff has lost $50,000, but we don't want to leave the defendant broke, either" factor.

Nebraska forbids a plaintiff's attorney from explaining to the jury that insurance is involved in the lawsuit. If the "i" word is even mentioned to a jury, the case is often a mistrial, and the lawyer who mentioned it is subject to sanctions. None of the Nebraska outbreak victims' juries would ever know that the defendants had insurance to pay for the plaintiffs' damages.

Special Treatment for the Hospital

Many years ago, Nebraska lawmakers passed legislation that limited a plaintiff's ability to sue the state of Nebraska. It is called the Nebraska Political Subdivision Tort Claim Act (NPSTCA). Essentially, if a private citizen injures another citizen, the victim can go to the courthouse and file a lawsuit for damages. In the end, the victim has a right to have a jury of his peers hear the case and determine how much money should be awarded to him.

Under the NPSTCA (and the Twelfth Amendment to the US Constitution), however, the state of Nebraska is afforded special protection from such lawsuits. If a government-run entity injures a citizen, that victim does not have the right to a jury trial. It may not be apparent at first, but this was devastating to the victims of the Nebraska outbreak.

When the hepatitis C lawsuits were filed, most plaintiffs named Dr. Javed, his nurses and the hospital as defendants. At the time of the Nebraska outbreak, the Fremont Area Medical Center was owned by Dodge County. Dodge County, as a political subdivision of the state of Nebraska, could not be sued in front of a jury because of the NPSTCA. This meant that each case essentially had to be tried twice. One courtroom battle would take place in front of a judge to determine if the hospital was liable, and then a second courtroom battle would take place in front of a jury to determine the liability and damages caused by the guilty parties.

Trials cost plaintiffs money. Not because of the plaintiffs' lawyers—as they only get paid if their clients win their cases—but because a plaintiff must pay for litigation costs. These costs are greatly exacerbated by Nebraska laws regarding medical expert witnesses (see below). They were expected to run between $40,000 and $50,000 per hepatitis C trial. These are upfront costs that the plaintiff has to pay before the trial begins.

This cost would come at a time when the plaintiff was already burdened with illness and income loss. These costs put the plaintiffs in jeopardy of not only walking away from the Nebraska outbreak with a terrible disease, but also with enormous debt if they lost their trial. Even in cases wherein the plaintiff settles his or her case out of court, these upfront costs often must be paid before defendants will agree to settle.

The Nebraska Political Subdivision Tort Claim Act doubled those costs, as now each plaintiff who elected to sue the hospital (and the majority did) would have to essentially try their cases twice—once against the hospital and once against the doctor and nurses. Plaintiffs and their lawyers laid awake at night wondering where they would come up with almost $100,000 to try their cases. On top of all that, Nebraska law would not allow them to recover those trial costs. In fact, Nebraska law prevented them from even mentioning to the jury that they had to pay those costs to put on their cases. The juries would not be allowed to know that if they awarded a plaintiff $100,000 for their damages, the plaintiff essentially walked away empty-handed.

The Expert Witness Rule

When a plaintiff calls a doctor to the stand to explain a complicated medical theory to a jury, the plaintiff incurs costs. It is uncommon for a doctor to agree to testify against another doctor in a medical malpractice action without being paid an enormous sum of money.

Often, expert doctors will only agree to testify if they are paid between $10,000 and $15,000 for their testimony before a jury. Their testimony is often limited to one or two days. Yet, Nebraska law does not force a doctor to offer opinions at trial without first being paid to do so. On top of that, expert witness doctors usually require that the plaintiff pay for pretrial opinions and airfare, lodging and meal expenses at the time of the trial. As a result, each plaintiffs' expert witness can cost a plaintiff $20,000 or more.

When I explained this over and over to the victims of the Nebraska outbreak, they were stunned. Some broke down and sobbed. One after another asked me one simple question: "Then why hire expert witness doctors at all?"

Logically, it made sense. These hepatitis C cases were not so complex medically that it would take a doctor to explain the facts to a jury. The way the plaintiffs contracted hepatitis C was straightforward. Healthcare personnel reused syringes on patients, and blood was passed from one victim to another. An expert wouldn't have been necessary if it weren't required by law.

Nebraska law prohibits a jury from awarding damages for medical injuries without a doctor testifying to explain the injury in detail. In the Nebraska outbreak cases, a plaintiff could not simply testify that he contracted hepatitis C from the cancer center. An expert had to be called to explain the mode of transmission, test results, treatment options and the victim's prognosis. In addition, the patient's medical records from his or her post-outbreak liver specialists were not allowed into evidence unless the physician testified to them.

As I explained this over and over to the victims of the Nebraska outbreak, they were devastated. A few even went as far as to proclaim that they would then waive their right to recover for pain and suffering, and only ask the jury to award them their lost wages and medical costs. Once again, I had the sad task of explaining that it would not work. Nebraska law even went so far as to prevent a plaintiff from recovering his or her out-of-pocket costs for medical treatment to fight their disease, unless an expert witness doctor was called to testify that those damages were "fair and reasonable." Upon hearing this news, one of my clients shook her head in disgust.

"It's too bad Nebraska law is not 'fair and reasonable,'" she said.

I could not disagree.

Nebraska Versus the Outbreak Victims

The foundation of our entire American judicial process is built around the principle that when a losing party walks out of the courthouse door, he or she feels that they lost a fair fight—and not because the state, or its attorneys, had conspired against them. Without this appearance of neutrality, our system does not work.

As the Nebraska outbreak litigation unfolded, the state performed many of the functions in the wake of the disaster that a state should:

1. The state epidemiologist conducted testing on all possible outbreak victims to determine who had been infected with the disease and how it had happened.
2. The Department of Health and Human Services investigated the outbreak and turned its results over to the Nebraska attorney general's office.
3. The Nebraska attorney general's office pursued the license revocation of Dr. Javed and Nurse Prochaska.

At the same time that the state was taking these actions, it was also actively defending the Nebraska Excess Liability Fund (NELF) against the claims of the outbreak victims. It was fervent in its defense of the NELF. Some of the most well-known insurance defense attorneys in the Midwest were hired by the state to protect it, and to make sure that the outbreak victims were compensated as little as possible for their infection with hepatitis C.

The state was extremely concerned that if the NELF were forced to pay the outbreak victims, the fund itself would go bankrupt. It was a fear that was widespread among the state's legal counsel. The more it looked like the victims should be paid, the harder the state fought to protect the NELF. It was soon apparent to the victims of the outbreak that their cases were in reality no longer against Dr. Javed, but were against the NELF, which held the purse strings.

Initially, the state's zealous defense of the NELF was simply disappointing to many outbreak victims and their attorneys. The victims believed that they had already gone through enough, and that the NELF should do its duty and pay for the victims' medical treatments, lost wages, etc. As time passed, however, it became apparent to many plaintiffs that the state was engaged in an apparent conflict of interests. On one hand, it was entrusted with protecting the victims' health and welfare. On the other hand, it was working against the victims by defending the fund. This appearance of conflicting interests became unnerving as one after another, the state's actions to protect the victims fell short of my expectations:

1. The state epidemiologist did not use the most effective hepatitis C test when testing potential victims (recall

Chapter 21). As a result, the state initially told approximately one-third of the outbreak victims that they did not have the disease and that no further testing was necessary. The mistake endangered victims' lives, and came at the time when the victims' statute of limitations was rapidly approaching. If the error had been caught much later, a number of victims would not have been able to recover from the state fund at all because the statute of limitations would have run. After the Nebraska outbreak litigation was nearing completion, the epidemiologist's office stated that their mistake was not intentional. They said they had simply followed the recommendation of the CDC and that their testing of victims was based on the current medical practices. The Nebraska outbreak made history because through it, doctors have learned that immunocompromised patients are not good candidates for antibody testing.

2. The Nebraska Health and Human Services investigations into the outbreak contained information about how the outbreak occurred (recall Chapter 23). Days before the license revocation hearings of Dr. Javed and Linda Prochaska, the state (working through the attorney general's office) entered into an agreement wherein Javed and Prochaska gave up their licenses to practice medicine. In essence, the state agreed to accept their guilty pleas on some of the charges and dropped other allegations against them since their admissions of guilt would lead to their license revocations. As a result, the state was not required to turn their investigative findings about the facts of the outbreak over to the outbreak victims. This information would have greatly benefited the outbreak victims, but would have obviously been detrimental to the state's simultaneous defense of the NELF. While there was never any clear evidence that the attorney general's office encouraged Javed and Prochaska to surrender their licenses, it was certainly oddly coincidental that they chose to relinquish them. Dr. Javed had made statements to the Pakistani press a month earlier that had challenged

Nebraska to take his license. Linda Prochaska was still working as a nurse when she volunteered her license and therefore gave up her means of supporting her family. While the state was clearly within its legal authority to accept their voluntary revocations and to therefore deny victims the right to see the results of their investigations, their actions still had negative repercussions for the victims. Since their injuries were the cause of the investigations, it was unfair that they were denied information about *how* they got injured. It was another example of how Nebraska law is unfair to plaintiffs.

3. No criminal charges were ever filed against any of the defendants in the Nebraska outbreak.

Irrespective of whether these state actions were legal, they were detrimental to the outbreak victims. In a system free of the appearance of conflicts of interest, these events would only have been seen as coincidental. In the Nebraska system, however, the state was not only the protector of the outbreak victims, but was also charged with the task of making sure that they did not recover from the NELF. (See Chapter 27, wherein the State Department of Insurance filed suit in Lancaster County, asking that court to hold that the state fund did not have to pay eighty-six of the eighty-nine outbreak victims.) Certainly, no evidence ever came to light during or after the Nebraska outbreak, which showed that there was ever any collusion between different departments of the state in an effort to conspire against the outbreak victims. As the state's efforts continued to work against the victims, however, I had to question the neutrality of the system. It is a clear example of how a state should not be involved in defending medical malpractice cases.

BOOK III

■

Coping with the Nebraska Outbreak

CHAPTER 34

■

The Cohort

Dr. Mark Mailliard's Study of the Cohort

At the time of the Nebraska outbreak, Dr. Mark Mailliard was an associate professor in the division of gastroenterology and hepatology at the University of Nebraska Medical Center. Many of the infected chose him as their liver doctor. He was very involved as an expert witness in the litigation.

At the time of this writing, Dr. Mailliard was conducting ongoing research into the Nebraska outbreak. The study had not yet been published in a medical journal at the time that this book went to print. The goals of the study were to describe the natural history of healthcare-acquired hepatitis C3a and evaluate immune factors in at-risk and chronically infected patients. The Nebraska cluster of patients represented a unique cohort because of age, conditions of exposure, concurrent chemotherapy and associated immunosuppression. The study of this unique group will add to the knowledge of the hepatitis C virus.

Dr. Mailliard collected data on the outbreak victims by reviewing their medical records and then comparing the data to a matched control group of non-infected cancer patients.

Sixty-four of the ninety-nine outbreak victims generously gave Dr. Mailliard permission to review their medical records. It is considered a large percentage of participants for such a study.

The study participants ranged in age from early twenties to eighties. They had a broad spectrum of cancer diagnoses. Of the sixty-four participants, approximately forty underwent interferon/Ribavirin treatment. Nearly eighty percent of those undergoing treatment achieved a "sustained virologic response," meaning that they no longer had a detectable virus in their system. The remaining failed treatment and did not achieve a sustained virologic response.

There has been one reported case of sexual transmission, whereby a victim gave the virus to a committed sexual partner.

Approximately sixteen percent of the study participants had significant liver disease. Three victims died of their liver disease. Several of the cohort underwent the rigorous treatment regimen and achieved a sustained virologic response but within a few years, died of cancer.

Other Persons Involved in the Nebraska Outbreak

Dr. M. Salman Haroon's oncology practice, Midlands Regional Cancer Center, earned inclusion into the Missouri Valley Cancer Consortium for conducting cancer research in January of 2007.

Dr. Tom McKnight continues to admit his patients to Fremont Area Medical Center.

Evelyn McKnight, Monica Weber, Valerie Wheaton, Jill Watson, Byron Schafersman and Bob Ridder have all celebrated at least six years of being cancer-free.

Glenn Doescher returned to work after recovering from a liver transplant.

John Hughes resigned as vice president of the Fremont Area Medical Center to become an administrator at a medical clinic in Iowa.

Fremont Area Medical Center's guilt or innocence of medical malpractice was never determined in a court of law. To date, the hospital has not issued a public statement of compassion to the victims. It is currently (2008) building a $17 million radiology facility.

Linda Prochaska works in a non-licensed capacity in the process improvement department at a hospital in Omaha.

Dr. Tahir Ali Javed resides in Pakistan with his wife and children, untouched by the outbreak he left behind. He is a high-ranking political figure in Pakistan, and has never been held accountable for his negligence. Neither the United States nor the state of Nebraska has called for his extradition so that he can stand trial for his part in the largest American outbreak of hepatitis C in history.

■

CHAPTER 35

The Victims' Emotional Journey, As Reported by Evelyn

"You know, how many emotions can you have? You know, it [the Nebraska outbreak] is just a terrible thing. I mean, I don't even know how to put it into context. I'm not sure I have words for it… I mean, it's sad."
—Michael Leibert,
president of the Fremont Hospital in sworn testimony on May 25, 2004

The Nebraska hepatitis C outbreak changed many people's lives. The victims were not the only people affected. Their families, the healthcare providers, legal representatives and state officials suffered as well. Even as this chapter is written, the experience of the Nebraska outbreak continues to color the participants' lives.

This chapter takes a look at the outbreak through the eyes of the victims. The authors conducted interviews with approximately thirty victims and/or their families. The interviewees bravely shared their stories with us, sometimes weeping as they spoke. The following quotes are from the interviews. Some names have been changed or withheld to protect privacy.

The Shocking First News of the Outbreak

In July 2002, the victims received a letter from Dr. Javed, saying he was leaving for Pakistan to care for his ailing mother. The next thing we knew, the newspapers were blaring the news of a potential outbreak of hepatitis C. It came as a shock to everyone.

"I learned about the outbreak through the Fremont and Omaha papers. I couldn't believe it," Melva recalled.

"The letter from the state [that encouraged testing] came to me as a shock," *Jan* said.

"It was the biggest shock of my life when I was told I was positive for hepatitis. [It was] hard to handle," *Maria* said. "I was shocked and bewildered by Dr. Javed and his nurse."

Betrayal

Once we realized that the news was true and that the consequences were long-lasting, our feelings turned to betrayal.

"I wonder who you *can* trust in the medical profession," Melva questioned.

Cancer patients often form strong bonds with their cancer doctors while they are going through chemotherapy. We put our lives in the hands of our oncologists, and the relationship is often very intimate. We shared our worries about our lives and deaths with Dr. Javed. We told him about our families' ability and inability to cope with our disease. He, in turn, demonstrated compassion, care and tender encouragement. Was he genuinely concerned, or was he a very convincing actor? Regardless of what was in his heart, his calculating betrayal was devastating.

We were scarred by several of our sacred institutions. It was unfathomable that we had been infected with hepatitis C through disregard of very basic standard procedure by medical professionals. We felt neglected by healthcare workers who didn't do enough to stop the outbreak, to our way of thinking. During the litigation process, we were disillusioned by some witnesses who were evasive, uncooperative and adversarial. We felt deep disappointment in the state for conducting the litigation process in a manner contrary to the victims' welfare. Lastly, we felt let down by our federal government when it refused to prosecute Dr. Javed for criminal negligence.

Loss of Privacy

Everyone deals with trauma in his or her own way. Some individuals want to share their stories with anyone willing to listen. Others don't want to tell a soul. In October 2002, our story was everywhere, all the time. Coffee shop conversation about the outbreak became a form of entertainment. "Some people are just kind of dumb and nosy," Eleanor wisely observed about the escalating gossip.

Suddenly, everyone asked us if we were "one of them" (with hepatitis C). Our privacy was violated daily. If acquaintances knew we had been treated at Javed's clinic, they asked what our screening results were. The question was posed in public settings such as the grocery store, church, the workplace and social gatherings. The media filmed us as we entered and left the blood-screening site. Mysteriously, some members of the media learned our names and hounded us for interviews. After we filed our lawsuits, a news story showed the stack of files at the courthouse. The names of some of the plaintiffs were legible and broadcast for the world to see.

Worries, Worries

The victims had many worries throughout the course of the outbreak and the resulting litigation. Would hepatitis C claim our lives after we had fought cancer so courageously? Would all ninety-nine die within a year, as Cheryl Gentry had? Was the outbreak caused simply by negligence or was terrorism involved? Would the hospital refuse us care in an emergency if we named them in a lawsuit?

We also had another fear. We were afraid of transmitting the disease to our loved ones. We knew the pain and suffering that our infection had caused us and we certainly did not want to pass it on. Grandparents who were victims limited their contact with their grandchildren. Coaches and teachers were reluctant to tend to the minor cuts of their young charges. Mothers worried that their toddlers would play in the trash where they had disposed of their bloody sanitary products.

"I received a call that my in-laws would not be coming to our house for Thanksgiving," *Vicki* said. "My father-in-law, who is infected, didn't want the rest of the family eating off the same dishes and forks that he had."

"I was crushed when I found out I had hepatitis C," Judy said. "It ended my work as a nurse. It was my life. I'm too afraid of infecting someone else to the point of being paranoid. I know all the facts of hepatitis C, but it doesn't matter. I carry Band-aids all the time in case I scratch myself or a hangnail bleeds. As a nurse, I was always an organ donor and they even took that away. I was in nursing for twenty-one years. I just can't go back to nursing. I'm so afraid of giving this to someone. I know it sounds paranoid. My work involves saving lives, not taking them."

Not only do we worry about infecting our loved ones through casual contact, we also worry about sexual transmission of hepatitis C. We would never in a million years want to infect the ones we love with this wretched disease. We continue to worry, though the experts say the likelihood of sexual transmission is slight. Through four years of lawsuit testimony, we heard time and time again that the odds of transmitting hepatitis C through sexual contact was one in a million. The experts made our fear sound irrational. However, our worries have not been unfounded. Shortly after the lawsuits were over, we learned that there had indeed been at least one case wherein an outbreak victim had passed the virus to a long-term sexual partner.

Other people also worried about getting the disease from us. Stigma was very real. Most people did not understand hepatitis C but they knew they didn't want it.

"It was kind of a hush-hush social thing that you shouldn't have," Vicki said.

One victim's wife, Rosemary, struggled with the temptation to tell her husband not to kiss the grandkids.

Judy's daughter-in-law would not let her visit a newborn granddaughter because Judy might give the baby hepatitis C. Her son sneaked the baby to Judy's house when his wife was out so that Judy could see her.

Dave admitted that the safety supervisor at work "treated it (hepatitis C) like AIDS." Patrons would leave local restaurants when they saw a victim enter rather than be served there. Siblings stopped having coffee together because the uninfected was afraid of contracting the virus from the victim.

Financial Strain

One of the most immediate concerns for many outbreak victims was how they would continue to support their families during their illness. As the horrors of interferon/Ribavirin treatment went on for six months, many victims became too sick to work. This left some without income. Some lost their jobs because they couldn't continue to work and as a result, lost their health insurance. Today, many outbreak victims cannot qualify for health insurance at normal costs because of their history of hepatitis C. Life insurance is all but impossible to obtain.

"Scot lost his health insurance when he lost his job. He then had to go on Medicaid and Medicare. Our church had a benefit for him and raised $10,000. All in all, it was awful," Marion recalled.

"I could not survive at all if it were not for my poor brother giving me money to help pay my bills and getting me some clothes that fit after I lost sixty-three pounds because of the interferon," Judy told us.

Community Reaction

Initially, everyone in the community was shocked and concerned. Community members were concerned about the victims and concerned about the reputation of the hospital. At first, there was a lot of media attention on a state and local level. Although it was the largest outbreak of hepatitis C in the history of the United States, it caused only a ripple of interest at the national level.

Many people were, and continue to be, concerned about the victims of the Nebraska outbreak. For the support and kind concern of these good people, we say, "Thank you." We couldn't have gotten through this ordeal without you. We hope you will continue to stand with us and work for positive change in our legal and medical systems and in our cultural reaction to hepatitis C and other types of disasters.

As time went on, many issues distracted the uninvolved citizens from concern about the Nebraska outbreak. The war on terror, the drought in the Midwest, Hurricane Katrina and the daily demands of life all took attention off our plight. The court-issued gag order resulted in minimal media coverage. The magnitude and complexity of the Nebraska outbreak also dampened interest. For the average individual, the Nebraska outbreak was too complicated, too embarrassing and too unfathomable to understand.

"Where are the rallies for hepatitis C survivors?" *Carol* asked. "Why aren't there fundraisers for research? When is the telethon?"

There is a strong Christian ethic in Fremont. There are churches of all denominations on every block of the main part of downtown. However, no community prayer service was held in support of the victims.

Doctors throughout Nebraska were afraid of an increase in malpractice premiums. Taxpayers imagined an increase in taxes because the hospital was a county entity and this rampant misperception was not addressed or dispelled by public leadership. State officials worried about bankruptcy of the Nebraska Excess Liability Fund.

Jill organized a community information session. She didn't think enough was being done to educate the community about hepatitis C. She hosted a forum focusing on the medical facts of the disease. As a long-time, loyal customer, she requested that her bank donate pencils for note-taking. She was surprised by the bank's response.

"No, we don't want to take sides," the bank told her.

Sometimes, people were even more hostile.

"Well," a woman told Joyce when she learned Joyce was an outbreak victim, "I suppose you are going to get a lot of money [from settlement]. I had cancer, too, but no one paid me a lot of money!"

Public Officials' Reaction

One of the most poignant disappointments following the Nebraska outbreak was the reaction of public officials. The only statement that came from a public official regarding the victims' circumstances was Dr. Tom Safranek's quote that they would live "perfectly normal lives." Virtually all the press releases by the state health department downplayed the seriousness of hepatitis C. Perhaps state health officials wanted to reassure us with their emphasis on the "normal course of hepatitis C being twenty years" and that "many victims do not even know they are infected."

However, without a counterbalance of facts about the potential for great harm, it felt to the victims as though their situation were being minimized and discounted. Ironically, as the state was seeking to lessen the seriousness of the outbreak, some victims had already died from the disease.

Other people in authority did not even acknowledge the tragedy. No one in an official position at the county, state or federal level ever made a public statement of compassion toward the victims.

"Where were the messages of condolence? Where were the support groups?" *Esmeralda* asked. "Where were the trauma counselors? Where were the candlelight vigils? Where were the public education efforts? Didn't we learn anything about how to respond to disaster victims after the Oklahoma City bombings, or Columbine, or 9/11?"

"We feel for the victims of the Nebraska outbreak and are dedicated to making sure this sort of thing does not happen again" would have been a comforting statement from government officials. Instead, there was only silence.

The Hospital's Reaction

Hospital officials were afraid of the damage the outbreak would cause to the hospital's reputation. The press releases by the hospital vehemently denied responsibility for the outbreak. The press releases did not at any time convey a message of concern for the injured. A statement of compassion would have done much to heal emotional wounds for the entire community. A statement such as, "We are saddened by the outbreak of hepatitis C in the community. We wish the victims good health and our heart goes out to them. We will investigate the situation thoroughly and do everything we can on our end to make sure such a thing never happens again" would have been very comforting to the victims and would have been a source of pride for everyone in the community.

Moreover, the hospital was in the best situation to help the victims in other ways. The victims would have appreciated free follow-up care and free hepatitis C screening for their families. It was not offered.

An Emotionally Responsive Way
of Resolving Malpractice Disputes

Other healthcare providers have found ways to settle malpractice disputes in a responsive and responsible way. At the same time that the adversarial and dissatisfying litigation of the Nebraska outbreak was taking place in Fremont, just down the road in Omaha, a hospital and a family who had lost a son to alleged malpractice collaborated to resolve their conflict in a way that provided healing for the family and process improvement for the hospital.

According to a story in the *Omaha World Herald* on August 29, 2007, a nineteen-year-old died on October 7, 2002 after an Omaha doctor allegedly missed an aortic dissection diagnosis. During negotiations for settlement with the young man's family, the involved hospital administrators offered to make a video that would keep the young man's memory alive and would hopefully prevent other deaths from aortic dissection. In the video, the hospital's doctors acknowledge the mistakes that they made in diagnosing aortic dissection and provide education to healthcare professionals on its diagnosis.

The video is posted on the hospital's Website and has been distributed nationally to educate other hospitals and doctors about aortic dissection. The video not only provided closure and healing for both the family and physicians, but it also led to process improvement within the hospital itself. In the video, the hospital administration show how they have changed their processes to make sure this mistake doesn't happen again. Furthermore, the hospital staff say in the video that since the process improvements have been instituted, they have properly diagnosed five cases of aortic dissection—and successfully treated those patients. The young man died, but thanks to the video and disclosure process, five patients (and five families) live on.

No Apology by Javed or Prochaska

The two main players in the Nebraska hepatitis C outbreak never apologized to the outbreak victims. The closest that Dr. Javed or Linda Prochaska came to an apology was at the Bob Ridder trial, during closing statements.

"[Linda] prays for the victims every day," her attorney told the jury.

The statement was very opportunistic; it was made just before the jury was about to decide how much money Nurse Prochaska's insurance company would have to pay the Ridders. As a result, some victims met it with skepticism.

"What is she praying for?" Esmeralda wondered. "That we all croak off?"

Complicated Grief

With the onslaught of losses, many victims experienced complicated or traumatic grief. The grief process was complex and prolonged. Basic belief systems were shattered. Nothing made sense anymore.

Some victims reported that they felt worse emotionally, rather than better, as time passed. The initial wave of shock at the news of the Nebraska outbreak had insulated them. As the shock and numbness wore off and reality set in, they felt bereft. Some continue to grieve.

Early in the outbreak, the infected were devastated by learning the names of other victims. Each new victim with hepatitis C was a knife to the heart.

When Cheryl Gentry died from hepatitis C, the victims were stunned. Cheryl Gentry was one of them. They read about Cheryl's final suffering and death in the newspaper. It shook them to their very souls.

"Cheryl and I used to have chemo together and she would sit in one chair and I would sit in the other and I have horrible thoughts of that room, dreadful. I prayed a lot," Eleanor mourned.

Time and again over the years, the victims were confronted by gut-wrenching losses. They experienced an additional wave of grief at every turn. News stories reported:

"Javed elected health minister in Pakistan."

"Cheryl Gentry dies of Hepatitis C."

"Seventeen more cases diagnosed."

"State sues to be excluded from lawsuits."

"Javed defies Nebraska to take his license."

The victims' belief in the quality of healthcare and the benevolence of local, state and federal government in the United States toward its constituents was rudely dashed. There was betrayal and abandonment at every turn. The litigation process was long, stressful, wearisome and ultimately unsatisfying.

Reaching Acceptance

In dealing with the hepatitis C infection, the victims had to come to terms with more than simply taking interferon treatments. For their own well-being, they had to come to terms with how the Nebraska outbreak changed their lives.

The process of coming to acceptance of the life-changing Nebraska outbreak experience was similar to working through the grieving process. Dr. Elisabeth Kubler-Ross described the grieving process in her 1969 book *On Death and Dying*. She described the stages of grief as denial, anger, bargaining, depression and finally, acceptance.

In the beginning, the victims were overwhelmed. The reaction was denial. Some couldn't bring themselves to say the words "hepatitis C" but talked about it as "an infection."

There were other kinds of denial.

"If he [Javed] knew about it, I think he was the kind of person who would not let it continue," Bill said. "I still cannot blame Javed. The man to me was a peach, a peach."

"I don't know, it just didn't bother me a whole lot. I didn't think about it [the Nebraska outbreak] much," Robert said.

"Experts tell us it is treatable, it has a ninety-nine percent cure rate!" *Oliver* proclaimed.

As time passed, many became angry.

"I hate what somebody has done to my body. [They] have violated my body to the nth degree. Are you trying to tell me you would not be bitter?" Bill argued. "It just eats on me that I have to give up my social life, because if you drink alcohol, it goes right to your liver."

"What was so upsetting was the fact that the hospital wouldn't take any responsibility for what happened. We trusted the doctors and nurses to make him well, not to infect him with a fatal disease," *Alexis* said of her dad.

"She just went downhill after they told her she had the hepatitis C," Max said about his wife. "She didn't care about living much. She blamed everybody, she blamed Javed, she blamed the hospital, everything."

"I was upset with the health department for not caring where I got the disease until over a year later," Carol complained.

Joyce explained her feelings this way: "I was not really angry at first. I got angry when I read Dr. Javed's reports. My [medical] reports were full of lies."

"To me, it was an outright crime," Oliver declared. "I cannot look at it any differently. I think those people involved knew better and if they didn't, they sure as heck should have."

"If they are responsible for Jim's death, I hope that they have a very sad life," Karla said passionately.

Many victims moved from one stage of grief to another and then back again. In bargaining, the victims imagined what the transgressors would have to do to earn forgiveness.

"I think the only one who could help us is Javed himself. Facing us and telling us why he tried to kill us," Judy remarked. "That is what I would like him to do for us."

"If he [Javed] asked for forgiveness, I might forgive," Max told us.

"Javed wouldn't even have to come back," Esmerelda explained. "If he would just send us a message that he was sorry, I could get over this. If the hospital would just say they were sorry and that they have taken steps to make sure it won't happen again, I would consider going back there for care."

Depression was another stage of grieving. Many began to suffer symptoms of depression and felt as though *they* were to blame.

"My personality has changed and I feel as though I really do not have anything to look forward to," Maria lamented.

"I look back in horror. It put me in bed for weeks. I didn't know what I was dying from," Jan added. "I had no strength, no desire to live."

"I shouldn't have let her [my wife] get a port put in," Max said, as though he could have possibly known what was to come.

"I feel like an idiot because I did not see it happening," *John* said, putting the blame on himself.

As time goes on, many of us reach a level of acceptance. Some of us were even able to find some good that came from the outbreak.

"One good thing, the outbreak got Javed out of our country. Now Pakistan has to put up with him," Esmeralda observed.

"The only thing better for me is that I have more time to spend with my kids and grandkids, which makes me happy," Judy commented. She had more free time because she became too ill from hepatitis C to keep working.

"My dad started changing," Alexis said. "He was more serious. He said kinder words. He kissed us all. I loved it, even though I knew he was dying."

"What good does it do to be bitter? [It] is all in the past," Eleanor observed.

We all had our own journey toward accepting what had happened to us. Some have truly "gotten over it" emotionally. Some never will.

One Woman's Journey

When I was diagnosed with hepatitis C, I began a long journey toward acceptance. My journey was similar to the others in that I had to work through the grieving process. There were many bumps, sharp turns and dead ends on my journey. Acceptance is not a one-time decision. As new limitations and lessons come up, I must continue to work toward accepting what happened to me and ninety-nine others.

I've tried all sorts of remedies to ease the emotional pain of the Nebraska outbreak. I've exercised, lifted weights, taken nature walks and practiced yoga until near-exhaustion. I've distracted myself with music, art, dance, drama, literature and sporting events. I've gone to counseling, written whole notebooks of my innermost anguish, and read scores of self-help and inspirational books. I've kept amulets and scripture sayings in my pocket and worn the miraculous medal around my neck. I've meditated, made religious pilgrimages, said novenas, prayed uncountable rosaries, and even sought the healing powers of an Incan shaman in Peru. All of these efforts were fruitful and taught me something that I needed to learn.

One other step on the journey was to admit that I make mistakes also. In retrospect, I made some regrettable decisions regarding medical treatment and litigation. My intentions were good and I did what I thought was right at the time. In thinking about the healthcare and government participants of the Nebraska outbreak, I think that most of them would say the same thing. I am sharing my mistakes here so that others may learn from them:

- I regret that I chose to be treated by Dr. Javed for the sake of convenience rather than be treated by our long-term associate, Dr. Soori.
- I should have stayed awake during chemotherapy and been vigilant about the safety of healthcare rendered to me.
- I regret that it took me a full year to work through the stigma of hepatitis C and become an active participant in the litigation process.
- I disregarded my lawyers' advice and visited with hospital representatives during ongoing litigation. These visits had negative consequences for me both as a plaintiff and a defendant.
- I made the mistake of signing the compromise regarding the twenty non-monetary points with its nebulous language regarding intent to damage the reputation of the hospital. In attempting to justify its attempt to stop publication of our book, the hospital claimed that this provision made me vulnerable to further lawsuits and this has hindered my patient advocacy efforts.
- I should have insisted on a neutral third party to oversee the implementation of the twenty non-monetary points.

Despite (or, more likely, because of) these lessons, I have realized some blessings. I am profoundly grateful for these blessings:

- After a long and painful separation, I reconnected with God in a more mature yet more intimate way.
- I have a deeper appreciation for the freedoms we enjoy in this country, especially the freedom of speech.
- Through patient advocacy, I have found a mission for my life that is richly satisfying.
- I came to a profound realization that there are many, many good people in this world.
- Although by nature I am a rather timid person, I developed a courage that I never had before.
- I found a compassion for and an identification with the marginalized in the United States: the sick, the unjustly injured, the homeless and the incarcerated.

- I have come to an acceptance of my limitations and through it have developed a life that has better balance. I work at balancing time for work, play, relationships and solitude.
- Knowing that sorrow can find me at any time, I actively seek and cherish joy.
- I am no longer driven to please other people at the expense of compromising deeply held values. I accept that my good intentions may not be recognized as such by other people, even those I consider to be genuinely good people.
- I have a new appreciation for the interconnectedness of life. I see that we are harmed by the misguided actions of some and blessed by the noble deeds of others. I was irreparably harmed by a young person's (the index case's) decision to abuse drugs a thousand miles away and thirty years ago. I have also been blessed beyond measure by the actions of many, many people who go out of their way to do good. There are people (such as lawmakers and health officials) who have been personally unaffected by the Nebraska outbreak but are striving to reform our health-care system because of it and the other outbreaks. Pondering the interconnectedness of all life has caused me to choose my own actions more carefully.

These personal blessings I may never have realized if I had not been a victim of the Nebraska outbreak. I sincerely hope that all the other participants in the Nebraska outbreak will realize some new blessing because of their experience.

The Struggle to Forgive

The question I have asked myself repeatedly is, "Do I forgive?"

I wrestled with the answer night and day for years. In the struggle to find the answer, it felt like I was being taken apart piece by piece and then put back together again. The miracle of the story is that I was put back together again.

Finally, I am able to say, "Yes, I forgive." I do forgive the transgressors, although I do not excuse them from accountability.

I know that some people did not want me to publish this book. I hope that in time *they* will forgive *me*. I hope that the book does so much good for patient safety that it will be easy for them to forgive me.

As I think about the emotional journey of the Nebraska Outbreak, this prayer pushes me toward forgiveness. It was found written on a scrap of paper in 1945, near the body of a dead child in Ravensbruck, a Nazi death camp where 92,000 women and children died.

The Ravensbruck Prayer
Lord, remember not only
the men and women of goodwill,
but also those of ill will.
But do not only remember all the suffering
they have inflicted upon us,
remember the fruits we have bought thanks to this suffering—
our comradeship, our loyalty, our humility,
the courage, the generosity,
the greatness of heart
that has grown out of all of this.
And when they come to judgment
let all the fruits we have borne be their forgiveness.
Amen. Amen. Amen.

CHAPTER 36

■

Hepatitis Outbreaks' National Organization for Reform

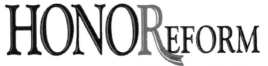

A Patient Advocacy Foundation

The Nebraska hepatitis C outbreak was not an isolated incident. Unfortunately, healthcare-associated outbreaks of hepatitis C continue to occur, even in 2008. In 2007 and 2008, over *70,000 Americans* have received letters urging them to get tested for deadly infectious diseases as a result of the unsafe medical practices of their physicians.

On February 27, 2008, health officials in Nevada announced that over *40,000 residents* were at risk of contracting hepatitis C, hepatitis B and HIV as a result of the reuse of syringes and vials at an endoscopy outpatient center. On April 28, 2008 health officials sent letters to an additional *10,000 Nevadans*, advising them to seek testing related to procedures at the same outpatient center. As of this writing, investigators have determined that approximately eighty-five cases of hepatitis C may be linked to improper procedures at the outpatient center. Ultimately, the Nevada outbreak may result in more cases of hepatitis C than the Nebraska outbreak, although the Nevada outbreak will have multiple sources of infection, whereas the Nebraska cases can all be traced to a single index case.

In New York City, health department officials urged over *4,500 patients* to get tested for hepatitis C as a result of the unsafe practices of an anesthesiologist who provided treatment during the course of endoscopy procedures. In Long Island, the New York State Health Department notified over *10,400 patients* and urged them to get tested for blood-borne diseases after receiving treatment from an anesthesiologist who practiced at a pain management clinic in Plainview. In Grand Rapids, Michigan, another *13,000 patients* were notified by the Kent County Health Department based on syringe reuse and other deficiencies related to possible exposure to hepatitis C, hepatitis B as well as HIV through treatments they received from their dermatologist.

These are examples of recent publicized outbreaks; it is unknown how many people are infected through undocumented healthcare transmission. Obviously, in the United States, we are continuing to make healthcare mistakes that lead to the transmission of disease and untold human suffering.

Because of the need to learn the lessons of the Nebraska hepatitis C outbreak, Travis, Tom and Evelyn formed the patient advocacy group entitled *Hepatitis Outbreaks' National Organization for Reform*—HONOReform. HONOReform is a public-benefit corporation that is organized and operated exclusively for the benefit of social welfare promotion as described in Section 501(c)4 of the Internal Revenue Code. A Section 501(c)3 corporation, HONOReform *Foundation* was incorporated for charitable and educational purposes. Evelyn's settlement award was the seed money for these foundations. Membership is open to everyone. Please visit the Website at www.HONOReform.org or www.HONOReformFoundation.org to learn more about our goals and to join in our patient advocacy effort.

HONOReform's slogan is, *"History unexamined is history repeated."* Its purpose is to learn from the hepatitis C outbreaks and the victim suffering that followed it, so that such tragedies may be prevented in the future. Without examination of these outbreaks, there will be even more suffering from preventable mistakes.

Through the activities of HONOReform, we work to foster:

- Policy changes and enforcement of current policy so that healthcare in all settings is truly safe
- A just and reliable medical malpractice system that provides for the needs of the medically harmed and their healthcare providers
- Compassionate leadership that recognizes the emotional and physical needs of disaster victims

Some of the specific things that we support are: a congressional hearing into the recent spate of hepatitis outbreaks, to understand and address their root causes; monitoring of private ambulatory-care clinics; enforcement and expansion of mandatory reporting laws; public access to licensure investigation reports; use of retractable needles and other "auto-disabling devices" to remove the human factor; safe healthcare practices, "I'm sorry" legislation; and transparency and accountability in malpractice events.

We are currently working with the CDC to launch **The One & Only™ Campaign**. The campaign is designed to educate patients on proper adherence to safe injection practices, to prevent disease transmission from needles, syringes and the misuse of multi-dose vials. The campaign works to empower patients to ask questions about basic infection control in any invasive treatment or procedures they may receive. Patients must understand and realize that reusing a needle or syringe places them at risk of contracting blood-borne illnesses that are life-threatening. These include hepatitis C, hepatitis B and HIV.

The campaign educates healthcare providers (doctors, nurses and anyone providing injections) on basic infection-control practices. Specifically, regarding the use of needles and syringes: *A needle or syringe never should be reused,* either from one patient to another or to withdraw medicine from a vial; *both the needle and syringe must be discarded* once they have been used; and it is *never safe to change the needle and reuse the syringe.* Regarding multi-dose vials: the Centers for Disease Control and Prevention (CDC) recommends *that single-use vials be used and that multi-dose vials of medication be assigned to a single patient, to reduce the risk of disease transmission.*

Promoting the goals of HONOReform is very rewarding. We spoke to an introductory nursing class at the Johns Hopkins University School of Nursing on patient safety issues. When we finished, the professor thanked us by saying, "Today you have spoken to about a hundred new nurses. But through your words, you will foster safety for thousands of patients."

It is words like these that comfort the hepatitis C outbreak victims. By telling and learning from the stories of people infected with hepatitis through healthcare, we can bring about healthcare safety for millions of patients.

Timeline of the Nebraska Hepatitis C Outbreak

January 5, 1998—Dr. Tahir Javed opened Fremont Cancer Center with a generous recruitment package from Fremont Area Medical Center (referred to as "the hospital"). He trained Linda Prochaska, RN, to work as the oncology nurse.

January 1998 through August 1999—The hospital laboratory personnel consistently rejected lab specimens and filed complaints with the laboratory director, Dr. Rodney Koerber, about the lab specimens drawn in the Fremont Cancer Center. Complaints included improper or no labeling and compromised integrity of samples. Dr. Koerber discussed reported improper procedures with Dr. Javed repeatedly. Approximately at the end of 1999, Dr. Javed moved the majority of his lab work to other pathology lab(s).

July 21, 1999—Gerri Means, RN (infection control nurse at the hospital), fielded a report that there was a poinsettia plant in the Fremont Cancer Center chemo hood.

August 4, 1999—Gerri Means fielded a report from lab personnel that Linda Prochaska drew blood from a patient in the Fremont Cancer Center. Linda was not wearing gloves and had visible blood on her hands as she went from patient to patient without washing her hands.

Summer 1999—The hospital initiated a vascular access device committee to address the uncommonly high incidence of clotted ports in cancer patients. The committee recommended a standardized flush procedure, among other things. The standardized flush procedure was not adopted by the Fremont Cancer Center.

November 8, 1999—Peg Kennedy (vice president of the hospital) wrote to Dr. Javed, requesting that he prohibit Linda Prochaska from administrating medication in the hospital proper.

Fall 1999–Spring 2001—Dan McGill underwent treatment at Fremont Cancer Center for colon cancer.

March 2000—The index hepatitis C3a case began treatment at the Fremont Cancer Center.

April 19, 2000–March 5, 2002—The hospital housekeeping department reported ten incidences of improper hazardous waste management in the Fremont Cancer Center to middle management. These reports included glass vials of blood in regular trash cans and blood leaking on the floor.

May 2000—Dr. Javed began an extramarital affair with Individual #7. His wife and children returned to Pakistan.

August 9, 2000—Dr. Javed was brought to the hospital emergency department by ambulance for a possible suicide attempt.

November 16, 2000–April 10, 2001—Evelyn McKnight underwent chemotherapy at Fremont Cancer Center.

December 2000—Heather Schumacher, RN, was hired by the Fremont Cancer Center.

February 5, 2001—Dr. Ralph Dinsdale called Gerri Means and Dr. Javed to discuss a cancer patient with no risk factors who had been recently diagnosed with hepatitis C.

February 14, 2001—Monica Weber reported to Gerri Means and Vice President John Hughes her observation of improper port flushes performed on her at the

Fremont Cancer Center. Gerri discussed the report with Dr. Koerber, Peg Kennedy and Deb Wohlenhaus (hospital safety officer).

February 21, 2001—Gerri Means gave a written report to Dr. Koerber of the reported improper port flush procedure along with a technical article that described an outbreak of hepatitis C in a pediatric oncology service in a different facility, where the disease was spread in the manner described by Monica Weber.

April 12, 2001—Leslie Mayberry, RN, and Marissa Winke, RN, of the Missouri Valley Cancer Consortium, conducted a site visit at the Fremont Cancer Center to determine if the cancer center would qualify to participate in clinical trials.

April 19, 2001—Leslie Mayberry and Marissa Winke returned to the Fremont Cancer Center to give their oral and written report of the site audit. Twenty-six serious violations jeopardizing the heath and safety of employees and patients were noted. The Fremont Cancer Center was not approved for inclusion in clinical research trials.

April 24 and 27, 2001—Gerri Means fielded two reports from hospital employees of patients' descriptions of the improper port flush procedure at the Fremont Cancer Center.

May 1, 2001—Mike Leibert (CEO of the hospital) and John Hughes (VP of the hospital) visited Dr. Javed in his office to discuss improvements in nursing procedure in the Fremont Cancer Center so that it could be approved to participate in clinical trials.

May 10, 2001—The hospital announced its plans for a new, $8 million facility, which included space for expanded cancer services.

May 16, 2001—Dr. Javed reviewed with Gerri Means a chart audit he had compiled on the now five known hepatitis C cases in his practice. The chart audit denied any responsibility by the Fremont Cancer Center for the five known cases.

June 1, 2001—Valerie Wheaton met with Vice President John Hughes and described improper port flushes done at Fremont Cancer Center. The description was the same as that outlined in the Missouri Valley Cancer Consortium audit report, which Hughes had received.

June 12, 2001—Through Heather Schumacher's efforts, the Fremont Cancer Center passed a second inspection by the Missouri Valley Cancer Consortium audit team, and was approved for inclusion in clinical research trials.

June 19, 2001—Valerie Wheaton called Vice President John Hughes and informed him that she had contracted hepatitis C at the Fremont Cancer Center.

June 22, 2001—Hospital administrators met at 9:00 a.m. to discuss Valerie Wheaton's report that she contracted hepatitis C at the cancer center. At 10:00 a.m., John Hughes met with Dr. Javed to discuss the situation. At noon, Linda Prochaska left employment at the Fremont Cancer Center. Gerri Means called Nebraska Health and Human Services to discuss the hepatitis C cases.

July 19–23, 2001—Dr. Javed impersonated two physicians to cancel or obtain test results on Individual #7.

February 8, 2002—Evelyn McKnight was diagnosed with hepatitis C.

February 2002—Monica Weber was diagnosed with hepatitis C and was referred to Dr. Ted Matthews for treatment.

April 15, 2002—Dan McGill died of hepatitis C.

June, 2002—Dr. Tom McKnight diagnosed three new cases of hepatitis C in patients who had been treated at the Fremont Cancer Center.

July 1–11, 2002—Dr. Tom McKnight met individually with Gerri Means and Dr. Javed several times to discuss possible causes of hepatitis C in the cancer patients. Dr. Javed denied any connection to procedures at the Fremont Cancer Center.

July 13, 2002—Dr. Javed left for Pakistan with the explanation that his mother was ill but said that he would return.

August 13, 2002—Dr. M. Salman Haroon took over oncologist duties at the Fremont Cancer Center.

September 10, 2002—Omaha gastroenterologist Dr. Ted Matthews called Dr. Tom McKnight to discuss his concerns about several patients diagnosed with hepatitis C with rare genotype 3a. Dr. Matthews then called the state epidemiologist, Dr. Tom Safranek. Nebraska Health and Human Services began an investigation of the cluster of hepatitis C cases the next day.

October 11, 2002—Nebraska Health and Human Services announced mass screening for former Fremont Cancer Center patients for hepatitis B, hepatitis C and HIV. Four hundred eighty-six patients participated and eighty-two were found to have hepatitis C3a.

November 4, 2002—Travis Bennington filed a lawsuit against the Fremont Area Medical Center to obtain a patient's medical records.

November 2002–January 2003—The eighty-six hepatitis C victims retained lawyers. In all, about thirty lawyers were retained.

Fall 2002—The FBI and the FDA investigated Dr. Javed and the Fremont Cancer Center. The investigation was closed without action one year later.

January 2, 2003—Dr. Javed was appointed as the minister of health for the Punjab region of the Islamic Republic of Pakistan.

January 2003—Jill Watson, who tested negative for hepatitis C during the state-run screening, tested positive using a more sophisticated test. The state health department retested the previous negative cases and found seventeen more cases of hepatitis C, bringing the total to ninety-nine.

March 7, 2003—Cheryl Gentry died of Hepatitis C.

Spring 2003—Judge Samson issued a gag order on plaintiffs and defendants in the litigation.

Spring 2003—The state of Nebraska (acting as administrator of the Nebraska Excess Liability Fund) filed suit in District Court. It alleged it was not responsible for malpractice awards for eighty-six of the eighty-nine plaintiffs. In October 2004, District Court Judge Merritt did not uphold the state's contention.

October 1, 2003—Dr. Javed voluntarily surrendered his license to practice medicine in the state of Nebraska. The Nebraska Health and Human Services' records of the investigation into Javed's licensure complaint were sealed from the plaintiffs.

March 22, 2004—Linda Prochaska voluntarily surrendered her license as a registered nurse. The licensure investigation records were sealed.

Fall 2004—Group settlement talks between plaintiffs and defense failed.

February 24, 2005—*Omaha World Herald* published the incendiary article "Taxpayers Largely Stuck with Hepatitis C Payouts."

June 7, 2005—*Annals of Internal Medicine* printed "An Outbreak of Hepatitis C Virus Infections among Outpatients at a Hematology/Oncology Clinic," which discussed an outbreak of hepatitis C in eastern Nebraska.

October 2005—Bob Ridder's case went to trial.

February 13, 2006—Attorneys representing the Nebraska Excess Liability Fund conducted a telephone survey in Dodge County, asking residents about their knowledge of and affiliation with Drs. Tom and Evelyn McKnight, for the purpose of requesting a change of venue.

March 22, 2006—The McKnights and the defense reached a settlement through mediation. The settlement included the hospital agreeing to implement twenty non-monetary stipulations.

May 9, 2006—Glenn Doescher, an outbreak victim, received a liver transplant at University of Nebraska Medical Center.

December 27, 2006—The last hepatitis C case, Glenn Doescher, reached a settlement with defense through mediation.

January 2007—Travis Bennington and Tom and Evelyn McKnight launched a patient advocacy group called **H**epatitis **O**utbreak of **N**ebraska **O**utreach & **R**eform—**HONOR**eform.

January 31, 2007—Fremont Area Medical Center refused to work with the McKnights on the agreed-upon twenty non-monetary points.

May 31, 2007—Tom and Evelyn McKnight met with several hospital board members and the CEO to request implementation of the twenty non-monetary points. The publication of the book was also discussed.

June 12, 2007—Fremont Area Medical Center received an unauthorized manuscript in the mail.

June 21, 2007—Fremont Area Medical Center asked for an injunction prohibiting the publication of this book. It also filed suit against the authors for defamation of character based on an unauthorized manuscript.

July 6, 2007—Dodge County District Court struck down the injunction prohibiting the publication of this book.

September 6, 2007—Fremont Area Medical Center dropped the defamation of character suit against the authors.

Information About Hepatitis C

This appendix is included as basic background information on the liver and hepatitis C. The information was obtained from The Hepatitis C Support Project (www.hcvadvocate.org) and the Centers for Disease Control (www.cdc.gov/ncidod/diseases/hepatitis/c/index) and is reprinted with their gracious permission.

Hepatitis C Virus Infection in the United States

Hepatitis C virus is the most common chronic, blood-borne viral infection in the United States. First identified in 1988, hepatitis C is the causative agent for what was formerly known as non-A, non-B hepatitis, and is estimated to have infected as many as 242,000 Americans annually during the 1980s. Since 1989, the annual number of new infections has declined by more than eighty percent, to approximately 41,000 by 1998.

A national survey (the third National Health and Nutrition Examinations Survey) of the civilian, non-institutionalized US population found that 1.8 percent of Americans (3.9 million) have been infected with hepatitis C, of whom most (2.7 million) are chronically infected with hepatitis C. These estimates of prevalence are likely conservative, because the survey excluded incarcerated and homeless person groups that have a high prevalence of hepatitis C infection.

Many of these individuals are not aware of their infection and are not clinically ill. However, the consequences of chronic liver disease from hepatitis C generally do not become apparent until ten to twenty years after infection.

What Is the Liver?

The liver is the largest internal organ in the body. It is reddish-brown and is about the size of a football. The really amazing thing about the liver is that if one-half of it is taken away, it will grow back in a few weeks.

The liver's job is to run over 500 functions to keep the body healthy. It is also a very important organ because it filters everything we eat and breathe—even things that get on the skin. The problem is that things such as alcohol, street drugs, cigarette smoke, toxic fumes, some herbs and even some medicines can damage the liver.

The liver helps the body by taking certain foods and turning them into chemicals that give the body energy and keep it healthy. The liver also stores many important things such as vitamins. The liver may be damaged by taking too many vitamins.

Healthy Liver Tips

- Stay away from toxic fumes or liquids.
- Stop drinking alcohol, smoking tobacco and taking street drugs. If you can't stop, try to cut back—talk with a doctor, family or friends about getting some help to stop.
- Talk to your doctor about vaccines to help protect the liver.
- Tell your doctor about all medicines you are taking, even if it's just an aspirin or Tylenol.
- Eat a healthy and well-balanced diet.
- Drink lots of water.
- Stay away from raw or undercooked shellfish.

What Are the Symptoms of Hepatitis C?

Some patients with hepatitis C have no symptoms but others can have many symptoms. The most common symptom is fatigue. Other symptoms are nausea and aches and pains in the muscles, joints, stomach and liver. Occasionally, fevers and night sweats are reported. Depression, anxiety, cognitive and memory problems occur. These types of symptoms can be very troubling and should be reported to a doctor to ensure that they are from hepatitis C and not from another illness or condition. Fortunately for most patients with these types of symptoms, it may mean that they are not getting any sicker from the virus—it may simply mean that the body is fighting the virus.

There are other symptoms if the liver is really damaged and scarred. The term for this condition is "cirrhosis." During cirrhosis, the liver cannot perform many of its important functions. There will be many warning signs and symptoms that the doctor will need to know about. For this reason, it is important for hepatitis-C-infected patients to have regular medical check-ups for observation and treatment of the symptoms.

Risk Factors for Infection

Individuals who injected drugs, even if they did so on only one occasion many years ago, are at highest risk for hepatitis C infection. Hepatitis C infection is rapidly acquired following the initiation of injection drug use and occurs from the sharing of needles, syringes or other equipment associated with drug use. Of persons injecting drugs for at least five years, sixty percent to eighty percent are infected with hepatitis C, compared to about thirty percent infected with HIV. The high rate of hepatitis C infection among injection drug users is also reflected in the high rates (fifteen percent to forty percent) of hepatitis C infection found among incarcerated persons. More than eighty percent of the nation's estimated 1.7 million current injecting drug users have been incarcerated.

Prior to the mid-1980s, there was a seven-percent to ten-percent risk of non-A, non-B hepatitis (hepatitis C) from blood transfusion. This risk declined by more than fifty percent between 1985 and 1990 as a result of implementation of blood donor screening for HIV and surrogate testing for non-A, non-B hepatitis. In 1990, specific blood and plasma donor screening tests for hepatitis C were implemented and by 1992, the risk of hepatitis C infection from a unit of transfused blood was reduced to one in 100,000. As of 2006, the risk of hepatitis C infection from a unit of transfused blood is one in 1,035,000... transfused units. Since 2002, all donations have been screened using molecular technology (nucleic acid testing), approved by the Food and Drug Administration (*Look It Up! A Quick Reference in Transfusion Medicine* by Mark E. Brecher, AABB Press, 2006).

Clotting factor concentrates (plasma-derived products used to treat individuals with hemophilia) also posed a high risk for hepatitis C infection prior to the use of donor screening tests and virus inactivation procedures that were introduced in 1985 and 1987. Except for one outbreak of hepatitis C from a single type of contaminated intravenous immunoglobulin, other plasma-derived products, including immune globulin for intramuscular administration, have not been associated with the transmission of hepatitis C in the United States. Currently, all immune globulin products undergo a virus inactivation procedure or test negative for hepatitis C prior to release.

Sexual exposures account for about fifteen percent of cases of hepatitis C.

Although the risk of transmitting hepatitis C infection through sexual inter-course is low, sex is a common behavior in the general population, a substantial proportion of the adult population has had unprotected sex with multiple part-ners, and there are a large number of persons with hepatitis C infection. While other types of exposures are more likely to transmit hepatitis C (e.g., transfu-sion from an infected donor), they account for a smaller proportion of infections because of the relatively small proportion of the population in whom these exposures have occurred.

Exposures resulting from hemodialysis, employment in the healthcare field and birth to a hepatitis-C-infected mother together account for about five percent of cases. About ten percent of people with hepatitis C infection have no recognized source for their infection.

While it is possible for hepatitis C to be transmitted from any percutaneous exposure to blood, exposures such as tattooing, body piercing or acupuncture have not been shown to place people at increased risk for infection. Higher rates of hepatitis C infection are not found among persons with these exposures alone and these exposures are rarely reported among new cases of hepatitis C.

Consequences of Hepatitis C Infection

About fifteen percent to twenty-five percent of persons with acute hepatitis C resolve their infection without further problems. The remainder develops a chronic infection and about sixty percent to seventy percent of these persons develop chronic hepatitis. Cirrhosis of the liver develops in ten percent to twenty percent of persons with chronic hepatitis C over a period of twenty to thirty years, and hepatocellular carcinoma (liver cancer) in one percent to five percent. For individuals with cirrhosis, however, the rate of development of liver cancer might be as high as one percent to four percent *per year.*

Lower rates of complications have been reported from studies of persons who acquired infection as children. However, longer follow-up studies are needed to assess lifetime consequences of chronic hepatitis C infection in different populations, especially among children.

Chronic liver disease is the tenth-leading cause of death among adults in the Untied States. It is estimated that forty percent to sixty percent of chronic liver disease is due to hepatitis C and another ten percent to fifteen percent is due to chronic hepatitis B. Hepatitis-C-associated chronic liver disease is the most frequent indication for liver transplantation among adults. Additionally, because alcohol use is one of the most important contributing factors to progression of chronic liver disease among persons with hepatitis C, it is important to identify infected individuals as early as possible so that they can be counseled to limit alcohol consumption and be offered treatment if appropriate.

Treatment for Hepatitis C

In 2002, a National Institute of Health Consensus Development Conference updated the guidelines for the medical management of hepatitis C. A combination of PEGylated interferon and Ribavirin is currently the most effective therapy and achieves a sustained viral response (SVR) rate of approximately forty-five percent in patients with genotype 1 and approximately eighty percent in patients with genotypes 2 and 3.

However, ten percent to twenty percent of treated patients do not complete therapy because they experience significant side effects. In addition, some patients may have conditions, such as severe cirrhosis, which prohibit treatment. Current antiviral therapy is not licensed for patients below age eighteen years.

Persons with chronic hepatitis C who continue to abuse alcohol are at risk for ongoing liver injury, and antiviral therapy may be ineffective. In addition, interferon therapy can be associated with relapse in people with a previous history of alcohol abuse; therefore, abstinence from alcohol is recommended during antiviral therapy. Interferon therapy should be considered with caution for patients who recently stopped alcohol abuse, and these patients require the support of alcohol treatment programs.

Patients with hepatitis C on methadone treatment have been successfully treated with interferon. However, there is limited experience with treatment of persons who are recovered injection drug users or who are active injection drug users. In addition, there is the concern that active injection drug users are at risk for reinfection with hepatitis C. When patients with past or continuing substance abuse are considered for antiviral treatment, such patients should receive drug treatment or care from substance abuse specialists or counselors.

Drug treatment is an important adjunct to care for many persons with hepatitis C. Persons with hepatitis-C-related liver disease should be vaccinated against diseases that may produce further complications or increase their risk of death. Susceptible persons with chronic liver disease should receive a hepatitis A vaccine since they are at increased risk of death from liver failure if they get hepatitis A. All persons with chronic liver disease should be vaccinated annually against influenza and should receive pneumoccocal vaccine. In addition, persons with continued risk factors for HBV infection should receive hepatitis B vaccine.

Co-infection

Co-infection with hepatitis C, HIV and/or hepatitis B is currently recognized as a serious problem and is more likely to be found among injection drug users and persons treated for hemophilia before the availability of inactivated clotting factor concentrates. Deaths from chronic hepatitis C among patients with HIV are expected to increase as advances with antiretroviral therapy extend the life span of these patients. Management of HIV infection in hepatitis-C-co-infected patients generally is similar to that for patients with HIV alone, although there is some risk of liver toxicity from the antiretroviral drugs. Hepatitis-C-co-infected patients should be evaluated to determine if they are candidates for antiviral treatment of their chronic liver disease. Because treatment and medical management of co-infected patients is complicated and rapidly evolving, such patients are best managed by healthcare providers with experience in treating both HIV and hepatitis C infection. More research is needed to determine the ideal management and treatment of co-infected individuals.

Persons for Whom Routine Hepatitis C Testing Is Recommended

- Persons who ever injected illegal drugs, including those who injected once or a few times many years ago.
- Persons who received a blood transfusion or organ transplant before July 1992.
- Persons who received clotting factor concentrates produced before 1987.
- Persons who were ever on long-term dialysis.
- Children born to hepatitis-C-positive women.
- Healthcare, emergency medical and public safety workers after needle sticks, sharps or mucosal exposures to hepatitis-C-positive blood.

Safety Tips to Prevent Transmission

- Cover any open cuts or wounds.
- Sexual transmission is low, but the use of condoms and barriers will help reduce the risk even more.
- Make sure that in healthcare settings, standard safety precautions are being carefully followed.

- Do not share needles or works (cottons cookers, ties) used to inject drugs, hormones steroids and vitamins. Wash hands before injecting.
- Do not share any straws to snort drugs or pipes to smoke crack. Or, better yet, don't do crack.
- Do not share any personal hygiene items such as razors, toothbrushes, nail clippers or pierced earrings. Cover personal items and keep them separate from other people you live with.
- Make sure tattoo and piercing equipment is sterile. For a tattoo, make sure that a new needle and ink pot is used for each person. For a piercing, make sure that a new needle is used and that the needle package is opened up in front of you.

Hepatitis C Facts

- One out of fifty Americans is infected with hepatitis C.
- A fourfold increase of chronic hepatitis C infections is predicted by 2015.
- Fifteen thousand deaths per year in the US are caused by hepatitis C.
- A threefold increase in the death toll caused by hepatitis C is predicted by 2010.
- Hepatitis C is four times more common than HIV in the US.
- One out of three people infected with HIV is also infected with hepatitis C.
- Hepatitis C is the most common cause of death in people with HIV.
- Thirty-five thousand new infections of hepatitis C happen annually in the US.
- The financial burden of hepatitis C in the US is estimated at $15 billion per year.
- The financial burden of hepatitis C in the US is estimated to increase to $26 billion per year by 2021.
- Hepatitis C is the leading cause of liver cancer in the US.
- Hepatitis C is the leading cause of liver disease in the US.

- There is no vaccine to prevent its spread.
- Treatment is only fifty-percent effective for the types of hepatitis C seen in the US.
- Eighty percent of individuals infected with hepatitis C have no signs or symptoms of the infection.
- Most people are infected for fifteen or more years before they are diagnosed.

■

Legal Documents and Other Evidence

FAMC / Javed Contract

Contract Package Highlights
August 12, 1997

$50,000 ## Signing Bonus
-- $25,000 to be paid to MD upon signed letter of intent.
-- $25,000 to be paid upon relocation
-- No repayment if final contract is signed.

$10,000 ## Relocation Expense Allowance
-- To be paid to MD as documentation is submitted.
-- Includes 2 househunting trips, moving expenses, temporary housing, other "allowable" expenses.
-- Professional "tail" insurance covered.
-- No repayment unless MD failure to meet contract terms.

$50,000 ## Business Start-up Loan
-- To be paid upon to MD 30 days prior to practice begin date.
-- To cover initial inventory, legal and accounting fees, etc.
-- Repayment of loan is necessary.
  If paid within 1 year.....interest free
  If paid within 2 years....first year interest free. 2nd year = 8%.
  If not paid within 2 years....8% interest from date of check.
  If MD agrees to practice additional 2 years....loan to be forgiven.

Income Guarantee Loan
$600,000/yr -- Definition: Collections from all non-chemo billings + chemo profit.
Gross Collections -- 2 year income guarantee to be paid to MD if monthly collections are less than minimum amount.
-- Interest free loan during the 2 year period.
-- Advance one month in lieu of last month.
-- Monthly calculations based upon MD gross billings.
  If less than guarantee....FAMC to pay MD up to guarantee amt.
  If more than guarantee...MD to pay FAMC up to prior subsidy rcd.
-- Final accounting at end of year 2. MD to pay FAMC up to total amount received if total is greater than or equal to the guarantee in total.
-- If physician reaches minimum amount within first 12 months, loan to be forgiven at: 50% at end of year 2; 75% at end of year 3; 100% at end of year 4.

$17.50/sq ft ## Rental Agreement
-- Equal to fair market value of furnished and equipped rental space.
-- To be paid monthly from MD to FAMC.
-- Approximately $2,579/month based upon 1,769 sq feet.
-- Physician has option to purchase all equipment/furnishings at fair market value at any time and rent will be adjusted accordingly.

The 1997 Recruitment Package

file
9C

From: ████████rkins
To: Gerri Means
Date: 7/21/99 2:43pm
Subject: Laminar Flow Hood information

Received a call from ██████████ last week reporting that Dr.
Javed has a pointsettia plant in his hood. She wondered if we
should alert him to the fact that there should not be plants
there. Deb visited with █████ about it & we decided to check
with you when you returned to see if there is any information
regarding Laminar Flow Hoods that we could forward to him for
educational purposes. Unable to find anything in the manuals in
our office. Since you don't do Safety Surveillance in his
office. wasn't sure how to handle it.

8-4-99 Contacted by ████████ - Lab that yesterday had
to go to Dr Javed's office (due to funeral & staffing)
Dr K. told her to be sure lab drawn from a venipuncture
(pt receiving chemo) & not the port. due to Type & Xmat
asked for gloves & Linda says "Oh we don't use them
Linda ended up doing draw from port —& had visible
blood on her hands & was no gloves.
Kay informed Dr Kerber of situation.
Informed Dr Kerber about email received about
laminar flow hood issue.
Office is rented from hospital so have no jurisdiction
on Dr J's employees.
Dr Kerber said there is a vascular access meeting
Aug 20. —perhaps issues can be addressed

Reports to the hospital infection control practitioner about cancer center
dangers—years before the Nebraska outbreak was uncovered.

Monday November 22, 1999

Doctor Javed,

As of today I am giving my 2 week notice. Due to many circumstances I am unable to continue to work for you. I feel I have given 100% to my job here and I do thank- you for what I have learned. I hope we are able to talk about why I am leaving but since we sometimes aren't able to , I am going to jot down a few thoughts for you.

When I was hired we spoke of numerous things that were going to take place in my position. I was under the impression that these things were understood when I took the job. 1) There would be paid holidays and vacations, 2) We would have a computer system within a year and I would be taking over your billing, 3) There was the possibility of hiring another office person, and I would take on more of an Office Managerial position. Basically none of these things have taken place.

Of course one of the biggest things that I have had to deal with is your nurse. I don't think you have any idea of the verbal abuse I have taken from her. I have tryed to smooth over many things with not only patients but people of the hospital when her temper has gotten out of control and her rudeness have taken over. I am able to get along with just about anyone, but Linda has now taken the role of running the office and treats me like I am some sort of idiot. I am not allowed to schedule patients without some remark or having to change times to fit her. If she wasn't so rude we could work this out but she has a way of making a person feel really useless. I really think you need to decide just who is the boss. There are many things that are not done to OSHA codes and I know you are aware of them, but don't seem to make her accountable. I also know many people and administration from the hospital have questioned her ways. From Linda having things her way, Rose has now taken on alot of her attitude and has become her little clone. They neither one can even say Good-morning as they walk right by my desk in the morning. Life is too short to stay in an environment where one feels extremely unwanted.

I wish you the best in your practice, I think you are a brilliant Doctor and are very much needed in this community.

Best of luck to you, and God Bless,

Karla

P.S. I trust that this letter will be kept confidential.

Javed's receptionist hands in her resignation letter.

From: Gerri Means
To: Deb Wohlenhaus
Date: 4/20/00 4:28pm
Subject: Javed's office

Diane Sukstorf called me this afternoon to tell me that last eveing when Facilities was in Dr Javed's office there was a small tube with a plastic apparatus laying on on of the chemo chair. She is questioning how to handle the "improper waste report" since normally it is sent to the manager (and a record is kept by HAZ MAT). She was going to contact the office today and inform them of this incident but does anyone else need this info (besides HAZ MAT)?

CC: Diane Sukstorf

From: Deb Wohlenhaus
To: Gerri Means
Date: 4/21/00 6:31am
Subject: Javed's office -Reply

not much else Diane can do but report through that manner, and note for her own records. We have no jurisdiction in that office, but I can pass info on to John Hughes, as he works closely with Dr. Javed, especially since FAMC is going to do some major reworking and remodeling in his area again.

The hospital emails.

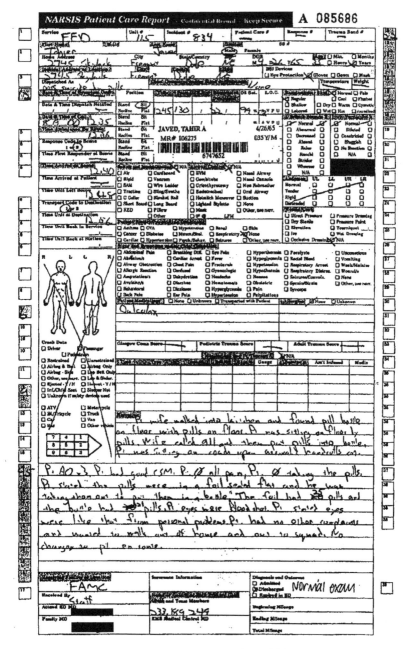

The hospital ER records of Dr. Javed's possible suicide attempt.

Appendix C

FREMONT AREA MEDICAL CENTER

EMERGENCY DEPARTMENT NOTE

NAME:	JAVED, TAHIR A		ROOM#: ER
ACCT#:	6747652	DOB: 04/26/1965	AGE: 35Y
MR#:	106275	PTSEX: M	PT TYPE: E
ATTENDING:	████ M.D.		ADMIT: 08/09/2000
DICTATING:	████ M.D.		

HISTORY: The patient is a 35-year-old physician who was brought to the emergency room apparently when the police called the rescue squad. The patient had apparently had a heated and emotional discussion with a friend earlier in the day. When his friend arrived at his home some tablets had been spilled and the friend got the idea that the patient had attempted an overdose. 911 was called and the police investigated, and the rescue squad brought Dr. Javed to the emergency room.

The patient denies taking any medications. The medications in question were Dulcolax. He denies any suicidal ideation. He does admit to some increased stress of late.

The patient has no history of depression or suicide. His only medical problems were a cholecystectomy a year ago which was done laparoscopically. He has otherwise been healthy. He is a nonsmoker.

PHYSICAL EXAMINATION: Shows normal vital signs. Head, Eyes, Ears, Nose, and Throat: Unremarkable. The posterior pharynx is benign. Neck is supple. Trachea midline. Thyroid is not enlarged. No bruits are heard in the neck. Lungs are clear bilaterally. Heart has a regular rate and rhythm without murmur or gallop. The abdomen is soft and nontender with normal bowel sounds. There is no organomegaly or mass. Genitalia and rectal were deferred. The lower extremities have full range of motion with good distal pulses. Cranial nerves II-XII are intact. Deep tendon reflexes are symmetrical. The fundi are normal bilaterally. Motor, sensory, and cerebellar function are intact. There are no pathological reflexes. His gait is normal.

ASSESSMENT: Normal examination without evidence of drug ingestion or suicidal ideation.

PLAN: The patient wishes to have a urine screen to provide objective evidence that there was no ingestion. Sample was gathered and the patient was discharged with no further recommendations.

```
\: jgw
/:    128
DD: 08/10/2000
DT: 08/10/2000     1851
ID: 000239438
cc: ████     M.D. (00128)
    T. A. JAVED, M.D. (00604)
>
```

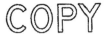

COPY

Dr. Aronson' ER report.

Date:	February 21, 2001
To:	Dr. R. K. Koerber Infection Control Chairman
From:	Gerri Means, RN-CIC Infection Control Practitioner
Subject:	Hepatitis C

After I receive a positive report from the lab on a patient with HIV, Hepatitis B or Hepatitis C, I review the patient's old medical records to determine if there is any correlation to blood transfusion products. (All positive cases for HIV, Hepatitis B and C are reported to the State Health Department by the ICP also).

Two patients recently were positive for Hepatitis C antibody and it was noted that they had breast cancer. Their surgeries had been done at FAMC but by different surgeons. There were no known blood transfusions or blood products given at FAMC. Both patients had ports and were being followed by Oncology (Dr. Javed).

On February 5, 2001, Dr. ▮▮▮▮▮▮called my office asking if I was conducting an investigation on the Hepatitis C cases. He reported that he had discussed his patient (who had recently had a positive Hepatitis C antibody) with Dr. Javed (she also has breast cancer). He has no idea where she got the disease since she hasn't had blood products and has no other known risk factors. He said that Dr. Javed had informed him that he has 4-5 Hepatitis C patients. I reviewed my bloodborne disease log again and can only identify three patients who are patients of Dr. Javed's.

After I informed you on February 5, 2001 about ▮▮▮▮▮ information, I compiled the list of names I have reported to State with Hepatitis C in the past year for you to review. I reviewed the history information again on these patients and still do not feel there is any association with blood transfusions or blood products. I also went back to employee injury reports related to blood and body fluid exposures and find no link.

On February 14, 2001, I had a person who has been receiving chemotherapy in Dr. Javed's office request a meeting with me to discuss "infection control" issues. Concerns were expressed about the office nurse "Linda" who is accessing ports and seldom wears gloves. Patients are lined up in chairs to receive their chemotherapy and this nurse goes between these patients without washing her hands.

This person reports that after Linda accesses the port, a needle with a syringe is used to draw back blood to check the patency and then the blood is pushed back into the port again. Having been a patient at FAMC, hospital nurses were observed discarding this needle/syringe with blood after the port was checked for patency.

The needle/syringe which had been used to check the patency (and previously had blood in it) is then used to draw off saline from a bag that is also used for other patients in the office. The port on this saline bag is not wiped off with an alcohol wipe prior to inserting the needle. The saline that is in the syringe is then pushed into the port. With the same needle and syringe (that was used to check patency and flush with saline), it is then put into a Heparin vial that is used on other patients also.

Hearing about this office practice, I am concerned that there might be contamination of the saline and/or Heparin if these multidose products have had a needle/syringe with blood introduced into them.

I am enclosing an article about a Hepatitis C investigation on a pediatric oncology service and pharmacy information from the APIC Text.

Gerri Means' memo to Dr. Koerber.

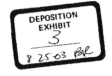

On February 14, 2001, I had a person who has been receiving chemotherapy in Dr. Javed's office request a meeting with me to discuss "infection control" issues. Concerns were expressed about the office nurse "Linda" who is accessing ports and seldom wears gloves. Patients are lined up in chairs to receive their chemotherapy and this nurse goes between these patients without washing her hands.

This person reports that after Linda accesses the port, a needle with a syringe is used to draw back blood to check the patency and then the blood is pushed back into the port again. Having been a patient at FAMC, hospital nurses were observed discarding this needle/syringe with blood after the port was checked for patency.

The needle/syringe which had been used to check the patency (and previously had blood in it) is then used to draw off saline from a bag that is also used for other patients in the office. The port on this saline bag is not wiped off with an alcohol wipe prior to inserting the needle. The saline that is in the syringe is then pushed into the port. With the same needle and syringe (that was used to check patency and flush with saline), it is then put into a Heparin vial that is used on other patients also.

On 4-24-01 ███████ called to find out what the hospital protocol is to access a port. She has a friend receiving chemo in Dr Javed's office who has a concern about the techniques used to flush the port - draw blood - change needle - then pull solution from a bag (syringe) that had old blood in it) She has talked to Dr Javed about this issue:

4-27-0' ███████████ called. had accessed a port in a pt expressing concerns about Radiology on ' techniques used in Dr Javed's office - needle changed on syringe (that had blood in it) Bag was almost empty & had to push on it to get enough solution (saline ? H2O) for the syringe. Advised ████ to talk to Dr Kauber. - the pt discuss concerns with Dr Javed ±/or John Hughs. pt:

Gerri Means' notes on her meeting with Monica Weber, and her handwritten notes on calls from Nurse Cline and Nurse Tilson.

**Missouri Valley
Cancer Consortium
CCOP**

Memo

To: ▮▮▮▮▮▮▮

From: ▮▮▮▮▮▮▮▮▮ Executive Director, MVCC

CC: Dr. Javed

Date: 04/19/01

Re:

▮▮▮▮▮▮▮▮

I was asked to accompany you to the Fremont Area Medical Center, specifically, the Cancer Center, to review the office process of Dr. Javed. The purpose of this meeting was to insure that the system utilized by Dr. Javed would be conducive to conducting clinical research in the office setting, with the support of the hospital personnel and the Alegent Health research office.

On April 12, 2001, I accompanied you to the office to spend time in observance of practice routines. I have enclosed a copy of my findings and recommendations for your review.

At this time, I do not recommend initiating clinical trials in Dr. Javed's office based on the issues that I have included in my initial report. Once the issues have been resolved and corrected, I believe we would be ready to institute clinical trials.

Of most concern are the practices by the nursing staff related to admixture and administration techniques. The current nursing practices are poor, and in violation of OSHA regulations. I believe that these practices could significantly influence the reporting and outcome of the research to be conducted, and therefore, I do not feel that the CCOP at this time would benefit from this situation.

Please review my findings and feel free to discuss them with me at any time. We have a meeting scheduled with Dr. Javed on April 19, 2001 to discuss these concerns and where to go with them from here.

I have discussed these issues in private with Dr. ▮▮▮▮▮▮▮▮ PI, Missouri Valley Cancer Consortium CCOP, and he is in agreement with my recommendation at this time.

MVCC report, page 1 of 5.

REVIEW OF PROCESS

OFFICE OF DR. JAVED

FREMONT AREA MEDICAL CENTER

CANCER CENTER

PHYSICIAN DICTATION:

Review of Dr. Javed's dictation indicates an excellent communication mechanism that is concise to the patient condition. Dictation is completed in a timely fashion and is on the chart in a timely manner.

From a clinical research standpoint, Dr. Javed will need to incorporate into his dictation practice the following:

Performance Score, toxicities and the grade, as well as attribution, a note of interval labs, tumor measurements if applicable, and in the initial discussion with the patient, the review of the consent process and patient understanding and agreement to participate.

OFFICE ROUTINE:

Observation of the routine of patient flow through the office appears to be conducive to conducting clinical research. Ample time is allotted between patients to accommodate the research process.

LAB WORK:

Labs (cbc) are completed in the office by the nursing staff, and ran manually in the office by a technician. Labs are reviewed and signed off by Dr. Javed. It was not clear to me how chemistries and other send out labs are handled.

XRAYS:

All radiological studies are completed in the Fremont Hospital, convenient for the patient, and easy access to reports and radiologists for measurements.

MVCC report, page 2 of 5.

Appendix C

MIXING AREA AND ADMIXTURE PROCEDURES:

There are serious violations of OSHA regulations related to the area in question, and serious improper admixture procedures observed. Specifically:

1.   OSHA violations observed:

Food and food supplies are set up on the same cabinet space where chemotherapy is stored, mixed, and set

There was not any protective equipment for admixture or administration in site. Specifically, no gowns or gloves

A pregnant tech was observed handling chemo-contaminated supplies and equipment without protective equipment

No spill kit in site, no eye wash in site

There was not observance of extravasation kit or procedure

Chemo-contaminated supplies were being discarded in the regular trash, unmarked

Blood and blood products not being handled by personnel wearing gloves

Chemo is being laid on top of open charts, thus contaminating the charts

There was no apparent signage indicating possible chemotherapy contamination

Staff was not wearing protective equipment, not washing hands, and eating/drinking in chemo mixing area

Admixed drugs were being stored in the cabinet without being labeled for dilution in mg/ml, and in date of admixture.

There was not observance of an emergency kit on hand in the event of anaphylaxis, or cardiac arrest related to drug administration.

Recommendations:

Remove all food, and related supplies and equipment immediately. It should all be considered contaminated and discarded. Equipment should be cleaned thoroughly before relocating.

Protective equipment should be ordered and staff mandated to wear gown and gloves whenever handling chemotherapy. A separate gown should be used for admixing, and this gown utilized by the person mixing, and discarded at the end of each day. This gown should not be worn beyond the mixing area. A separate gown should be worn when administering chemotherapy.

The pregnant technician should be kept out of the chemo area as much as possible, and should be mandated to wear protective equipment.

MVCC report, page 3 of 5.

An emergency kit needs to be developed if not already done so to be utilized in the event of an emergency. In addition, the center needs a chemo spill kit, and an extravasation kit available to the staff, if not already available.

There should be specially marked trash bags for which the staff discards chemo contaminated waste. It should not be put into the general trash.

Staff should be wearing protective equipment when handling blood and blood products,

There should be signage indicating that there is chemotherapy in the area, alerting other staff and family members to potential contamination.

Staff should not have food/drink in the area of mixing.

2.   Admixture violations observed:

Staff not wearing gown and gloves to mix, did not wash hands after mixing, observed eating/drinking in chemo mixing area

No underpad to absorb drips or spills in bottom of hood...there were dried chemo drips in the bottom of the hood

The chemo waste bucket was inside the hood, as well as a pile of syringes, thus contaminated

There was no use of alcohol wipes in site. RN was observed removing a used vial of chemo from the cabinet, and inserting a needle into it without wiping it off first with an alcohol wipe

Syringe used to draw up chemotherapy was not discarded; it was laid on the cupboard next to the patient's chart. The RN informed me that she reuses the syringe for additional medications when needed by the patient. This syringe should have been discarded immediately after it was used. The countertop is presumed contaminated

There were needles left in vials of sterile saline. The RNs attached previously used syringes from multiple patients to the same needle in the vial for drawing up saline for patient use. The vial should be presumed no longer sterile with an uncovered needle left in the vial. There is poor nursing technique and risk of infection associated with this procedure, as well as cross contamination by multiple patients to this vial

There were dirty syringes laid on the countertop next to the patient chart. The syringe had blood in it, and was not covered but open ended. This syringe should have been discarded. It is contaminated and there is bacterial growth associated with leaving it open. The nurse informed me that she uses this syringe to flush patient ports and IV lines. This is the syringe that is attached to the needles that are in the vials of saline

There was a nurses' aide observed drawing up and administering neumega and GCSF products. While she may have been taught to do this procedure, she was observed drawing up multiple syringes at one time, of two different drugs, and none of the syringes were labeled with the patient name. At one point, she walked out with three syringes in her hand for patient administration. Although she may be reliable, this practice sets up for the patient to receive wrong dose or drug

Tubing is not primed with IV solution prior to admixing the chemo

MVCC report, page 4 of 5.

Chemo is admixed by drawing solution from the IV bag

None of the bags were labeled with the patient name, or the drug and dose that was in the bag

Drugs were observed being admixed incorrectly, with the wrong amount of diluent. The drug was cloudy in the vial, and was obviously not in solution, yet was drawn up and put into an unmarked bag. Another drug was observed being admixed incorrectly by not allowing the drug to go into solution prior to drawing up

Drugs were put back on the shelf for future use without being marked for dilution in mg/ml, or the date of dilution. Some drugs are only stable for a matter of a few hours, and this was not being taken into consideration

It was reported to me that the RNs reinject the 3-5cc discard that is pulled off of a port or catheter prior to drawing specimens. They are reinjecting small clots, fibrin, and bacteria, and this practice in all aspects of catheter care is unacceptable, placing the patient at high risk for infection and blood clots along and in the catheter

Recommendations:

These issues can be considered violation of OSHA standards as well, as practices do not protect the employee or the patient. This is a tremendous liability for Dr. Javed as well as the hospital.

I would recommend that Dr. Javed get immediate assistance of a pharmacist or RN trained in the admixing and administration of chemotherapy to assist the staff until the staff can be properly trained in these areas.

The RNs are observed not only using poor chemo admix and adminstration techniques, but also poor basic nursing techniques.

At minimum, the RNs should have the following basic training:

Chemotherapy certification

Training by an experienced pharmacist or RN on correct admixing techniques

Port and catheter management training

Infection control training

They should be encouraged to become ONS members if not already, and to seek the publications available to them on all aspects of oncologic nursing practices

MVCC report, page 5 of 5.

Appendix C

Missouri Valley Cancer Consortium

A Community Clinical Oncology Program Funded by the National Cancer Institute

Board of Directors

Lincoln Cancer Center

Oncology Hematology West, P.C.

Creighton Cancer Center

Creighton Cancer Center
Principal Investigator

Consultants in Radiation
Oncology, P.C.

— Alegent Health Midlands
Cancer Center

Medical Oncology/Hematology

Hematology & Oncology
Consultants, P.C.

Components

**Alegent Bergan Mercy
Cancer Center**
7500 Mercy Road
Omaha, NE 68124
(402) 398-6064

Creighton Cancer Center
601 N. 30th Street, Suite 2565
Omaha, NE 68131
(402) 280-4364

**Alegent Immanuel
Cancer Center**
6901 N. 72nd Street
Omaha, NE 68122
(402) 572-2988

The Cancer Resource Center
4600 Valley Road
Suite 336
Lincoln, NE 68510-4844
(402) 483-2827

To: Tahir Javed, M.D.
     Fremont Area Medical Center

From: ███████ RN ████
     Executive Director
     Missouri Valley Cancer Consortium

Re: Follow-up of Issues

Date: April 23, 2001

Dr. Javed,

I want to thank you again for your interest in clinical trial research, and for your receptivity to the issues we discussed last week. I realize that the meeting was difficult for you and your staff.

To review, after we met, ████████ and I met with your staff. I did spend a great deal of time explaining my concerns, and relaying them to your staff from a standpoint of safety for the patients and staff, and from the concern of patient outcomes. It was not my place to judge or criticize, but to point out areas of deficiencies that could ultimately affect the outcome of the clinical research to be conducted.

Unfortunately, we were not able to develop a plan with your staff for correcting the issues at hand, as you had requested. I believe that Heather and Rose were quite overwhelmed by the information, and Linda appeared unwilling to discuss options, and was obviously angry that we were there. I am aware of the sensitive nature of the issues, but it would be a shame to miss out on research opportunities on the basis of staff who are unwilling to learn and improve patient care processes. I left it with Linda that she and the staff have full support of the CCOP staff to help as a resource to improve your situations, and that she should get back with either Laura or myself as to how she would like to proceed. As of today, we have not heard from her.

Again, my purpose is to ensure that if clinical trials are to be conducted at your office, the processes must be conducive to quality data outcomes. The mixing issues lead me to believe that your patients are not receiving correct doses of medications as ordered; the safety issues are OSHA requirements, not mine or anyone else's. The Missouri Valley Cancer Consortium prides itself on quality patient care at all levels. Therefore, we will have to wait until issues in your

MVCC offers help, page 1 of 2.

clinic are restored to a higher level of nursing care and drug management before we can begin research work.

Please contact either ████████████ or myself at your earliest convenience as to your plans. I have honored your request to keep this information private, and to allow you and your staff time to digest and begin process improvements. You have full support of the system to help you however and wherever we can. I hope you will not let these issues set you back from participation. I look forward to hearing from you soon.

Sincerely,

████████████████ RN

MVCC offers help, page 2 of 2.

Appendix C

Met from 1430-1520 c̄ Dr Javed

at one point wanted hospital help + then didn't.

= resources & limited space it can't be done

hospital vs. private practice.

5 page report.

"FAMC Pharmacist don't know anything"

- when things are right - need to stay on course

- only 3 neutropenic sepsis pts on 3 yrs. then A to now in 5 mos.

- 10 x daily - (then said he wasn't back there).

- they are knowledgeable.

ery serious OSHA violations

θ alcohol wipes

- θ gloves, gowns
  ot mixing correctly, nothing labeled.

blood on syringe

- shelf life
  splatters in hood
  mixing → drinking coffee → pts.
  θ hand washing

- Asked Linda if had spill kit
- OSHA guidelines.
- wouldn't answer questions.

Dr Javed requested a copy not given to Administration yt untle he had time to correct problems. Respect his privacy.

- Dr Javed upset that I sat in - rifts between hospital nurses + his nurses.

mB offered classes, training pharmacist. for nurses to come to Creighton Clinic + spend a day.

he left...
need back in

FAMC 000865

Cathy Spelling's notes from the MVCC inspection.

296

interested in chemo class).

concerned - only one concerned

– she's not in charge & made very clear to her

– wants help

– internet research

  – books

  anything she could get her hands on

– made copies - took to Linda + ███ over weekend.

Friday

– He was upset at the findings however he doesn't seem to want to make changes – he's not interested in changing things.

– He told Linda to order an OSHA manual.

When she asked if she should wear gowns & gloves. You can wear that astronaut suit if you want to.

– Then - ust asked Linda if she should go to a class - Linda stated you don't need to do that - I'm teaching you everything you need to know.

– "I'm doing what the doctor is telling me to do.

Cathy Spelling's notes from her visit with Heather.

Missouri Valley Cancer Consortium

A Community Clinical Oncology Program Funded by the National Cancer Institute

To: Mr. Hughes
        Fremont Area Medical Center

From: ████████ RN   ████████
        Executive Director, MVCC-CCOP

Re: Clinical Trial Participation with Dr. Javed

Date: May 1, 2001

Mr. Hughes,

I have been working with Dr. Javed, ████████ RN, and ████████ RN (Alegent Health) on the establishment of a clinical trial program at your institution.

I have spent time with Dr. Javed and his staff reviewing processes to assure that the environment is conducive to conducting quality research work. I believe that Dr. Javed is not only interested, but has the experience and knowledge to conduct clinical trials. However, as I discussed with Dr. Javed, there are a number of serious issues related to nursing care processes that I found unacceptable practice in any patient care setting, and specifically, in the area of oncology nursing practice. I indicated to Dr. Javed that the poor nursing care would undoubtedly directly affect research outcomes, and therefore, we could not agree to begin clinical trial work until these issues have been resolved or improved. I offered full support of the CCOP staff resources to assist with process improvements and nursing education.

I spoke with Dr. Javed this morning, and he indicated to me that he has met with your administration a couple of times regarding my issues of concern, and the consensus at this time is to wait to begin clinical trial work until the new Cancer Center is built and established, where he felt the environment would be more conducive to conducting research.

At this time, the CCOP will not pursue this issue any further with Dr. Javed. However, I am extremely concerned about the poor nursing care practices that I observed in the area. I feel there is a moral and ethical issue to at least make you aware of what I had observed, and to reiterate to you that these poor practices are in breech of OSHA regulations, and that the poor care is undoubtedly affecting patient outcomes, and the quality of your cancer program reputation.

I have enclosed a copy of my report to Dr. Javed for your review. Again, I offer the full support of CCOP staff resources to assist as needed. If you feel the need for additional discussion on this issue, please feel free to contact me at the CCOP office. My number there is (402) 398-8010. Thank you.

Winke's letter to the hospital.

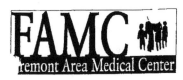

Here for life!

May 4, 2001

Tahir A. Javed, M.D.
Fremont Cancer Center, PC
450 East 23rd Street, Suite 1
Fremont, Nebraska 68025

Dear Dr. Javed:

Thank you for taking the time out of your busy schedule to meet with Mike Leibert and me in my office on Tuesday. I appreciate your efforts and your expertise as we work together to achieve our common vision of an exceptional cancer center in our community.

I look forward to meeting with you next week as we put together the action plan that will put the cancer program in a position to offer protocols through the Missouri Valley Cancer Consortium. Your willingness to be an active participant in the process is a vital element in the success of this effort.

Just to let you know, I have asked ▮▮▮▮▮▮▮▮ FAMC's Director of Marketing and Public Relations, to provide me with a mechanism to survey the oncology patients in our community. I expect to hear from her before our meeting next week and I will provide more details at that time.

As always, if you have questions or if I can be of assistance, please do not hesitate to contact me.

Sincerely,

John C. Hughes, CHE
Vice-President, Professional Services

cc: Mike Leibert

DEPOSITION
EXHIBIT
186
2/4/04

The hospital's letter to Javed.

Appendix C

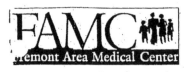

Here for life!

R. K. Koerber, M.D.
Medical Director of Laboratory

Javed —

This was given to me by Gerri means. Im sorry I took so long in getting it to you but Im behind. Some of these things were talked about before — but some of the information may be of concern to you.

The Hospital Infection Control Committee has no authority in this issue but we would be happy to discuss it at any time if you wish.

Rod K.

FAMC 000082

Gerri Received 5-14-01   Gerri does not know what date Dr. Koerber sent this.

Nebraska 68025 • (402) 721-1610

Dr. Koerber's handwritten note to Javed.

Appendix C

May 14, 2001 *Given to Gerri Means by Dr. Javed*

Hepatitis C Positive

PATIENT NAME:
DOB: 2/18/32
DIAGNOSIS: Right breast cancer and Hepatitis C positive status.

Risk Factor: Patient states that in December of 2000 she was <u>stuck by a hyperdermic needle lying in a trash can at a movie theater.</u>

Patient received chemotherapy from 4/27/99 to 8/10/99. Received six cycles of CMF. Since then she has come for a port flush which was removed in April.

_____ and _____ seen on 4/28/00 on the same day; however _____ was seen at 10:00 am for a port flush only _____ came at 3:00 pm for Procrit shot (given subcutaneously). No saline was used for port flush. Otherwise, there is no overlap of visits to suggest contamination.

PATIENT NAME:
DOB: 6/11/49
DIAGNOSIS: Left breast cancer and Hepatitis C positive status.

Patient received chemotherapy from 3/3/2000 up to 6/28/2000 with six cycles of CAF.

_____ had one visit at _____'s time, however during this time _____ had come for a port flush, _____ had come for Procrit shot. No contact. She reported two times for a port flush on 8/9 and 11/15/00, the same days _____ was here for fluids and chemotherapy. However, again, port-a-cath flush does not involve saline and there is no risk of cross contamination.

PATIENT NAME:
DOB: 3/29/61
DIAGNOSIS: Rectal cancer and Hepatitis C positive status.

Risk Factor: Hepatitis C, <u>history of IV drug abuse.</u>

Patient received chemotherapy as an outpatient from 7/19 to 12/6/2000. Currently, she has been coming for port-a-cath flushes.

On 9/7 she was here the same day as _____ however _____ was present only for a port-a-cath flush with <u>no risk of contamination.</u>

PATIENT NAME:
DOB: 6/11/56
DIAGNOSIS: *consult (visit)* Polycythemia and Hepatitis C positive status.
Date of visit: 11/15/00 and 11/27/00.

On 11/27/00 patient had a bone marrow aspirate and biopsy done by me. <u>No risk of contamination</u> of other members of the staff or patients.

No port - No lab

an 11-26-22   Known Hepatitis C + appear 10 yrs - mylodysplastic.
Goes to Dr. McKnight office for Lab   Drew blood only 1x May 20. 2000 at Dr. J's.
Bon 5-22-00   10-31-00

Javed makes excuses.

301

Appendix C

Summary of meeting in Dr. Javed's office on May 16, 2001:

Dr. Javed arranged a meeting with Gerri Means, RN-CIC from Infection Control at FAMC to review the information he has collected from the chart reviews he had conducted on the five known Hepatitis C positive patients seen in his office practice.

Although Dr. ████████ previously had told Gerri there were no known risk factors for ████████ that would associate her with a blood borne pathogen, Dr. Javed has information from the patient that relates she had been stuck by a needle in a trash can at a movie theater in December 2000.

Gerri shared information about concerns received from patients and/or family members about techniques utilized with port draws (i.e., using a syringe which had previously had blood in it from the port draw and then using this syringe to access the saline bag). These people had expressed concerns about the difference in procedures utilized in the office and the hospital personnel. According to Dr. Javed, the protocol has been reviewed with the office staff and he also spent a day last week observing chemotherapy administration.

From the chart reviews done by Dr. Javed, he could not identify a day when these five known hepatitis C patients would have had a potential cross contamination with the saline. He noted that there have been changes made in the office (i.e., individual syringes drawn up with saline). I was told the chemo drugs are done under the hood but they do have some specific drugs that are drawn up directly from the vial, so this may lead to questions about the hood usage for drug preparation.

Gerri has encouraged those people who have contacted her about the office practices to discuss their concerns with the physician. Dr. Javed does want open communication with his patients/family, so he asked Gerri to communicate directly with him on any issues that might come thru her office.

He noted that due to space, there does get to be problems with storage, food consumption, etc. Arrangements have been made by Dr. Javed to have the office staff attend an OSHA meeting in June in Omaha.

Gerri Means' notes from her meeting with Javed.

Appendix C

June 22, '01 9am
Met with Mike, John H, Reg K, Dr Kaeber,
[redacted] + Gerri
Discuss Appendix C - newest pt who came to John
- she did not have lab done at FAMC.
John Reviewed report C [redacted] on
    Missouri Alliance Cancer Consortium's issues
Gerri to make State aware of issue - called [redacted]
    ([redacted])

Chris discussed situation with Dr Safranek
    Only keeping count of number of cases reported.
Advised to talk to
    [redacted]
        Director of Investigations
        402 471 4964

John to talk to Dr Javid - 10am
Noon - told Linda is no longer working.

4:15 Diane Facilities reports there is a food
    tray that has been in Dr Javid's office
    with mold growing
    Also have a "bag issue" - Chemo bag in
    a receptacle with black bag
    Advised to talk to John.

DEPOSITION
EXHIBIT
185
2/4/04

FAMC 000078

Gerri Means' notes from the June 22, 2001 meeting.

303

᷐ahir A. Javed, M.L.
Hematology & Oncology

FREMONT CANCER CENTER, P.C.
450 E. 23ʳᵈ Street, Suite #1
Fremont, NE 68025
Phone: (402) 727-3410 Fax: (402) 727-3616

Memorandum

Date: June 22, 2001

From: Dr. Tahir A. Javed, Medical Director

To: Linda Prochaska, Personnel File

Today I invited Ms. Prochaska to my office and relieved her of nursing duties at the Fremont Cancer Center. On various occasions during the past year and a half, I have had the opportunity to discuss the general code of conduct and health and safety issues with her. On multiple occasions, as documented in previous memos, I have stressed upon her the importance of taking proper safety precautions in the nursing management of patients. Disciplinary procedures from the Fremont Cancer Center Policy and Procedure Manual have been discussed with her. OSHA regulations, chemotherapy administration and disposal, portacath flushing policy, and universal safety precautions, such as hand washing; wearing of gloves, and usage of protection equipment had been reviewed.

Ms. Prochaska had been clearly informed that any deviation from these regulations and policies would not be tolerated. On June 20, 2001 Ms. Prochaska was seen accessing a port without gloves. I reminded her that she must wear gloves when taking care of patients. I also informed her that latex-free gloves were available if she had allergies. On June 21, 2001, I observed that Ms. Prochaska was not properly labeling chemotherapy/NS bags. She was violating FCC policies. This was a clear demonstration of insubordination, which comes under Group II offenses as stated in the FCC Policy and Procedure Manual. Therefore, she has been terminated as an employee of FCC as of noon, June 22, 2001.

Javed fabricates a memorandum to his own files.

JAVED'S ONCOLOGY CLINIC/FREMONT CANCER CENTER ONCOLOGY
CLINIC HISTORY WITH THE FREMONT AREA MEDICAL CENTER
LABORATORY, VASCULAR ACCESS DEVICES AND INFECTION CONTROL

On February 21, 2001, Geri Means typed a memo to me regarding concerns about two
patients with Hepatitis C who had been treated in the Fremont Cancer Center Oncology
Clinic (FCC), a concern about another patient with Hepatitis C brought to her attention
by Dr. ███████, and additional concerns about nursing practices in port access
during chemotherapy by a "person" who states she had been treated at the FCC. I
informed Geri Means that if these concerns and alleged violation of nursing practice were
related to the FCC, then this was not a hospital infection control issue since the hospital
Infection Control Committee had no authority over the employees of the FCC or, for that
matter, any of the private clinics in the community. Furthermore, since the concerns
were related to the private clinic setting rather than the hospital Outpatient or Inpatient
Departments, there was nothing that could be done at the medical staff level regarding
peer review for Dr. Javed.

I was given the impression by Dr. Javed that the issues, if any, would be resolved; and
about this time a registered nurse, Heather Shepard, was hired. I met her at Tumor
Board, which she attended regularly. Heather seemed very interested in nursing
technique and on occasion came to the laboratory to ask specific questions about
protocol, especially for bone marrow preparations. This furthered my impression that Dr.
Javed had taken steps toward improving professionalism and nursing practice within his
clinic.

I subsequently learned that registered nurse ████████████ had also communicated
with Dr. Javed on numerous occasions while he was making rounds on the fourth floor.
She expressed specific concerns about the nursing practices of LP and the possible
adverse effects for patient welfare. ███ did not have access to the clinic, and thus no first-
hand observations were available. ███ did, however, communicate her concerns to the
Missouri Valley Cancer Consortium (MVCC). An on-site clinic inspection was a
prerequisite for participation in cancer therapy protocols of the MVCC.

On April 19, 2001, MVCC nurses met with Dr. Javed following an on-site inspection of
his clinic and informed him that nursing practices within his clinic were poor and in
violation of OSHA regulations, and that his office was not eligible to participate in
protocol work.

On April 24, 2001 and April 27, 2001, additional patient concerns were expressed to
Gerri Means regarding careless nursing practices of LP in Dr. Javed's clinic.

At this point, there was substantial concern of suboptimal infection control techniques in
the FCC (patients' statements and MVCC conclusion) and nearly all of the information
implicated one employee (LP).

Dr. Koerber's summary of Javed's clinic, page 1 of 3.

At this time, I repeated all of the concerns to Dr. Javed; and I gave him a copy of the previous memo dated February 21, 2001, from Geri Means to me to be absolutely certain that there was no question about what was trying to be conveyed to him regarding nursing practices within his clinic.

Dr. Javed subsequently met with Geri Means on May 16, 2001, and the MVCC declared the clinic eligible for protocol work. On June 19, 2001, the clinic office staff completed OSHA training in infection control.

I reviewed my files concerning the Laboratory's relationship with LP, and after this review it was clear that there was an aggregate pattern of behavior established by LP that did not bode well for future compliance with rigorous infection control standards once she was free from the scrutiny of OSHA and/or MVCC inspectors.

My impression of LP's aggregate pattern of behavior is summarized specifically as follows:

Within the first four to six weeks after the FCC opened, Dr. Javed ordered a blood transfusion to be given in the FCC; and this request, when brought to my attention, was unequivocally denied. LP's response to this denial was rude and arrogant.

I also received complaints from Laboratory personnel regarding LP's rude conduct in communicating with the Laboratory. There were numerous areas of concern regarding nonspecific orders, lack of history, incorrect specimen requirements, improper labeling and lack of compliance with established procedures and policies (see attached).

In 1999, a Vascular Access Device (VAD) Task Force was formed because of questions regarding the reliability of coagulation studies drawn from ports. It came to the attention of the VAD Task Force that LP had drawn blood from patients' ports in the Radiology Department of the Fremont Area Medical Center. The VAD Task Force concluded unequivocally that this practice must cease immediately. Dr. Javed was contacted, and a letter was written to him signed by me on August 4, 1999.

I subsequently contacted Dr. ████, general surgeon and medical staff liaison officer, who agreed that the alleged substandard nursing practices in the FCC were not a medical staff issue since all of the alleged violations, to the best of our knowledge, had occurred solely within the setting of the FCC. Because of increasing concern on the part of the administration, Geri Means, Dr. ████, and myself a meeting was called on June 22, 2001, at 9:00 a.m. in the administration conference room on second floor. In attendance were Mike Leibert, John Hughes, Peg Kennedy, Deb Wohlenhaus, Geri Means, Dr. ████ and me.

We discussed the numerous patient complaints and the conclusions of the MVCC. It was the consensus of the members of this meeting that Dr. Javed needed to be informed of all of our concerns and all of the patient concerns expressed to us.

Dr. Koerber's summary of Javed's clinic, page 2 of 3.

Although we understood and respected the independent status of the FCC, it was clear that the future of the new cancer center could be threatened with the continued employment of individuals such as LP.

John Hughes agreed to meet with Dr. Javed later on that morning at 10:00 a.m., and LP left the building around noon that day.

Geri Means notified the State of Nebraska Department of Epidemiology with our specific concerns regarding careless nursing practices, and the situation was discussed eventually with Dr. Safranek. We were told that the State only keeps count of the number of cases reported and advised us to talk to the Director of Investigations.

Sincerely,

Rodney K. Koerber, M.D.
Medical Director of the Laboratory

Dr. Koerber's summary of Javed's clinic, page 3 of 3.

July 2, 2002
11am - Dr Javed's office.

Received a call from Dr Javed requesting
I meet him in his office to discuss 2 hepatitis
C cases.
Informed during the meeting that Dr McKnight
has come to him with concerns of Hepatitis C
in patients that have been patients in his office.

Names:

Pt # 1 ▓▓▓▓▓▓▓ chemo 4-2001 → 9-4-01
abnormal liver functions Hep C 6-5-01

Pt # 2 ▓▓▓▓▓▓▓ Chemo 11-17-00 → April 2001
Hep profile neg 6-7-01 Hep C 2-02

Pt # 3 ▓▓▓▓▓▓▓ chemo Febr. March. April 2001
Hep profile neg 6-1-01 Hep C 6-24-02

Pt. # 4 ▓▓▓▓▓▓▓ chemo finished Dec '01
Hep C 6-19-02

He wanted to know if I'd been seeing an increase in
hepatitis C in the hospital. I knew I did not have
these names on my lime list.
He was going to make contact with some specialists
(in East Coast) to further investigate the various genotypes
& Reminded that Dr McKnight ▓▓▓▓▓▓▓▓▓▓▓▓▓▓

Javed and Gerri Means discuss more hepatitis C victims, page1 of 2.

He said he had 2 patients he would use as
a "Control" that have elevated enzymes.

    - 4-19-02 enzymes High.
    Chemo 4-10-02

    Chemo 7-24-01 → 1-18-02
    Dec 2001 - abdominal pain
      Enzymes neg.
  Liver function still high in Dec 200.
  January 2002 normal.

Javed and Gerri Means discuss more hepatitis C victims, page 2 of 2.

July 10, 2002
Dr. Javed's office - 5:15pm.

Note: Prior to meeting I have been reviewing patients records - my line listing. and new names given to me on July 2. Is there some ~~some~~ common factor, ie surgeon, anesthesia, all new cases are Dr McKnight's patients - what do they have done at that office?

Brought to meeting a "rough" time table. These patients had chemo when "Linda" was working. Had copies of articles of cross contamination. Questioned how many doses could be drawn from a saline bag. Was it used more than one day? Does procid require any dilution? How ~~were~~ Heparin vials handled? Review port a cath flush

Asked him to share with Dr McKnight that I was informed of the 4 new cases that were his patients

Advised him to make contact with the State Health Department (Dr Safranek). Also gave him information about the CDC Hepatitis C division.

Gerri Means' timetable of infections, page 1 of 2.

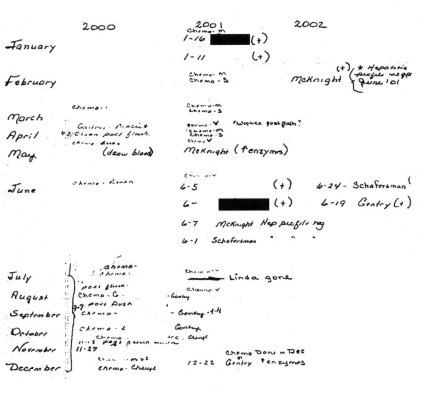

Gerri Means' timetable of infections, page 2 of 2.

Tahir A. Javed, M.D.
Hematology & Oncology

FREMONT CANCER CENTER, P.C.
450 E. 23rd Street, Suite #1
Fremont, NE 68025
Phone: (402) 727-3410 Fax: (402) 727-3616

July 12, 2002

Dear Ms. Jill Watson:

Due to a family emergency, I have to immediately go overseas.

During my absence, Dr. Janet Pieck will be covering the Cancer Center. Dr. M. Salman Haroon, my new partner, will be covering for oncological and hematological emergencies. His office phone number is 712-322-4136.

Dr. Pieck may be reached at 402-727-3580. Dr. M. Salman Haroon will start full-time practice at the Fremont Cancer Center on Tuesday, August 13th, but is available for any questions, follow-ups, and new consultations. If you desire to choose another oncologist for your care, please let my office know and we will mail your medical records accordingly.

Please contact my office staff at 402-727-3410 if you have any questions or concerns.

Thank you for your support and understanding.

Yours sincerely,

Tahir A. Javed, M.D.

Javed's "family emergency" letter.

312

Tom's notes about Hepatitis C

9/16/02: discussed with Mr. Leibert in his office; there was a consensus report from Alegent. FAMC infectious disease dept (including Dr. Koerber) were aware of report and failed to report Prochaska or Javed's negligence to state licensing bureau.

9/17: discussed with Dr. Koerber in his office: he had several visits with Javed and the deficiencies in the Cancer Center. Koerber went over Alegent report with Javed previous to July 2001. In July 2001 Koerber and John Hughes (FAMC) went to Javed and demanded that Prochaska be fired. Koerber also said there was a questionable charge regarding his personal life pending against Javed.

9/18: visited with Mr. Leibert in his office: Leibert had been in contact with Javed and requested that he return to practice within two weeks. Leibert had also been in contact with Javed's attorney. Attorney indicated he was told of the Hep C outbreak by Javed before he left for Pakistan in July, 2002.

9/24: met with Mr. Leibert at my office at the request of Leibert in the evening: Leibert mentioned Haroon was considering leaving Javed's office and Leibert wanted by support to keep Haroon here. Leibert stated "the hospital has some liability because Javed was acting as oncology director." FAMC knew about the problems with break in sterile technique but they had not been reported to FAMC medical staff committees nor to state licensure.

9/27: met with Dr. Haroon: he indicated he had minimal to no contact with Javed at present. He was unaware of any of aforementioned difficulties before he began to work in Fremont. Also indicated he was aware that Javed had other agendas in Pakistan (e.g., running for political office).

9/30: Mr. Leibert said John Hughes had found on the internet that Tahir A. Javed MD was running for political office in Pakistan.

10/2: visited with ██████████, RN: she was aware of Alegent consensus report. She had discussed this with hospital infectious disease and Javed on more than one occasion. She was told she was "just being hard on Prochaska".

Hospital and Javed had information about break in sterile technique several months before Prochaska was terminated. Cathy reported several other nurses who worked on a temporary basis also report breaks in sterile technique and some refused to return to work there.

10/3: Javed's office staff told my office manager that Javed had taken his diplomas off his wall before he left for Pakistan.

10/8/02: hospital staff meeting with Dr. Safranek. He said the window of problems was 3/2000- 12/2001. Question was asked: "how do we know when to set the end point of the window?" He replied "problem employee was terminated July, 2001. They allowed a window for Hep C conversion after the termination."

Appendix C

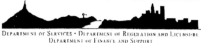

NEBRASKA HEALTH AND HUMAN SERVICES SYSTEM

DEPARTMENT OF SERVICES · DEPARTMENT OF REGULATION AND LICENSURE
DEPARTMENT OF FINANCE AND SUPPORT

STATE OF NEBRASKA
MIKE JOHANNS, GOVERNOR

October 11, 2002

Dear Sir/Madam:

This letter is addressed to individuals who received care from Dr. Tahir Javed at his medical oncology clinic between March 1, 2000, and December 31, 2001. Public health officials at the Nebraska Health and Human Services System (NHHSS) have recently identified several people in the Fremont area with hepatitis C virus (HCV). Investigation of this problem, including the specific method of HCV transmission is on-going. Based on current information, all of the affected persons appear to have been cared for in the office of Dr. Tahir Javed.

Hepatitis C virus causes an infection of the liver. The infection is treatable in most cases. In most people this infection causes no symptoms. Eventually some people experience symptoms such as fatigue, loss of appetite and a yellowing of the skin. While some people clear the virus from the body and are no longer infected, others remain infected for an extended period of time. Transmission through routine household exposure is extremely rare. It is important that individuals who have contracted this virus be identified.

Laboratory tests can identify both previously and currently infected patients. Based on information from this on-going investigation, the risk for transmission among patients at Dr. Javed's clinic appears confined to those who received care between March 1, 2000, and December 31, 2001. We recommend that persons cared for at the clinic during this time period be tested for HCV. Standard public health practice calls for including tests for hepatitis B and HIV under these circumstances.

The Fremont Area Medical Center (FAMC), working in conjunction with the NHHSS, has established a testing clinic. The FAMC clinic will be located at 410 E. 22nd street in Fremont (the building previously occupied by Drs. Anderson, Beacom, McKnight, Otten and Sellon). Blood draws in the clinic will be offered from *Thursday, October 17 through Friday, November 1, 9:00 a.m. until 5:30 p.m.* The blood test performed at the FAMC clinic will be free of charge. You will be notified of test results within 14 days after your blood draw. Please call 402-941-7020 (this is a local call in Fremont) to schedule your blood draw. We have shared this information with the medical community serving the Fremont area. Your primary care physician is prepared to answer questions and to provide patient care and referral services when indicated for those seeking such assistance.

Included with this letter is a fact sheet about HCV. In addition, the Centers for Disease Control has a website (http://www.cdc.gov/ncidod/diseases/hepatitis/c/index.htm) which is an excellent source for additional information about HCV. Hospital and medical staff in the Fremont community are working closely with public health experts to provide the highest level of care for persons affected by this situation. Beginning Monday, October 14, nursing staff from the NHHSS and the Fremont Area Medical Center will be available by telephone at 402-941-7020 from 9 AM to 5:00 PM to address additional questions you might have regarding this situation. Your participation in this screening will help us clarify this situation and assure that all patients receive the best medical advice and treatment. Thank you in advance.

Sincerely,

Thomas J. Safranek MD

Thomas J. Safranek, M.D
State Epidemiologist
Nebraska Department of Health and Human Services

DEPARTMENT OF HEALTH AND HUMAN SERVICES REGULATION AND LICENSURE
PO Box 95007, Lincoln, NE 68509-5007 Phone (402) 471-2133
An Equal Opportunity/Affirmative Action Employer

The state's letter to potential victims.

Appendix C

NEBRASKA HEALTH AND HUMAN SERVICES SYSTEM

STATE OF NEBRASKA
MIKE JOHANNS, GOVERNOR

DEPARTMENT OF SERVICES • DEPARTMENT OF REGULATION AND LICENSURE
DEPARTMENT OF FINANCE AND SUPPORT

October 31, 2002

Dear Sir/Madam,

I would like to thank you for helping with the Fremont area Hepatitis C investigation by having your blood tested.

I am happy to inform you that your blood has tested **NEGATIVE** for all three of the blood borne pathogens tested for: Hepatitis B, Hepatitis C, and HIV. Based on this information we are confident that you **ARE NOT** infected with these agents. No further testing or medical care is necessary with regards to this situation.

If you have any further questions regarding your tests, please contact your primary care doctor who will be able to address your concerns. Thank you again for your assistance in helping us address this problem.

Sincerely,

Thomas J. Safranek, M.D.
Nebraska State Epidemiologist

DEPARTMENT OF HEALTH AND HUMAN SERVICES REGULATION AND LICENSURE
PO BOX 95007, LINCOLN, NE 68509-5007 PHONE (402) 471-2133
An Equal Opportunity/Affirmative Action Employer
PRINTED WITH SOY INK ON RECYCLED PAPER

The state's letter to some victims.

Appendix C

Mr. Jon Bruning
Office of the Attorney General
2115 State Capitol
Lincoln, NE 68059

Dear Mr. Bruning,

Seven months ago, it was determined that 81 people were infected with Hepatitis C through the Fremont Cancer Center. The outbreak was investigated by the Nebraska Dept of Health and the Center for Disease control. Complaints were filed against the medical licenses of Tahir Javed MD and Linda Prochaska RN. Nebraska Dept of Health and Human Services Dept of Regulation and Licensure investigated these complaints and their reports were given to you for your ruling.

Mr. Bruning, as a citizen of Nebraska, I am asking that you make a prompt ruling on the licenses in question. May I remind you that one of the major goals of the Attorney General's office as stated on your website is to "protect the public health and safety of Nebraskans by vigorously pursuing disciplinary actions against health care professionals who endanger the public by violations of health regulations or drug laws". Please meet this goal by making a prompt ruling.

Sincerely,

Grassroots campaign form letter.

Appendix C

THE DEPARTMENT OF HEALTH AND HUMAN SERVICES
REGULATION AND LICENSURE
STATE OF NEBRASKA

STATE OF NEBRASKA,   )
)
            Plaintiff, **COPY**)
)   **PETITION FOR**
v.   )   **DISCIPLINARY ACTION**
)
TAHIR ALI JAVED, M.B.B.S.,   )   69-30722
)
            Defendant.   )

The Plaintiff alleges as follows:

ALLEGATIONS COMMON TO ALL CAUSES OF ACTION

1.   Jurisdiction is based on NEB. REV. STAT. §71-150.

2.   On October 8, 1997 the Defendant Tahir Ali Javed was issued a license to practice medicine and surgery by the Nebraska Department of Health and Human Services Regulation and Licensure (hereinafter "Department"), and at all times relevant herein, has been the holder of that license (#20624).

3.   The Department is the agency of the State of Nebraska authorized to enforce the provisions of the Uniform Licensing Law regulating the practice of medicine and surgery.

4.   The Nebraska Board of Medicine and Surgery has considered the investigation of this matter and made its recommendation to the Attorney General to file disciplinary proceedings against the Defendant's license to practice medicine and surgery.

5.   From January 1, 1998 until July 13, 2002 the Defendant owned and operated a medical practice as a sole practitioner under the name the Fremont Cancer Center, 450 East 23rd Street, Fremont, Nebraska.

6.   From January 1, 1998 until July 13, 2002 the Fremont Cancer Center was the site of the Defendant's medical office and was the primary site where he practiced medicine and surgery, specializing in oncology.

The state's petition to revoke Javed's license to practice medicine.

318

Appendix C

ALLEGATIONS COMMON TO THE FIRST TWO CAUSES OF ACTION

7.   From January 1, 1998 to June 22, 2001 no other medical doctor regularly practiced at the Fremont Cancer Center, and the Defendant was responsible for the operation of the medical office, including all medical treatment.

8.   The Defendant employed at his medical office a registered nurse on a full-time basis from December 21, 1997 to June 22, 2001, and an additional registered nurse on a part-time basis from January 2001 through March 2002. The Defendant provided all oncology training to the registered nurses. From January 1998 until after April 19, 2001 the Defendant instituted few written infection control polices or procedures for the operation of the clinic.

9.   The registered nurses employed by the Defendant were assigned by the Defendant to administer chemotherapy as part of their usual duties, including preparing medications and chemotherapy agents, accessing implanted vascular access devices (hereinafter IVADs), drawing blood from IVADs, flushing IVADs, and infusing the medications and chemotherapy agents.

10.   From the time the clinic opened the registered nurses failed to follow basic infection control requirements. Improper acts included: (1) Taking single-use disposable syringes and drawing blood from patients, reusing the syringes to obtain saline from a source common to all patients, and then reusing the syringes to flush the IVADs with the saline; and, (2) re-injection of patients' discard blood into the same patients.

11.   From January 1998 to at least June 22, 2001 every patient of the Defendant, whose chemotherapy treatment at Fremont Cancer Center included accessing an IVAD, was exposed to risk of harm due to the failure of the staff to follow basic infection control practices when providing treatment.

12.   The provision of chemotherapy is a basic and integral part of an oncology practice. The above improper acts of the registered nurses employed by the Defendant occurred during chemotherapy treatment in the oncology treatment room and patient examination rooms, while under the supervision of the Defendant. The Defendant at all times was responsible for the medical oncology treatment of all of the patients and had access to the oncology treatment room and patient examination rooms.

FIRST CAUSE OF ACTION

13.   Paragraphs 1 through 12 are incorporated by reference.

14.   The Defendant's actions in failing to have sufficient procedures in place, in failing to provide sufficient training to staff, or in failing to exercise appropriate oversight, any or all of which allowed the continued and repeated acts of improper infection control during therapy, resulted from the lack of or inappropriate direction or lack of or inappropriate direct supervision of a licensed health care provider employed by the Defendant and constitutes "unprofessional conduct" in violation of Title 172 Nebraska Administrative Code, Chapter 88 – Regulations Governing the Practice of Medicine and Surgery and Osteopathic Medicine and Surgery, §013.21.

15.   Violation of the regulations defining "unprofessional conduct", as defined by the Board of Medicine and Surgery pursuant to NEB. REV. STAT. §71-148 (22), is grounds on which disciplinary measures may be taken against the Defendant's license pursuant to NEB. REV. STAT. §71-147 (10), and pursuant to 172 NAC §88-012.03J.

SECOND CAUSE OF ACTION

16.   Paragraphs 1 through 12 are incorporated by reference.

17.   The Defendant's lack of supervision of the basic care his medical practice provided and his failure to correct the improper basic infection control practices subjected patients to a serious risk of harm, which constitutes the practice of the profession with gross negligence.

18.   Practice of the profession with gross negligence violates NEB. REV. STAT. §71-147 (5) (d), and, Title 172 Nebraska Administrative Code, Chapter 88 – Regulations Governing the Practice of Medicine and Surgery and Osteopathic Medicine and Surgery, §12.03E (d).

19.   Violation of any of the provisions of NEB. REV. STAT. §71-147 is grounds on which disciplinary measures may be taken against the Defendant's license.

20.   Violation of any of the provisions of 172 NAC §88-012.03 is grounds on which the Department may discipline a license.

ALLEGATIONS COMMON TO THE THIRD THROUGH FIFTH CAUSES OF ACTION

21.   On and before November 22, 1999 the Defendant's receptionist, who was trained as a dental hygienist, informed the Defendant of the improper infection control practices being used by the registered nurses employed by the Defendant.

22.   Individual #1 was infected with Hepatitis C Virus (hereinafter HCV) genotype 3a prior to becoming a patient of the Defendant. Individual #1 became a patient of the Defendant on February 12, 2000, and the Defendant was aware that Individual #1 was infected with HCV when Individual #1 became his patient. This patient did not receive in-office blood draws or chemotherapy in Defendant's office until May 2, 2000.

23.   HCV genotype 3a is the least common form of HCV in the United States representing approximately five percent (5%) of the reported cases.

24.   On February 5, 2001 the Defendant learned that Individual #2, a patient of the Defendant, had developed HCV genotype 3a.

25.   On February 15, 2001 the Defendant learned that Individual #3, also a patient of the Defendant, had developed HCV.

26.   On or about March 1, 2001 the physician director of infection control from the Fremont Area Medical Center (hereinafter referred to as FAMC) notified the Defendant that patients of the Defendant had questioned FAMC's infection control nurse about the propriety of certain medical practices occurring in the Defendant's office, including reusing syringes that were once blood-filled to obtain saline from a large bag of saline and using that saline to flush patients' IVADs.

27.   On April 12, 2001 representatives from the Missouri Valley Cancer Consortium (hereinafter referred to as the Consortium) went to the Defendant's office for the purpose of evaluating whether the Defendant's office could meet the standards to allow participation for conducting clinical research. At that time one of the representatives of the Consortium, who was a registered nurse, observed the improper infection control practices referred to in paragraph #10, above, being performed by the full-time registered nurse employed by the Defendant.

28.   Prior to April 19, 2001 representatives of the Consortium notified the Defendant orally, and on April 19, 2001 notified him in writing of the improper infection control practices that the Consortium's registered nurse had observed being performed by the full-time registered nurse employed by the Defendant.

29.   Also on April 19, 2001 the representatives of the Consortium met with the Defendant and his staff, including the registered nurses employed by the Defendant, and discussed methods of correcting problems observed.

30.   On April 23, 2001 the representatives of the Consortium informed the Defendant of their concern that they were unable to develop a plan with his staff for correcting the issues they had identified. Specifically they indicated that the part time registered nurse and one other staff member were overwhelmed by the information, and that the full time registered nurse appeared unwilling to discuss options to correct the practices.

31.   Between April 23, 2001 and May 1, 2001 the Defendant met with representatives from FAMC to discuss the concerns raised by the representatives of the Consortium.

32.   On May 1, 2001 a representative of the Consortium informed a representative of FAMC in writing of the specific concerns about poor nursing practice and their opinion that the poor practices were affecting patient outcomes. Representatives of FAMC met with the Defendant on May 1 and May 4, 2001 concerning this report.

33.   On May 16, 2001 the Defendant met with the infection control nurse of FMAC and discussed ongoing concerns voiced to her by patients of the Defendant about techniques utilized with IVADs.

34.   On June 5, 2001 the Defendant learned that Individual #4, a patient of the Defendant, had developed HCV.

35.   On June 8, 2001 the Defendant learned that Individual #5, also a patient of the Defendant, had developed HCV.

36.   On June 22, 2001 the full time registered nurse's employment with the

Defendant was terminated; and the Defendant instituted new procedures concerning infection control and other safety standards.

37.   As a result of failing to follow basic infection control requirements, ninety-nine patients of the Defendant who were exposed between May 2, 2000 and June 22, 2001 have been diagnosed with HCV genotype 3a; including three patients whose first exposures occurred after April 19, 2001.

38.   HCV is a viral liver disease that causes inflammation and scarring of the liver and stops the liver from working causing harm to the individuals who contract it.

39.   As a result of the infection with HCV genotype 3a the ninety-nine patients have been harmed, including Individual #6, who died as a result of the HCV genotype 3a infection.

THIRD CAUSE OF ACTION

40.   Paragraphs 1 through 12 and 21 through 39 are incorporated by reference.

41.   The Defendant between November 22, 1999 and June 22, 2001 was repeatedly placed on notice of the improper infection control practices occurring in his office, as set out above. In each instance the Defendant failed to take steps to protect his patients, and in each instance that he failed to act he placed additional patients at risk. Failure to protect his patients from a serious risk of harm constitutes the practice of the profession with gross negligence. Practice of the profession with gross negligence violates NEB. REV. STAT. §71-147 (5) (d), and, Title 172 Nebraska Administrative Code, Chapter 88 – Regulations Governing the Practice of Medicine and Surgery and Osteopathic Medicine and Surgery, §12.03E (d).

42.   Violation of any of the provisions of NEB. REV. STAT. §71-147 is grounds on which disciplinary measures may be taken against the Defendant's license.

43.   Violation of any of the provisions of 172 NAC §88-012.03 is grounds on which the Department may discipline a license.

FOURTH CAUSE OF ACTION

44.   Paragraphs 1 through 12 and 21 through 39 are incorporated by reference.

45.   The Defendant between November 22, 1999 and June 22, 2001 was repeatedly placed on notice of the improper infection control practices occurring in his office, as set out above. In each instance the Defendant failed to take steps to protect his

patients, and in each instance that he failed to act he placed additional patients at risk. Failure to correct improper practice after repeatedly being made aware of the improper practice constitutes the practice of the profession in a pattern of negligent conduct. Practice of the profession in a pattern of negligent conduct violates NEB. REV. STAT. §71-147 (5) (e), and, Title 172 Nebraska Administrative Code, Chapter 88 – Regulations Governing the Practice of Medicine and Surgery and Osteopathic Medicine and Surgery, §12.03E (e).

46.   Violation of any of the provisions of NEB. REV. STAT. §71-147 is grounds on which disciplinary measures may be taken against the Defendant's license.

47.   Violation of any of the provisions of 172 NAC §88-012.03 is grounds on which the Department may discipline a license.

FIFTH CAUSE OF ACTION

48.   Paragraphs 1 through 12 and 21 through 39 are incorporated by reference.

49.   The conduct and practice of the Defendant between January 1998 and June 22, 2001 was outside the normal standard of care in the State of Nebraska and has resulted in harm to at least ninety-nine patients including death to at least one patient. Conduct or practices outside the normal standard of care in the State of Nebraska which is or might be harmful or dangerous to the health of patients constitutes "unprofessional conduct" in violation of Title 172 Nebraska Administrative Code, Chapter 88 – Regulations Governing the Practice of Medicine and Surgery and Osteopathic Medicine and Surgery, §013.18.

50.   Violation of the regulations defining "unprofessional conduct", as defined by the Board of Medicine and Surgery pursuant to NEB. REV. STAT. §71-148 (22), is grounds on which disciplinary measures may be taken against the Defendant's license pursuant to NEB. REV. STAT. §71-147 (10), and pursuant to 172 NAC §88-012.03J.

ALLEGATIONS COMMON TO THE SIXTH THROUGH TENTH CAUSES OF ACTION

51. During May of 2000 the Defendant began a sexual relationship with Individual #7, which relationship continued until approximately July 1, 2001. On or about April 1, 2001 the Defendant began to provide medical treatment to Individual #7 and created a physician-patient relationship, billing Individual #7 for at least some of the services.

52. During the time the Defendant maintained a physician-patient relationship with Individual #7 he intentionally provided Individual #7 with a false diagnosis, telling the individual that the individual had a fatal disease. He told Individual #7 not to seek other treatment because other providers would inform Individual #7's insurance company and Individual #7 would not be able to obtain insurance again.

53. During the time the Defendant maintained a physician-patient relationship with Individual #7 he failed to keep and maintain adequate records of the treatment and services.

54. The personal and professional relationships between Individual #7 and the Defendant were terminated no later than July 1, 2001.

55. Between July 19 and July 23, 2001 the Defendant contacted a clinical laboratory in Omaha, Nebraska on two occasions, and by impersonating two different physicians attempted to cancel certain laboratory tests for Individual #7 ordered by Individual #7's then treating nurse practitioner.

56. On July 23, 2001 the Defendant contacted the above-mentioned clinical laboratory and obtained the test results on Individual #7, an individual with whom he had no current physician-patient relationship.

SIX CAUSE OF ACTION

57. Paragraphs 1 through 6 and 51 and 52 are incorporated by reference.

58. The Defendant's action of intentionally providing a false diagnosis to Individual #7 during the time he maintained a physician-patient relationship with Individual #7, and influencing Individual #7 not to seek other treatment, constitutes

grossly immoral or dishonorable conduct evidencing unfitness for practice of the profession of medicine and surgery in this state.

59. Grossly immoral or dishonorable conduct evidencing unfitness for practice of the profession of medicine and surgery in this state is in violation of NEB. REV. STAT. §71-147 (2); and, Title 172 Nebraska Administrative Code, Chapter 88 – Regulations Governing the Practice of Medicine and Surgery and Osteopathic Medicine and Surgery, 12.03B.

60. Violation of any of the provisions of NEB. REV. STAT. §71-147 is grounds on which disciplinary measures may be taken against the Defendant's license.

61. Violation of any of the provisions of 172 NAC §88-012.03 is grounds on which the Department may discipline a license.

SEVENTH CAUSE OF ACTION

62. Paragraphs 1 through 6 and 51 and 52 are incorporated by reference.

63. The Defendant's action of intentionally providing a false diagnosis to Individual #7 during the time he maintained both a sexual relationship and a physician-patient relationship with Individual #7, and influencing Individual #7 not to seek other treatment, constituted sexual exploitation of Individual #7.

64. Sexual exploitation of a patient constitutes "unprofessional conduct" in violation of NEB. REV. STAT. §71-148 (18); and Title 172 Nebraska Administrative Code, Chapter 88 – Regulations Governing the Practice of Medicine and Surgery and Osteopathic Medicine and Surgery, §13.23.

65. Violation of the statute or of regulations defining "unprofessional conduct" is grounds on which disciplinary measures may be taken against the Defendant's license pursuant to NEB. REV. STAT. §71-147 (10), and pursuant to 172 NAC §88-012.03J.

EIGHTH CAUSE OF ACTION

66. Paragraphs 1 through 6 and 51 through 53 are incorporated by reference.

67. The Defendant's action of not keeping adequate records of treatment and service for patient Individual #7 constitutes "unprofessional conduct" in violation of NEB. REV. STAT. §71-148 (19); and, Title 172 Nebraska Administrative Code, Chapter 88 –

Regulations Governing the Practice of Medicine and Surgery and Osteopathic Medicine and Surgery, §013.24.

68.   Violation of the statute or of regulations defining "unprofessional conduct" is grounds on which disciplinary measures may be taken against the Defendant's license pursuant to NEB. REV. STAT. §71-147 (10), and pursuant to 172 NAC §88-012.03J.

NINTH CAUSE OF ACTION

69.   Paragraphs 1 through 6 and 51 through 56 are incorporated by reference.

70.   The Defendant's action of impersonation of other physicians in an effort to interfere in the treatment of an ex-patient and in obtaining the test results on an individual with whom he had no current physician-patient relationship constitutes practice of the profession fraudulently.

71.   Practice of the profession fraudulently violates NEB. REV. STAT. §71-147 (5) (a), and, Title 172 Nebraska Administrative Code, Chapter 88 – Regulations Governing the Practice of Medicine and Surgery and Osteopathic Medicine and Surgery, §12.03E (a).

72.   Violation of any of the provisions of NEB. REV. STAT. §71-147 is grounds on which disciplinary measures may be taken against the Defendant's license.

73.   Violation of any of the provisions of 172 NAC §88-012.03 is grounds on which the Department may discipline a license.

TENTH CAUSE OF ACTION

74.   Paragraphs 1 through 6 and 51 through 56 are incorporated by reference.

75.   The Defendant's action of obtaining the test results on an individual with whom he had no physician-patient relationship constitutes willful violation of confidentiality between a physician and patient and constitutes unprofessional conduct in violation of Title 172 Nebraska Administrative Code, Chapter 88 – Regulations Governing the Practice of Medicine and Surgery and Osteopathic Medicine and Surgery, §013.02.

76.   Violation of regulations defining "unprofessional conduct", as defined by the Board of Medicine and Surgery pursuant to NEB. REV. STAT. §71-148 (22), is grounds on which disciplinary measures may be taken against the Defendant's license pursuant to NEB. REV. STAT. §71-147 (10), and pursuant to 172 NAC §88-012.03J.

ALLEGATIONS COMMON TO THE ELEVENTH AND TWELFTH
CAUSES OF ACTION

77.　By the end of June of 2002 the Defendant knew that seven of his patients in addition to Individual #1 had been diagnosed with HCV, and that they had developed the HCV after Individual #1 had started receiving treatment in the Defendant's office. The Defendant also knew that three of those individuals shared the specific genotype 3a that Individual #1 had, and that the HCV genotype for the other four individuals had not then been determined.

78.　On July 2, 2002 the Defendant met with FAMC's infection control nurse to investigate the cause of the HCV infections. On July 10, 2002 the Defendant met for a second time with the infection control nurse. At that time, that individual reminded the Defendant of the requirement of reporting cases to the Department of Health and Human Services Regulation and Licensure.

79.　On July 11, 2002 another Fremont, Nebraska area medical practitioner informed the Defendant that that practitioner had four patients who had been diagnosed with HCV genotype 3a. The practitioner also informed the Defendant that the practitioner knew that the four patients had in common the fact that they had received treatment in the Defendant's office.

80.　On or about July 13, 2002 the Defendant left the United States.

81.　The Defendant sent a letter to some of his patients informing them he was leaving immediately to go overseas due to a family emergency. This letter was prepared on July 12, 2002, but was not mailed until July 13, 2002, and not received by the patients until after the Defendant had already left the United States.

82.　The above referenced letter indicated that during the Defendant's absence Dr. Pieck would provide medical coverage, and Dr. Haroon, who had been engaged to become the Defendant's partner in the Defendant's medical practice, would be covering for oncological and hematological emergencies.

83.　The Defendant had not contacted Dr. Pieck about providing medical coverage prior to sending the letter; nor had Dr. Pieck agreed to provide the coverage.

84.　On July 13, 2002 Dr. Haroon was still practicing in the state of Iowa, and was not scheduled to begin full-time practice at the Fremont Cancer Center until August 13, 2002.

85.   On July 13, 2002 Dr. Haroon did not have admitting privileges at the local hospital.

86.   At no time prior to leaving the country did the Defendant inform Dr. Haroon of any aspect of the HCV infections in the Defendant's patients.

87.   Since leaving the country the Defendant has failed to provide appropriate information necessary for the continued care of the patients of his practice, or to participate in their care.

ELEVENTH CAUSE OF ACTION

88.   Paragraphs 1 through 12, 21 through 39, and 77 through 87 are incorporated by reference.

89.   The Defendant's actions as set out above constitute patient abandonment which constitutes grossly immoral or dishonorable conduct evidencing unfitness for practice of the profession of medicine and surgery in this state.

90.   Grossly immoral or dishonorable conduct evidencing unfitness for practice of the profession of medicine and surgery in this state is in violation of NEB. REV. STAT. §71-147 (2); and, Title 172 Nebraska Administrative Code, Chapter 88 – Regulations Governing the Practice of Medicine and Surgery and Osteopathic Medicine and Surgery, 12.03B.

91.   Violation of any of the provisions of NEB. REV. STAT. §71-147 is grounds on which disciplinary measures may be taken against the Defendant's license.

92.   Violation of any of the provisions of 172 NAC §88-012.03 is grounds on which the Department may discipline a license.

TWELFTH CAUSE OF ACTION

93.   Paragraphs 1 through 12, 21 through 39, and 77 through 87 are incorporated by reference.

94.   The Defendant's actions as set out above constitute patient abandonment. Patient abandonment is conduct or practice outside the normal standard of care which is or might be harmful or dangerous to the health of the patient, and constitutes "unprofessional conduct" in violation of Title 172 Nebraska Administrative Code,

Chapter 88 – Regulations Governing the Practice of Medicine and Surgery and Osteopathic Medicine and Surgery, §013.18.

95. Violation of regulations defining "unprofessional conduct", as defined by the Board of Medicine and Surgery pursuant to NEB. REV. STAT. §71-148 (22), is grounds on which disciplinary measures may be taken against the Defendant's license pursuant to NEB. REV. STAT. §71-147 (10), and pursuant to 172 NAC §88-012.03J..

PRAYER

WHEREFORE, the Plaintiff prays that the Chief Medical Officer set this matter for hearing, order appropriate disciplinary action concerning the Defendant's license to practice medicine and surgery in the State of Nebraska pursuant to NEB. RE. STAT.§71-155, and tax the costs of this action to the Defendant.

STATE OF NEBRASKA
Plaintiff,

BY:　JON BRUNING
　　　Attorney General

By:　_____
Roger Brink, #10429
Special Assistant Attorney General
P. O. Box 95026
Lincoln, NE 68509-5026
Tel. (402) 471-4050
Attorneys for Plaintiff

January 25, 2004

Mr. Jon Bruning
Office of the Attorney General
2115 State Capitol
Lincoln, NE 68509

Dear Mr. Bruning,

Once again I am writing you to request a ruling on the complaints against the nursing license of Linda Prochaska, RN. Following is a brief review of the facts of the case. Pertinent supporting documents are attached.

- A cluster of Hepatitis C cases in the Fremont area were reported to Nebraska Health and Human Services in September, 2002. These cases were investigated and the Health Department asked 612 patients of the clinic to be tested. It was found that 82 Nebraskans tested positive for the disease.

- On October 10, 2002 my husband (a family physician) and I filed a complaint against the license of Tahir Javed, MD and Linda Prochaska, RN with the Nebraska Health and Human Services. Numerous other complaints against these licenses were filed by victims, professionals and community members about this same time.

- A thorough investigation was conducted by Nebraska Health and Human Services and the Center for Disease Control. It was determined that unsterile technique related to infection control practices at the Fremont Cancer Clinic was responsible for the Hepatitis C outbreak. The proper channels of licensure investigation were followed and the reports were given to you for your ruling early in 2003.

- A grassroots letter writing campaign was conducted to request you to make a ruling on the license in question in March-July, 2003. Hundreds of letters by Nebraskans were sent to you requesting prompt action.

- In March, 2003 Cheryl Gentry, one of the victims, died of liver failure related to Hepatitis C.

- In June, 2003 17 more cases of Hepatitis C related to the outbreak were confirmed. The total of cases is now 99, making it the largest outbreak of Hepatitis C on record.

Evelyn's letter to Jon Bruning, requesting action on Linda Prochaska's license.

- On July 29, 2003 a petition was filed for disciplinary action against the license of Dr. Javed by Nebraska Health and Human Services. Subsequently, his license was revoked on Oct 1, 2003.

Mr. Bruning, as you know, n o action has been taken regarding the license of Linda Prochaska, RN. She continues to work as a nurse in an Omaha hospital even though it has been shown that her egregious negligence results in the largest American outbreak of Hepatitis C in history. I strongly urge you to make a ruling now since the investigation regarding allegations against her license has been complete for more than a year. As stated on the website of the Nebraska Attorney General a major goal of your office is to "Protect the public health and safety of Nebraskans by vigorously pursuing disciplinary actions against health care professionals who endanger the public by violations of health regulations or drug laws".

I trust that you will make a ruling immediately, before the health of more Nebraskans is put in jeopardy and that I will not need to contact you again or seek legal or media resources to coerce you in this matter.

Sincerely,

Evelyn V. McKnight
4119 N. Somers Ave
Fremont, NE 68025

Making Sense of News
Patriotic Chronicle

14 November 2003 | 10:07:14

Here is a Pakistani Doctor's novel way of Jihad: To kill the Kuffar (infidels), he uses no guns or bomb., his weapons are plain, planned negligence and his largest, hapless American sick people, among whom he spread Hepatitis C virus. An UNPRECEDENTED case of gross, criminal negligence that can put the whole medical profession to shame has been committed.

Health minister denies charges of grave misconduct

By: Khalid Hasan and Waqar Gillani

LAHORE: Punjab Health Minister Dr Tahir Ali Javed, who was practicing in Nebraska before moving to Pakistan after winning an assembly seat from Narowal, is being held responsible here for being linked to the largest known Hepatitis C outbreak in the US. Dr Javed denied the charges against him. He has been formally accused by the State of Nebraska of what one official called "unprecedented negligence and misconduct". Dr Javed faces scores of allegations in a petition for disciplinary action filed against him in July and announced by state health regulatory officials. Eighty of his affected patients have filed suits against the Pakistani doctor. Health investigators have linked poor infection-control practices at Dr Javeds former cancer clinic in Fremont, Nebraska, to 99 cases of Hepatitis C diagnosed over the past two years. One patient has died. The petition, filed by a special assistant in the State Attorney Generals Office, outlines 12 reasons for discipline or revocation of Dr Javeds Nebraska medical licence. Most of the counts allege that Dr Javed used poor infection-control practices at the clinic and abandoned the cancer patients in his care last summer. "The conduct in this petition is unprecedented in our memory," said Richard Nelson, the director of regulation and licensure for the Nebraska Health and Human Services System. According to the petition filed against Dr. Javed, he was repeatedly informed as early as November 1999, months before the first known hepatitis-infected patient came to the clinic for treatment that his nurses were reusing syringes used to draw blood and saline. Although the practice put his patients at risk for blood-borne diseases, he allowed the practice to persist.

An article from a Pakistani newspaper.

333

April 22, 2003

Mike Leibert
2434 Peterson
Fremont, NE 68025

Dear Mike,

I am sorry we were not granted our request to meet with FAMC administrators and board of directors to discuss our recommendations for policy and procedure changes. I wanted to share my story with you face to face and discuss ways of improving healthcare at FAMC. I have enclosed the statement that I prepared for that meeting. I hope you will take the time to read it.

Mike, I know this is a difficult time for you as well. I ask that you approach the months ahead with courage and honor. You have the power to make wise, compassionate and just decisions in FAMC's response to the Hepatitis C outbreak. As you ponder the advice from your legal representatives, please consider what is honest, noble and just. The emotional and physical healing of 81 people, people who had put their faith in FAMC, depends upon your decisions. Please consider your choices carefully.

Thank you for your time, Mike. My best wishes for your strength and courage.

Sincerely,

Evelyn V. McKnight
4119 N. Somers Ave
Fremont, NE 68025

Evelyn's initial letter to hospital officials.

Appendix C

October 23, 2005

Dear Mr. ▆▆,

Thank you for your reply to my letter regarding requested steps that need to be implemented before I consider settling my lawsuit against FAMC. I was disappointed to read that of my twenty requests, one (#13) was agreed with, eight (#4, 5, 9a, 9b, 9c, 9d, 9e, 9f) were refused and eleven (#1, 2, 3, 6, 7, 8, 10, 11, 12, 14, 15) were answered with a very qualified possibly. Given this response, I must conclude that the discussion has derailed at this point. If the Board of Trustees and/or administration change their mind about any points, I would be happy to reopen the discussion.

In the meantime, I have instructed Mr. Miller and Mr. Brown to continue their preparations for the court trial.

Sincerely,

Evelyn V. McKnight, AuD
4119 N. Somers Ave
Fremont, NE 68025

Evelyn's letter in response to the rejection of her non-monetary points.

Appendix C

September 20, 2006

Evelyn McKnight, Au. D.
4119 N. Somers
Fremont, NE 68025

Dear Evelyn:

With the execution of the settlement agreement, it is my understanding that I now have the opportunity to share some of my thoughts with you regarding the Hepatitis C situation in Dr. Javed's office. First, I wanted you to know that your efforts and commitment to the mediation process involving your lawsuit were very much appreciated. After such a difficult mediation process, my feelings were very mixed with some relief, some regrets and some disappointment.

All said, however, the mediation process was without a doubt the best for the community. A trial would have been divisive in the community given the adversarial nature of our legal system. Regardless of who would have "won" from a legal perspective, such a trail would have ultimately been detrimental to the overall welfare and health of the community.

For the past three years Shirley and I have prayed not only for the physical healing of the Hepatitis C patients but we have also prayed for reconciliation in the community. There is so much work to be done in terms of providing health and medical services to our community. I believe that the ability of Dr. McKnight's practice and the hospital to work together is critical to the overall welfare of community we live in and care about.

There has seldom, if ever, been a day during the last three years where my thoughts have not turned to Dr. Javed and the Hepatitis C patients. I recognize that we will never be able to fully comprehend either the physical or emotional aspects of your disease. It is sincere our hope, however, that the mediated settlement will be the beginning of a reconciliation process.

Sincerely,

Michael Leibert

Letter from the hospital's president after Evelyn settled her lawsuit.

336

October 4, 2006

Mike Leibert
2434 Peterson
Fremont, NE 68025

Dear Mike,

Thank you for your letter of September 20, 2006. I appreciate your thoughtfulness and prayers.

I am ambivalent about the position that the mediation process was better for the community than a trial. It would be better for the overall welfare and health of the community to explore both sides of the issue and for the community to understand and appreciate the suffering of 99 of its members; if the way to do that is through a trial then so be it. It is imperative that we study the disaster so that we learn the lessons inherent in it. If we do not – if we continue to make the same mistakes that were made that allowed the Nebraska Outbreak to occur – then we will be responsible for a greater tragedy than 99 cases of Hepatitis C and the several deaths that resulted from the Nebraska Outbreak. The ultimate overall welfare of the community will be served for everyone – not just the hospital, not just the victims – if we explore the issues surrounding the Nebraska Outbreak.

In terms of reconciliation in the community, reconciliation is a two way street. For full, satisfying reconciliation for both sides, there must be good will extended from each side to the other. In other words, the defendants must extend good will to the plaintiffs and the plaintiffs must extend good will to the defendants. In our situation, plaintiffs are asked to heal, to forgive, and to "get over it". We have not been extended an apology by Prochaska and Javed: I sincerely doubt that this will happen. However, we would appreciate an expression of compassion and concern from you as the CEO of the county hospital, the primary healthcare provider in the area. I am not asking for an apology or an admission of guilt; what I am asking for is an acknowledgement of the suffering of your fellow citizens of Dodge County, concern for our welfare and wishes for our recovery. This expression of concern would have best served the community if it had been offered at the outset of the Nebraska

Evelyn's response to Leibert.

Outbreak; but it is still necessary and has merit now. Without an "official" expression of good will towards the victims, reconciliation is one sided, shallow and incomplete.

I wish you well, Mike. I hope that we all will grow in wisdom and integrity from this horrific event.

Thank you for the chance to dialogue. If you would like to meet in person, I would be most interested.

Sincerely,
Evelyn V. McKnight